*f*P

ALSO BY ROBERT JAY LIFTON

―――――

Superpower Syndrome: America's Apocalyptic Confrontation with the World

*Who Owns Death: Capital Punishment, the American Conscience,
and the End of Executions* (with Greg Mitchell)

*Destroying the World to Save It: Aum Shinrikyo, Apocalyptic Violence,
and the New Global Terrorism*

Hiroshima in America: Fifty Years of Denial (with Greg Mitchell)

The Protean Self: Human Resilience in an Age of Fragmentation

The Genocidal Mentality: Nazi Holocaust and Nuclear Threat
(with Eric Markusen)

The Future of Immortality—and Other Essays for a Nuclear Age

The Nazi Doctors: Medical Killing and the Psychology of Genocide

Indefensible Weapons: The Political and Psychological Case Against Nuclearism
(with Richard Falk)

The Broken Connection: On Death and the Continuity of Life

Six Lives/Six Deaths: Portraits from Modern Japan
(with Shuichi Kato and Michael Reich)

The Life of the Self: Toward a New Psychology

Living and Dying (with Eric Olson)

Home from the War: Vietnam Veterans—Neither Victims Nor Executioners

Boundaries: Psychological Man in Revolution

Death in Life: Survivors of Hiroshima

*History and Human Survival: Essays on the Young and the Old, Survivors
and the Dead, War and Peace, and on Contemporary Psychohistory*

Revolutionary Immortality: Mao Tse-tung and the Chinese Cultural Revolution

*Thought Reform and the Psychology of Totalism:
A Study of 'Brainwashing' in China*

EDITED BOOKS

Crimes of War: Iraq (with Richard Falk and Irene Gendzier)

In a Dark Time: Images for Survival (with Nicholas Humphrey)

Last Aid: Medical Dimensions of Nuclear War (with E. Chivian, S. Chivian, and J. E. Mack)

Beyond Invisible Walls: The Psychological Legacy of Soviet Trauma (with Jacob D. Lindy)

Crimes of War (with Richard Falk and Gabriel Kolko)

Explorations in Psychohistory: The Wellfleet Papers (with Eric Olson)

America and the Asian Revolutions

The Woman in America

HUMOROUS BIRD CARTOONS

Birds

Psychobirds

WITNESS TO AN
EXTREME CENTURY

A Memoir

ROBERT JAY LIFTON

FREE PRESS

New York London Toronto Sydney

Free Press
A Division of Simon & Schuster, Inc.
1230 Avenue of the Americas
New York, NY 10020

First Free Press hardcover edition June 2011

FREE PRESS and colophon are trademarks of Simon & Schuster, Inc.

For information about special discounts for bulk purchases,
please contact Simon & Schuster Special Sales at 1-866-506-1949
or business@simonandschuster.com.

The Simon & Schuster Speakers Bureau can bring authors to your
live event. For more information or to book an event contact the
Simon & Schuster Speakers Bureau at 1-866-248-3049 or
visit our website at www.simonspeakers.com.

Manufactured in the United States of America

1   3   5   7   9   10   8   6   4   2

Library of Congress Cataloging-in-Publication Data

Lifton, Robert Jay
Witness to an extreme century : a memoir / by Robert Jay Lifton.
p. cm.
1. Lifton, Robert Jay, 1926– 2. Historians—United States—Biography
3. Psychiatrists—United States—Biography 4. Political activists—United States—
Biography 5. History, Modern—20th century. 6. Military history, Modern—
20th century. 7. Genocide—History—20th century. 8. Nuclear warfare—
History—20th century. 9. Radicalism—History—20th century.
10. War and society—History—20th century. 11. Social change—
History—20th century. I. Title.

CT275.L4343A3 2011
973.02092—dc22
[B]   2010046148

ISBN 978-1-4165-9076-7
ISBN 978-1-4165-9718-6 (ebook)

To Ken and Natasha
To Kimberly, Jessica, Lila, and Dmitri
And to BJ

CONTENTS

PREFACE

I HAVE SPENT MUCH of my life listening. During interviews people have described to me in painful psychological detail their encounters with some of the defining acts of the late twentieth and early twenty-first centuries. In Hong Kong I listened to Chinese and Westerners who had been subjected to Chinese Communist thought reform, in Hiroshima to Japanese survivors of the atomic bomb, in New York City (and New Haven, Connecticut, and Gainesville, Florida) to American veterans of Vietnam who turned against their war, in Germany to Nazi doctors who had participated in a reversal of healing and killing, and in Israel, the United States, and countries throughout Europe to survivors of Auschwitz. I became a witness to the events I studied.

In response to that listening I began to do my share of talking. I developed an early habit of dictating notes closely describing not only the content of each interview or conversation but my own impressions, emotions, and associations. I called this a research diary, but the notes also became a bumpy narrative of my life as a researcher and activist, and of the extraordinary environments in which I have found myself. I have extended that talking into sustained conversations over years and decades with friends and partners in dialogue. And all of my books and articles have taken shape through dictated, and many redictated, drafts before they reached the typewriter or computer.

This volume is a culmination of nearly six decades of listening and talking. It is in no sense a systematic account of my research studies; I tried to provide such accounts in earlier books. Rather it is a highly subjective story of my life experience in connection with the work I have done, and of the historical worlds I have inhabited. I've tried to record my findings as accurately as possible, but that does not mean I have been neutral. I've been moved by victimized people I encountered and have spoken out publicly against the forces responsible for their suffering. That identification with survivors of cruel events has in fact been a major source of my social activism. After what I had heard and seen, it became quite natural—indeed urgent—for me to take stands against mind control, nuclear weapons, American warmaking, and Nazi-like cruelty and genocide. To be sure, I've brought to the work such inclinations toward protest, but these were deepened and clarified in ways that did not permit me to stay silent. I felt that I had gained special knowledge of the impact of these abuses, which could inform my witness, and that I was able to make use of my unusual vantage point to become an advocate for peaceful paths to justice and political decency. My always imperfect balance between scholarship and activism is a central theme of this volume.

There has always been something logical about my writing a memoir. Friends have often suggested it, pointing to work I have done in various places on issues that matter and to encounters and friendships with compelling people along the way. I considered the idea, but for years resisted it. It's not that I haven't been introspective—in addition to all those self-examining notes, I've long kept records of my dreams and associations to them. But as a person used to plunging ahead into new projects, I feared that a memoir would immerse me too much in the past. Also, as one who wrote mainly about other people, I did not quite know how to proceed with a book mainly about myself. I had to find a way to do two things: to simultaneously look back to the past and ahead to the future, and to locate myself in settings and ideas that had significance of a larger kind. As every writer discovers, structure is key. Mine for this volume should have been obvious, but it took me some years to come to it. I finally realized that the foundation I needed lay in the four most significant events I had confronted: Chinese thought reform, the atomic bomb in Hiroshima, the Vietnam War, and the behavior of Nazi doctors; and that all of these had immediate importance for present national and world dilemmas. With that realization, I could first imagine the project, and then embrace it.

It helped me a lot that I did not have to depend entirely on my memory. That was because of the collection of my papers at the New York

Public Library. Organized by its curator, Melanie Yolles, in more orderly fashion than I ever could have, the collection gave me marvelous access to hundreds of thousands of pages of research interviews, personal notes, and pre-computer correspondence. I made many all-day visits to the manuscript room in the 42nd St. branch, which I came to greatly appreciate for its aura combining contemporary efficiency (helpful, businesslike responses to requests) and antiquated quietude (no conversations, no cell phones, nothing but a smattering of earnest seekers working at quaintly old-fashioned but fully serviceable desks and lights). There I felt myself to be a medieval monk poring through ancient texts and folios—only in this case the texts and folios consisted mainly of my own words and actions.

What I read mostly felt familiar, though frequently deviating quite a bit from my memory—since memory is a rendering of the past from the perspective of the present. And on occasion I could be quite surprised by finding experiences of which I had absolutely no recollection. I could even at times feel myself to recover whole segments of my life that had been lost. Without that library collection, I'm not sure I could have embarked on the memoir at all. It provided me with an anchor in my own recorded historical actuality. Yet I also learned as I proceeded that I could not allow myself to be buried under the weight of those pages; and that the memoir, like all writing and thinking, had to be actively re-imagined from that factual anchor.

I look back at the man (and sometimes boy) of the past, and at the world of that time, through the prism of the man I am now, living in contemporary history. When a friend asked me which self I was writing about, my answer was that I could in no way avoid addressing both of them at the same time. Doing that has changed me, though I'm not sure exactly how. It has something to do with putting me in touch with fragments of my self, associated with different environments and historical moments, which have, however haphazardly, found some continuity and managed to blend. That in turn has given me an intimate awareness of the flow of personal and social change.

I do not consider these struggles to be what Freud called "self-analysis" (in connection with his pursuit of psychoanalytic insight into his own life). I see it instead as an effort to connect my developing understanding of extreme events with my own feelings and behavior—that is, to connect self and evolving doctrine. (I believe Freud was doing much the same in seeking from his own early life experience corroboration for his theory of childhood sexuality as the source of neurosis). The process can be convoluted, and one requires a certain amount of gallows humor concerning the world's absurdities and one's own contradictions. But that connection between self and doctrine is crucial both to the theorist who seeks conviction about his theories, and to the activist who wishes to behave honorably in the face of what he has learned.

Age has also mattered. I began the volume at close to eighty, knowing that I had limited time and energy to complete it. At issue has been not so much Buber's famous, still profound question, "If not now, when?" as whether or not to mobilize my finite resources for this particular project. The present volume is my way of answering that question.

So I have structured the book around those four crucial research studies, along with a fifth section on their reverberations in me and in others, and on my special relation to Wellfleet and the forty-five years of Wellfleet meetings I have convened on psychology and history. In each of these sections I have included especially memorable experiences in the research, as well as my more general intellectual struggles of the time. From my Hong Kong work on thought reform there is the searing image of a Dutch priest reduced to believing in his own false confession of espionage, but also at that time my discovery of mentors (especially Erik Erikson and David Riesman) and experience of the excitement of intellectual friendships. From my Hiroshima work I retain a life-changing image of the survivor who looked out at his former city to discover that "Hiroshima had disappeared," a memory that contributed directly to my antinuclear passions, particularly in the physicians' movement.

Antiwar veterans brought me devastating images of the slaughter of Vietnamese civilians at My Lai, which I could incorporate into my public testimony about "atrocity-producing situations," and ultimately into civil disobedience in opposing the war.

For my German section I retained images of Auschwitz as "a separate planet," from the perpetrators, Nazi doctors, and survivor-victims, Jewish and Polish; I also describe powerful friendships with people who have given much of their lives to exposing truths about Nazism and genocide, including Jewish American scholars such as Raul Hilberg as well as many non-Jewish Germans, notably Alexander and Margarete Mitscherlich. And in the last section, interspersed with the Wellfleet ambiance, is my longstanding dialogue and friendship with Norman Mailer.

This is a highly personal book, but not one mainly concerned with intimate family ties. To be sure, my parents, grandparents, children, and grandchildren all make appearances, and my wife BJ shares with me almost the entire journey. But even when family members remain in the background they are very much present in the interstices of my being. My narrative remains personal in a different way, having to do with my intellectual and ethical struggles—where they have taken me and where they still lead.

Part One

Discovering the World—and its Totalism

1

The Decision

IN LATE APRIL of 1954, when I was twenty-eight years old, I took a long walk through the streets of Kowloon, a crowded part of Hong Kong. Those streets were teeming with people as I passed shops of every kind, from small noodle stands to elegant dress stores with European mannequins, along with endless houses and small factories. My mind was on neither the people nor the buildings. I was painfully preoccupied with the important life decision I was trying to make.

My wife, BJ, and I had been living in Hong Kong for about three months, staying in a comfortable bohemian garret room we had negotiated at the then modest family-oriented Miramar Hotel. I had been interviewing both Westerners and Chinese who had been subjected on the Mainland to a remarkable process called "thought reform." The reformers employed considerable coercion, sometimes violence, but also powerful exhortation on behalf of a new Chinese dawn, seeking to bring the beliefs and worldviews of participants into accord with those of the triumphant Communist regime. I could observe that thought reform was by no means a casual undertaking but rather a systematic and widespread program that penetrated deeply into people's psyches and raised larger questions about the mind's vulnerability to manipulation and coerced change.

Hong Kong was supposed to be just the second stop on a leisurely round-the-world trip, which began in Japan, where I had arranged to be discharged from the military after two years of service as an Air Force psychiatrist. But that trip was interrupted by interviews arranged by people I met in Hong Kong with Western missionaries and teachers, and Chinese students and intellectuals who had been put through thought reform, and by my deep absorption in—one could say obsession with—those interviews. But now I was getting anxious. Our money was running out, and I was experiencing a sense of duty, a feeling of necessity to return to America for the serious business of psychoanalytic training and pursuit of my psychiatric career in general—that is, to get back to the structures of real life. I was very reluctant to leave Hong Kong but could not seem to imagine staying. BJ was game either way. Hence my solitary walk.

As I circled ever more widely from the hotel, walking away from the harbor to places that seemed quieter and a little less populated, I found myself coming to a decision. I rushed back to make my announcement to BJ. We had to leave and make our way home. It was impossible to stay.

Yet somehow the next morning, I was, with BJ's help, working on an application for a research grant to remain in Hong Kong. "You did not make the decision—the decision made you" is the way a friend put it when I told him the story. My profound inner desire was to stay, but I could not quite accept that desire—could not see myself as one who would do so—because it seemed to be a kind of transgression, a rejection of an expected career and a safer life.

It was just a decade after the end of World War II, and American psychiatry had been reenergized by the influence of psychoanalysis and had become an admired and lucrative profession. I had never doubted that I would be part of this surge, that I would combine psychiatric practice with a certain amount of related teaching and research. Remaining indefinitely half a world removed in a British colony did not seem to be a way to do that. At the same time I was not only fascinated with the interviews themselves but drawn to the larger historical world in which I found myself. I was having lively discussions with knowledgeable American, European, and Chinese scholars, journalists, and diplomats. These "China watchers" conveyed to me their insights on the appeal and excesses of the Communist revolution, and were in turn eager to hear my impressions, as a psychiatrist, of a thought reform process they found psychologically confusing. It was a heady immersion into immediate historical forces, and I wanted to sustain that immersion. I was aware of Hong Kong's antiquated status as a British colony in which there was limited contact between Europeans and the predominantly Chinese population. But I was nonetheless drawn to the place with its ferries and hills and relationship to the surrounding sea, as well as its partial access to the often mysterious events occurring during the early years of Chinese Communist governance of Mainland China. That partial access had special importance at a time when the United States did not recognize Communist China and there was little communication between the two nations.

My intellectual excitement about thought reform was accompanied by a sense of adventure, of plunging into realms that seemed uncharted. But I was also frightened by that impulse. It seemed dangerous, bound up with too great a risk, which is why I went through the motions of rejecting my desire to stay. BJ's support did much to help me overcome my anxiety. She never looked upon staying in Hong Kong as a transgression.

A Military Gift

How I came to be doing those interviews in Hong Kong is a bit of a story and has much to do with the military. I sometimes say that the military liberated me from a conventional life and I have never shown it much gratitude. Soon after the onset of the Korean War in June 1950, America instituted a special draft of doctors, as they were in short supply in the military. My draft board allowed me no time beyond my completion of the second year of my psychiatric residency at the Downstate Medical Center of the State University of New York, in June 1951. I was told that I had the choice of either enlisting in one of the services as a medical officer or being drafted into the Army as a private. I chose the Air Force for my medical enlistment for reasons I cannot completely recall, but which I believe had to do with having relatively more freedom in that service and a greater likelihood of working only in psychiatry. In any case, I made my one trip to the Pentagon, where I maneuvered through its labyrinthine ramps and archways to take and pass my physical examination.

Just a few months before my 1951 enlistment, I fell in love and began for the first time to think of my future as including another person. BJ was working in television after having graduated from Barnard College as an

English major, and was beginning to write. We met in a casual New York fashion—on a "double-blind date" in which each of us had been "fixed up" with someone else. BJ and I were quickly drawn to one another and, during the period between my enlistment and my first military assignment, we traveled together through France and Italy. That assignment was to a hospital at Westover Air Force Base, not far from Springfield, Massachusetts. There were four other psychiatrists in that hospital unit, all at about my level but a few years older, the one who arrived first serving as chief. The work was ordinary but valuable for me in gaining experience beyond the limited world of residency training. And BJ and I were able to stay together near the base in a little cabin on a small pond (all part of a dingy motel that seemed perfect for us), where she wrote children's stories and plays.

Our small idyll was rudely interrupted by a requisition for a psychiatrist to be sent overseas. The choice of which one had to be made by our then chief, Benson Snyder, who was to become a leading Boston psychoanalyst and teacher, and is still a good friend. Ben chose me because I was the youngest, the lowest in seniority (as the last to arrive), and the only one who was not married. My first reaction was resentment: I was happy the way things were, and did not want to be sent anywhere. Over the years Ben and I have joked about how that initial resentment gave way to deep gratitude to him for making a choice that so influenced my life. As I remember, I was permitted to make a request as to where I wished to be sent, and rather conventionally asked for Paris, but was hardly surprised when the orders came through for Tokyo. Now BJ and I were faced with our own choices. We were intent on staying together. So we married, in early 1952, in Cincinnati, which was her hometown, and our nervous three-day "honeymoon" consisted mainly of travel arrangements (to northern California, where I was to report for my flight to Japan) and other preparations for my overseas service. At the time I was much more upset by our separation than by any thought of physical danger ahead.

We were not separated for long, as she arranged to travel to Tokyo as a correspondent accredited to two American magazines, as opposed to enduring a wait of about a year or so, which was standard for a wife joining her officer husband in Japan. But our reunion was all too brief, as the Air Force in its wisdom sent me immediately to Korea—not as punishment for my wife's appearing in this unconventional way, but to make clear that her doing so would not deter them from their prior military planning. I then served for six months as command psychiatrist with the Fifth Air Force at Taegu, a medium-sized city in South Korea well behind the lines. What was remarkable was that I was the only Air Force psychiatrist in all of Korea—there were, of course, many Army psychiatrists, but in the Air Force only me. The Air Force would fly me to other bases to evaluate anyone who seemed to be in psychiatric trouble. Often as not the problem would consist of a kitchen worker threatening another with a knife, or an airman becoming withdrawn or depressed and unable to perform his duty. For more serious problems—for instance, pilots who refused to fly—referral would usually be made to "regular" Air Force medical officers (not necessarily psychiatrists), those with career commitments to the service who did flying time of their own. Those regular officers, committed as they were to command, would do everything possible to keep such pilots at duty. "Reservists" like myself, by contrast, were more likely to give precedence to individual psychological needs and to send such pilots back to the States for treatment.

During my six months as a flying psychiatrist in Korea, BJ settled into Tokyo, moving in with a Japanese family and continuing her writing, which now included feature stories for English-language Japanese newspapers. She also befriended a number of Japanese university students and with them formed the English-language "East–West discussion group," which provides perhaps the most amazing statistic of this volume in that it continues to meet fifty-eight years later. We could observe how students from Tokyo University who spoke so ardently of rebellious democratic principles or Marxist views of history evolved into leading Japanese diplomats or participants in the Japanese "economic miracle" (and subsequent decline).

These were the last days of the American occupation, and I had no trouble telephoning BJ almost every night from Korea. More than that, I could hitch rides on planes heading from Taegu to various Japanese cities. I would call to arrange a romantic rendezvous at, say, an inn in Kyoto or a hotel in Tokyo or Nagoya. (We would later advise friends that one of the two secrets to a long marriage was to live in separate cities during the first six months. [The second secret was to subscribe to two copies of *The New York Times*].) But despite those exciting reunions, I was happy to be sent back to Japan, where we could rent a Japanese-style house in the middle of rice paddies between the base at Tachikawa, to which I was assigned, and the Tokyo metropolis. We managed to spend a great deal of time in Tokyo, and my involvement with the city was furthered when I was asked to set up an outpatient clinic to handle general problems of Air Force personnel there, an opportunity that I happily embraced.

For me discovering Japan meant discovering the world. It was partly a matter of encountering a culture so different from my own, and partly the remarkable experience of the Japanese in undergoing the pain, confusion, and, for some, liberation associated with war, defeat, and occupation. Through the minds of the university students—only later did I realize that they were just five or six years younger than I was—I got a powerful sense of the country's shifting historical currents, and the degree to which young people especially were involved in struggles with change. Those struggles encompassed everything in Japan, whether involving cultural tradition, experience in families, or political beliefs and policies. Through BJ's work we also met a number of writers, painters, and potters who taught me much about the interweaving of creative work and social upheaval. And I began what was to be my longest Japanese friendship, with Takeo Doi, then a young psychiatrist at Tokyo University, who did some of his training in the United States.

For more than a half century, Takeo and I were to share idiosyncratic ideas about how individual people in both Japan and the United States combined deep conflict with innovation and achievement. We also found ways to help one another psychologically in our complicated personal journeys through the two cultures (including his opposition to his American psychoanalyst's pressure to undergo the kind of character change that would enable him to adapt more easily to Western professional practice). Takeo was to become a leading figure in Japanese psychiatry, noted for his nuanced work on the psychology of dependency in the mother–child relationship and throughout the society, work which had much relevance for Western cultural experience as well. Takeo was to deepen my understanding of everything I experienced in Japan, whether in connection with young people, Hiroshima survivors, or members of Aum Shinrikyo—always doing so with a kind of sardonic humor that made me aware that there was still much more to learn.

What I observed during those early days in Japan led to my preoccupation with the interplay of individual lives with the larger fluctuations of history, a theme I came to refer to as "individual psychology and historical change." In a couple of letters to friends I mentioned a possible future project of doing a study of Japanese youth as exemplars of that theme, so it is conceivable that I would have returned to Japan for some such project, even if I had not been swept up by what happened next.

During the summer of 1953, long after I was back in Japan, BJ finally managed to obtain the credentials for work as a correspondent in Korea that she had been seeking during the time I was there. She went there anyway and did some writing about events surrounding the armistice that brought an end to the war. It had been both a civil war and a military activation of the Cold War, expanded all too broadly by President Truman and his secretary of state Dean Acheson. Most Americans, myself included, were unaware of its dimensions of killing and dying, which were to rival those of the later Vietnam War. By the time I and BJ reached that country, early Communist victories had been reversed by a MacArthur-led surge, which had then been turned back by the intervention of Chinese "volunteers," culminating in a protracted stalemate at Panmunjom and the 38th Parallel.

In late August of 1953, during one of our telephone calls (now she was on the Korean end, calling me in Japan), she spoke excitedly about what was called "Operation Big Switch," the repatriation of American prisoners of war from Chinese Communist captivity in North Korea. She said that there were beginning observations and reports about the American soldiers having been subjected to a psychological process that left them confused and sometimes expressing the views of their former Communist enemies, and that psychiatrists were interviewing them upon their return. We agreed that it would be very interesting for me if I could arrange to be assigned to the project. I immediately contacted Colonel Donald Peterson, the medical officer in charge of all psychiatric personnel in the Far East. He had heard me discuss some of my impressions of the conflicts of the few combat pilots I had examined, was well disposed toward my work, and quickly arranged the assignment for me.

I joined the team of psychiatrists interviewing the returning men at the South Korean port city of Inchon, in Panmunjom, the "no-man's land" separating North and South Korea, where the men had been received. But I did most of my interviewing on a troop ship called the *General Pope*, joining the repatriated men on a fifteen-day voyage from Inchon to San Francisco. This sea voyage was useful to the men as an interlude between their hypercontrolled prisoner-of-war experience and the demands of the American environment to which they were returning. Like other psychiatrists on board, I conducted individual interviews with them—ninety in all—to determine their mental status and to decide whether any form of therapy was indicated.

The men had been held in prisoner-of-war camps administered by the Chinese and subjected there to a process their captors called "thought reform." There had been sensationalized accounts of "brainwashing" in China itself, but little was known about the actual workings of thought reform. I could identify its two basic components as confession-extraction and "reeducation." The confessions were produced by pressures, threats, and actual deprivations, which in the extreme conditions of the camps could be life-threatening. Confessions were inseparable from coercive forms of group study, involving eight to twelve or more POWs, in which Chinese mentors put forward their Communist interpretation of the American war against "the people" of Korea and China, and of the "capitalistic worldview" that brought on the war. The reeducation process included constant criticism and self-criticism in the service of the demanded change in POWs' personal attitudes and beliefs; and the self-examination could apply to not just these large issues but the smallest everyday misdemeanor. Consider the document, labeled "Confession and Self-Criticism," given me by one of the men I interviewed on the ship, containing what he wrote while in the camp:

> This morning after breakfast my plat leader came into my
> quarters and told me to clean up the yard. I saw that the plat
> leader was right in telling me to clean up the yard because it is
> his duty to see that it gets done. Instead of obeying my superior,
> I not only forgot about my work but another hour later I was
> caught in another co. I realize that if this were not the Chinese

people's Volunteers, if this were a Japanese or German POW camp, I would surely be punished to a terrible degree, maybe even to death. Because of the Chinese people's Lenient Policy in the care of POWs my punishment for this crime will be very light. I promise and guarantee that in the future I will try my very best to obey all the rules and regulations set forth by the Chinese people's Volunteers. If in the future I do make any more mistakes I will come to the Chinese and confess all my crimes. When I leave here, I will go and tell my plat leader how sorry I am that my disobedience has caused so much ill feelings among the Chinese and myself. I will then complete the job the plat leader assigned me to.

Signed

[name and serial number]

Those seen as resistive to the process were labeled by the Chinese as "reactionaries" and threatened with permanent incarceration or death, while those who were more responsive were considered "progressives" and sometimes given slight improvements in their treatment in ways that could contribute to survival. A handful was sufficiently affected by the reeducation to decide to remain with their captors by going back with them to Communist China.

I conducted twelve group therapy sessions on the voyage, which gave many of the men an opportunity to share feelings about their experiences and their former captors in ways that they could not permit themselves to do within the accusatory and fearful atmosphere of their imprisonment. Just as, during their incarceration, they had got through their experience by partial withdrawal—or as they put it, "playing it cool" or "putting my mind in neutral"—they continued to use these dissociative defenses on the ship and undoubtedly in their lives well beyond that voyage. Their openness was further constrained by the military setting, in which the men had to be concerned about being punished anew for something they did back there or said now.

Overall, I found the men to be deeply confused, still showing considerable apathy and withdrawal. They could, occasionally and sometimes inadvertently, express Communist views, but mostly they were resentful toward the Chinese for the pain they had caused, and in some that resentment could extend to the American military for having put them in that situation and for not showing enough understanding of their ordeal. As I later wrote, "The average repatriate [on arriving at Inchon] was dazed, lacked spontaneity, spoke in a dull, monotonous tone [and] . . . at the same time was tense, restless, clearly suspicious of his new surroundings." Nor did most of the men show great enthusiasm at arriving in San Francisco or being greeted there by family members or former military buddies. Their eyes often expressed what was called a "thousand-mile stare."

I had mixed feelings about those interviews and group sessions. I felt sympathy for the men and was concerned that our reports might not be confined to appropriate medical channels and be used for disciplinary purposes. So I limited my comments to psychological observations. At the same time I was deeply interested in the process of thought reform and its being applied across the board to American prisoners of war. It was clear that the reeducation had mixed results and that there had been much self-protective playacting and withdrawal on the part of the men. Still, the Chinese had managed, at least temporarily, to gain considerable control over the minds of many of the POWs. And even the absurd lengths to which they would go in producing childlike confessions suggested the commitment of the reformers to their project. I was frustrated, however, by the military setting and the relatively superficial quality of the interviews and group therapy I had been able to conduct. I wanted to learn more about the thought reform process.

I flew back to Tokyo, where BJ awaited me. But we did not leave Japan for almost another three months, as I had decided to write an article for a psychiatric journal on my experiences with the repatriated American soldiers. The paper that resulted, "Home by Ship: Reaction Patterns of American Prisoners of War Repatriated from North Korea," was published in the *American Journal of Psychiatry* in April 1954. It was of no great brilliance, but was probably the first article to be published on the subject of thought reform in a scholarly journal. I had stayed to write it because the experience had been important to me, and I wanted to record it. I also wanted to place myself somewhere on the map of my profession—to move ahead and be noticed. So began a pattern of feeling impelled to write something, getting well behind schedule, but staying put to see it through. I had no idea of what I was getting into.

The Vortex

As I immersed myself in the Hong Kong interviews, I realized that the thought reform to which the POWs had been exposed was an export version. Now I was hearing about a much more profound and systematic process, as applied on the Chinese Mainland. I was fascinated by it on two levels. The first was the nitty-gritty experience I would study with each Chinese or Western person I talked to, which led immediately to fundamental psychological questions about ways in which minds can be manipulated and changed, and about capacities to resist such manipulation. Also involved were important distinctions between coercive and therapeutic approaches to bringing about change. These questions were at the heart of my profession and have significance for the way we live in general. But there was another level to thought reform: its visionary or transcendent characteristic, the specter of hundreds of millions of Chinese—in their neighborhoods, schools, and places of work—caught up in a compulsory movement of purification and renewal. What did it mean for such an extreme ethos to dominate an entire vast society?

Intellectuals and students experienced the quintessential version of thought reform. It was the version that the Chinese Communists evolved over decades and that served as a major tool, a psychological underpinning, of their entire revolution. Then, in late 1951, two years after their takeover, and three years prior to my study, the regime mounted a national thought reform campaign aimed especially at intellectuals, creating what an observer called "one of the most spectacular events in human history [in which] tens of thousands of intellectuals . . . [were] brought to their knees, accusing themselves relentlessly at tens of thousands of meetings and in tens of millions of written words."

The overall narrative was always the same: the "old society" in China, or any noncommunist state anywhere, was evil and corrupt because of the domination of the "exploiting classes"—landowners and capitalists and bourgeoisie—and everyone exposed to such a society retains "evil remnants" or "ideological poisons," which must be eliminated to create a truly revolutionary society. In effect, what had to be destroyed was all mental life separate from or prior to the revolution, to be replaced by truly revolutionary mental life. Later I came to view the process as an apocalyptic cleansing of all the past—a *psychological* apocalypticism in which all prior products of the human mind had to give way to a new collective mind-set that was pure, perfect, and eternal. I was drawn into this vortex, not as a participant but as a critical explorer entering strange and unfamiliar territory.

The Things I Carried

What did I bring to my study of thought reform? Professionally, I was caught up in the exciting post–World War II American psychoanalytic honeymoon period. Psychoanalysis underwent considerable expansion after both world wars because it seemed to offer, as other schools of thought did not, understanding about the experience of soldiers in combat. But the American embrace of psychoanalysis during the decades after World War II was unique. It had much to do with the sanctuary our country could offer refugee European practitioners. But it also had to do with a deep-seated American enthusiasm about the possibilities for reshaping the self, given our history of people creating "new lives" through changing frontiers and through emigration from the "old world." I had read a certain amount of Freud in college and medical school. And during my psychiatric residency I began to take in the writings of contending schools within psychoanalysis. These included classical practitioners who held closely to Freud, "ego psychologists" who sought to diminish the focus on instinct or drive by emphasizing the formation of the individual self or ego, and "neo-Freudians" who moved further from the master in stressing cultural influences and collective behavior. But I was conflicted about my reactions to psychoanalysis. On the one hand I considered it one of the great revolutions of modern thought. On the other, I felt appalled by its frequently dogmatic tendencies, especially among its classical exponents, but also by the agitated hairsplitting among advocates of the various schools. And I was troubled by the heavy-handed prose of so much psychoanalytic writing, which seemed drowned in its own concepts.

I struggled with this ambivalence toward psychoanalysis during my two years of psychiatric residency training. My best teachers by far were psychoanalysts, and I learned a lot from them about what we called "dynamic psychiatry," which emphasized such basic psychoanalytic principles as unconscious motivation and the importance of childhood development. But I felt I always had to sort out what they said and differentiate between real insights and a quick tendency to invoke traditional concepts (such as the "Oedipus complex") to explain just about everything. I engaged in extensive conversations with other residents who had similar doubts, and struggled to translate psychoanalytic jargon into ordinary language. I had neither the experience nor the knowledge to provide much alternative theory. But I had a certain critical sensibility that included a strong aversion to dogma of any kind, especially that related to all-or-none beliefs and emotions, an early manifestation of what I would later call an allergy to totalism.

There was a certain parallel in my evolving political convictions. My parents and their friends were liberal Democrats, and I can remember my excitement when, at the age of six in 1932, my first-grade teacher announced that Franklin Delano Roosevelt had been elected president. My family, and everyone else around me, had made it clear that this was a big moment. Through my childhood we all held strongly to Rooseveltian liberalism, which, as my father made clear, was both "good for the Jews" and a form of larger social justice. At the same time, I now realize, my parents had a "don't rock the boat" mentality. Their parents had come to this country, in the late nineteenth century, fleeing their shtetl outside of Minsk to escape pogroms and avoid service in the czarist army. My mother and father, born in this country, were grateful for its sanctuary, and were intent on being fully American. That meant distancing themselves not only from the old country (which they had been told much about though never had seen) but also from the poverty they had seen too much of throughout their childhoods in the Lower East Side of Manhattan. While exposed to Yiddish in their families even before English, they would use it only when they did not want my sister and me to understand what they were saying.

I became aware early that Jews were always vulnerable to abuse, especially with the emergence of the Nazis, and I'm sure I was not free of more searing unconscious terror, having to do with persecutions, transmitted over Jewish generations. I had occasional brushes with Italian or Irish kids who came from outside our middle-class Jewish neighborhood in the Crown Heights section of Brooklyn and made anti-Semitic remarks. But I experienced our neighborhood as a protective environment and that gave me a sense of belonging. It provided our mostly Jewish friends, and also Ben and Sol's Delicatessen, where we went at least once a week for lox and bagels and corned beef and pastrami sandwiches—in no way superior to other nearby Jewish delicatessens but somehow *our* Jewish delicatessen.

I also had a touch of what a friend called a "Jewish Huck Finn childhood," which mostly had to do with the Brooklyn Dodgers and Ebbets Field, where they played, and became for me and a number of friends a "field of dreams." On frequent game day afternoons a few of us would hang around outside the stadium and then, during the late innings, "sneak in"—run wildly past the turnstiles and into the aisles opening up on the glorious vista of the large baseball diamond, and quickly find seats to settle into for the remainder of the game. We were never stopped or caught, and only much later did I realize that it was the policy of the guards to turn the other check and let the kids in with only an inning or two remaining. We, mostly well-behaved middle-class youngsters, could have the satisfaction of a successful transgression.

Sports in general, along with my studies, seemed to dominate my childhood. My father did not play at them much himself—though he was proud of having been student manager of the basketball team while an undergraduate at the City College of New York—but encouraged me to do so. I became a passable athlete, playing endlessly at stickball, baseball, football, basketball, and tennis—whether in the Brooklyn streets, a schoolyard, a local park, or the Jewish summer camp I attended from the ages of six to fifteen. I can remember thinking as a child that adult life must be very boring because it did not seem to include spending much time playing a game with a ball. I believe there was a kind of tandem between my passion for sports and my energy toward my studies. I was always a conscientious student and had a strong early interest in mathematics and history. My father's life experience was influential here as one of many bright Jewish kids from poor families guided by sympathetic teachers to the elite Townsend Harris Hall high school as a path to free higher education at City College. He delighted in telling me how many of the kids he grew up with became obscure stand-up comics or members of the Jewish Murder, Inc., with the implication that only education had saved him from such a fate.

But I had other family exposure of a very different kind, in the form of my maternal grandparents' version of Orthodox Judaism. It seemed to consist of suffocating rules about not just what one could eat and the sets of dishes to be used, but concerning just about every form of behavior, along with agitated intolerance for anyone who did not follow these rules. On those occasions that I was coerced into going to my grandparents' synagogue, everything was chanted in a language I could not understand, nor was there ever any attempt to explain to me the purpose or meaning of any ritual or prayer. I remember one strange incident that came to signify that kind of religion for me. A man selling Christmas trinkets managed somehow to gain entry into my grandparents' apartment. After he was angrily shown the door, my grandmother spent what seemed to be hours blessing and purifying the contaminated areas of the floor on which he had trodden, and attached booties to her own shoes to avoid stepping herself in those areas. Yet she and her husband were kind and modest people who happened to be caught up in an absolutized form of religion. My parents broke away from such religious practice, my mother with a certain nostalgia for Jewish ritual, and my father with an articulated (though not to the grandparents) disdain that legitimated my own discomfort. I now see that version of Orthodox Judaism as a childhood encounter with what I would later know as totalism.

I was just sixteen years old when I entered Cornell University in 1942, having been permitted to "skip" grades in primary school (a common practice then in relation to good students with ambitious parents), and having attended a rapid-advance junior high school program (gaining another year). At Cornell I was subject to wartime academic acceleration and did the equivalent of three years' work in two years before entering medical school. I was a biology major, as preparation for medical school, though I was more drawn to courses in history and literature. Eventually I became editorial page director of the *Cornell Daily Sun*, the student newspaper, and made the university tennis team.

But especially in the beginning I was lonely and somewhat confused, and trying to act older than I was took its toll. I can remember, a few months after I arrived at Cornell, sitting in an Ithaca movie theater close to tears in response to Bing Crosby's rendering of "White Christmas" in the film *Holiday Inn*. My response had little to do with Christmas, which I had never celebrated, or with missing my family (I wanted to be away from it and on my own), but with the sadness and longing in a song that was to become a staple of kitsch popular culture and at the time expressed much of the American mood at the beginning of our involvement in World War II. So I joined a Jewish Greek-letter fraternity, where I could become part of a small community, though often at odds with its atmosphere. I even found a girlfriend and became social chairman—I'm not sure how or why, but I was undoubtedly compensating for my social awkwardness. I have uncomfortable memories of too many evenings of drinking beer together and singing the inane songs college kids sang with their fraternity brothers in those days, but I have to admit now that the experience helped me to get along better with people in general.

My inner conflicts also led to painful failures. One had to do with tennis. As a neophyte reporter on the *Daily Sun* I was assigned to the tennis team and would sometimes practice on the court with its members. The coach became increasingly gloomy as he saw his team decimated by wartime enlistments. In a less than gracious invitation he said to me one day: "Since you're covering us anyhow, why don't you just join the team?" I was expected to be no more than a reserve, but on one occasion, when several regulars became unavailable, had to be a last-minute replacement in a doubles match. I remember the match going on endlessly in the alien small-town setting of State College, Pennsylvania (where Penn State is located); my abject humiliation as I missed shot after shot; my feelings of guilt toward my partner and the team; and the coach's plaintive despair as he cried out, "Bob, just try to play *half* as well as you do in practice!" While I wasn't a very good player—I would improve with my passion for the game over subsequent years—I think my collapse had to do with my sense of being illegitimate as a member of the team and perhaps, because of my age and immaturity, as a student at Cornell in general.

At the *Daily Sun* things were better. I advanced from sports to interviews of notable professors to editorials. But that did not mean that I had acquired wisdom. I remember one editorial I wrote in the spring of

1944, toward the end of my stay at Cornell, called "How new will the better world be?" The title was more catchy than my argument, which was something along the lines that, after winning the war, we could improve the world considerably and prevent future wars by making full use of existing institutions (I'm sure I emphasized the United Nations) rather than by dreams of overturning everything. The editorial was the work of a naïve young man (then turning eighteen) who was a bit carried away by his own rhetoric. I also wrote a few humor columns, inspired by the formidable presence of Kurt Vonnegut, just before he went off to war. Vonnegut was a charismatic figure at the paper (I always thought of him as editor in chief though he was actually associate editor), even then notable for his mordant satire. Decades later we became friends and shared occasional dinners and antinuclear and antiwar platforms. He taught me much about combining passion with a sense of absurdity but everything began with that glancing encounter at Cornell.

My editorials gained some attention on campus, and I was approached by the head of the student radio station concerning the possibility of joining his group and making a regular editorial commentary. I liked the idea, and was told that the next step was a radio tryout, which would be more or less a formality. But when reading various materials and responding to questions on this simulated broadcast, I was hesitant and uncertain, stumbling badly over my words and aware of making a dreadful impression. The radio person was tactful and said something to the effect that we should wait awhile before making any decision, and I was aware that my radio career at Cornell had come to an end.

But the most costly performance of that kind occurred when I was interviewed for Cornell Medical College, considered one of America's best. Though the medical college was in New York City, it was part of the same university, and two senior faculty members came to Ithaca specifically to interview premedical students there who were presumably given special consideration. While I don't recall much that happened during my interview, I distinctly remember feeling flustered, failing to look the men in the eye or address them by name, and being extremely inarticulate about explaining myself in connection with my interests, medical or otherwise. While medical schools then had Jewish quotas, it was surely my poor showing in that interview that did me in.

It is frequently said, in relation to physical growth during adolescence and young adulthood, that we need time to learn to inhabit our bodies. But we also need to learn how to inhabit our minds. I had sufficient intellectual curiosity to reach out toward some kind of public expression concerning the world but, unformed as I was, at critical moments I was unable to be verbally coherent. Later, precisely that verbal dimension was to become central to every aspect of my work and life, whether as a researcher, writer, speaker, activist, or partner in dialogue. When asked why I dictate all of my writing, I sometimes say that where others have a hand–brain connection (in producing words on their computer or typewriter), mine is a larynx–brain connection. Alfred Adler, the early Freudian disciple and dissident, would consider my sequence a clear example of his general principle of achievement compensating for earlier weaknesses.

I've never been quite clear about how I came to choose medicine as a career. I was not one of those who had long imagined himself wearing a white coat and a stethoscope and saving people's lives. In fact I remember once fainting in a movie theater while watching a gory medical scene in a film about Dr. Kildare, a prominent cinema hero of the time. But I was affected by being thrust into the reversal of roles with my older sister, a kind of premature therapeutic responsibility because of her early psychological confusions, depressive tendencies, and generally erratic behavior. In that sense becoming a physician and a psychiatrist were ways of mobilizing myself as an adult for what the child had been asked to do. An important influence was my father's year of military duty (after his graduation from City College in 1918, at the end of World War I) in the Army Medical Corps. He told me a number of times about the frustration of his fervent wish to become a doctor by his terrible financial situation at the time. So he became a businessman, dealing in household appliances. But throughout my childhood he took pride in cooperating closely with doctors in overseeing medical treatment in our family. Rather than being a scholar, he had a lively, restless intelligence and a pragmatic focus on knowledge as necessary to dealing with any situation. I was hardly unique in unconsciously carrying out unfulfilled parental ambitions, and in reflecting the immigrant Jewish sequence from poverty to business to the professions.

My mother was very much part of the equation. She was proud of being a high school graduate, spoke of many learned people in her family, and lovingly insisted that my attraction to schoolwork would lead me to great things. Not only did she embrace the Jewish pride in producing a medical offspring but she invoked a near-mythical shtetl ancestor, after whom I was partly named, known as a powerful healer. My middle name, Jay, was an Americanized version of Chaim Yacov, the name of her grandfather, whom she, with the help of many tales she had heard from the old country, increasingly likened to me, his ostensible namesake. Chaim Yacov was a great student of the Torah from early childhood, and so tall as a boy that when married at the age of thirteen he was given as a wedding gift a coat with a large seam to allow for his continuing growth. I too was always tall (eventually reaching six feet two) while everyone in between, including my parents, was quite short. Chaim Yacov would have become a rabbi, the story went, but the shtetl was too small to support one, so instead he became its wise man, called upon to give spiritual or material advice to anyone in need of it. My beloved Aunt Ida (my mother's slightly older first cousin) further embellished the stories with eyewitness accounts, as she had actually known Chaim Yacov as a child in the shtetl. At first I did not know what to make of these stories, but I soon came to enjoy them with full recognition of their mythic romanticization. I did not have him in mind when I chose to attend medical school, or when I quickly gravitated toward psychiatry. But he was surely inhabiting me as a faraway healer-hero and a link to an often vague Jewish past in a young person taking his plunge into an American future.

Much later, during my general internship at the Jewish Hospital of Brooklyn in 1948–49, and my two subsequent years of psychiatric residency, I was drawn into a social circle that first complicated and then clarified my politics. The group was centered around "Yip" Harburg and his wife, Edeline. Harburg was my father's best friend, a man he simply loved. The two had similar backgrounds of Lower East Side poverty as second-generation immigrant Jews and had been classmates at City College. They then became partners in a small business that eventually failed in the Depression, which released Harburg to do what he was meant to do, write brilliant socially conscious song lyrics. "Brother Can You Spare a Dime" became one of the most powerful cultural renderings of the Depression, to the extent that many thought it had contributed to

Franklin D. Roosevelt's election in 1932. Not long before completing this memoir, I was reduced to tears by a revival of Yip's great romantic-progressive musical, *Finian's Rainbow*. I was also joyfully amazed to learn that a Yip Harburg postage stamp was being issued, though hardly surprised that the phrase printed on it was not "Brother, can you spare a dime?" but (from his lyrics for the film *The Wizard of Oz*) "Somewhere over the rainbow skies are blue."

The Harburgs' Central Park West apartment was a gathering place for theater people and film writers, including many who had been "blacklisted" during those days of McCarthyite persecution. There was lots of music and singing, and I can still hear Yip's own raspy but haunting rendering of his lyrics from *Finian*. Those I met at the Harburgs' apartment or the summer place they rented from friends in Katonah, New York, included I. F. Stone, the legendary journalist; Leo Huberman, co-editor of the *Monthly Review*; Paul Robeson, the extraordinary actor, singer, and athlete who, after decades of American persecution, gravitated to the Soviet Union; and Henry Wallace, who was at the time running for president against Harry Truman and Thomas Dewey as the candidate of his own newly formed Progressive Party. I once participated in a tennis doubles game that included Robeson (quite old at the time but athletically graceful) and Wallace (a terrible but good-humored player). At the center of everything was Yip himself, one of the world's great charmers, who much resembled his leprechaun character in *Finian*. I sometimes felt dully conventional in a world of such lively and creative people, but was always accepted as one of them.

Much of the conversation at the Harburgs' was thoughtful and knowledgeable, but I began to notice that some of those present expressed romanticized views of the Soviet Union. I still remember one exchange in which someone was waxing poetic about the glories of Soviet policies toward workers, declaring (with how much irony I cannot recall) "Everybody is given three weeks' vacation to visit the Black Sea." Someone else asked in return, "But what if you don't like the Black Sea?"—to which there came the reply: "*Everybody* loves the Black Sea." I would discuss with my friend Murray Levin (who often joined me at the Harburgs' and was later to become a prominent political scientist) the unwillingness of some people in the group to acknowledge the infamous Soviet purge trials of the late thirties. Murray and I tried to carve out a more balanced perspective toward both the Soviet Union and our own country.

So where did all this leave me politically at the time? That was not completely clear, but I knew that I wanted to be critical of much American behavior while retaining my affection for my country, and at the same time to reject Soviet abuses and separate myself clearly from Soviet supporters on the left. So I cast my first presidential vote, in 1948, for Henry Wallace. Wallace had been an admirably progressive vice president and secretary of commerce under Roosevelt, and disagreed with Harry Truman's Cold War policies. When forced out by Truman, Wallace ran a passionate, if hopeless, third-party campaign, during which, as I later learned, he was a bit blind to communist manipulation within his movement. I have sometimes asked myself whether, knowing what I do now, I would have voted instead for Harry Truman, as my father told me he had. My answer tends to be no. While chastened by the 2000 presidential election against supporting a third-party candidate in a way that enhances the conservative cause, I would be reluctant to cast a vote for the man who made the decision to drop atomic bombs on Hiroshima and Nagasaki (all the more so in the light of a recent scholarly view that, had Roosevelt not replaced Wallace with Truman as his vice presidential candidate in 1944, Wallace might well have decided against using those atomic bombs). I would also be hesitant to support a president who would deal with the Korean crisis by involving us in such large-scale warfare, and had in addition initiated the "loyalty oaths" that were a precursor to McCarthyite persecution.

It turned out that I myself was not unnoticed by the FBI in those days. Soon after Robeson came to my apartment as a guest at a small party, I was told by workers at a garage in the same building that agents had come around asking them what they knew about me. When I enlisted in the Air Force soon afterward, I couldn't help but wonder whether this limited association with Robeson would cause me trouble.

The parallel themes in my evolving professional and political formation had to do with opposition to the status quo and with an allergy to totalism, accompanied by much uncertainty. Professionally, that allergy was to dogmatic psychoanalysis, which had rapidly become its own status quo (any psychiatric resident worth his or her salt in those days gravitated to psychoanalytic training). But I was also drawn to the intellectual ferment of the psychoanalytic movement and was far from clear about how I would resolve this contradiction. My political allergy toward totalism was easy enough to express in connection with the Nazis—everyone was opposed to them—but was an issue I had to struggle with in connection with the dogma and practice of communism. While I never shared the visionary embrace of communism characteristic of many people around me and a sizable number of American and European intellectuals, I often felt close to such people and could be somewhat caught up in their momentum. I was groping for principles consistent with more imaginative psychoanalytic thought and with radical noncommunist social criticism. I brought this strongly felt but by no means fully coherent constellation of influences and beliefs to my encounter with thought reform.

2

———

Method and Reach

S TAYING IN HONG KONG meant settling in to a long-term study of a
process that had immediate relevance for the Chinese Communist
revolution as well as fundamental significance for individual and collective psychology. Combining in my work those various levels was part of
the fascination I felt for the subject. I was also struck by the intensity of
what I was encountering: an elderly European bishop leaning forward
in his hospital bed and declaring that the Communist reform process
was so powerful that it was part of "an alliance with the demons," and
a young Chinese woman still recoiling from the group hatred she had
experienced at a university in Beijing and yet wondering if she had been
"selfish" in leaving. I knew that I required a systematic method of investigating my subject, one that would yield results that were both reliable
and meaningful.

From the beginning it seemed to me common sense to go about things
by talking to people who had been put through thought reform, to make
use of an interview method. All the more so as I had been trained in such
a method during my two years of psychiatric residency and had already
applied it, in limited fashion, in my work with prisoners of war. So I chose
two groups of people—Westerners caught up in Chinese prisons, and
Chinese intellectuals and university students—solely because they had
been exposed to intense versions of thought reform. The way that the

process was carried out differed greatly in the two groups: to produce confessions, imprisoned Westerners were frequently subjected to physical brutality and torture, not the case with the Chinese in educational institutions. The Chinese, in turn, were more susceptible to exhortation about their country's future and guilt about their own privileged status. Yet Westerners could also be vulnerable to that exhortation and Chinese could feel deeply threatened by the new regime should they fail to make adequate progress. Both, that is, were put through coercive forms of confession extraction, criticism, self-criticism, and "struggle" (focused and unrelenting verbal assault mostly by fellow thought reform participants). I had no previous experience with either group of people I interviewed, but I did have that important encounter with prisoners of war at Inchon and on the *General Pope*. I seemed to acclimate quickly to the Hong Kong environment, which was at that time a small enough place for me to be in touch with most of the people who received and helped those subjected to thought reform in China itself: with Western consular officials, representatives of religious orders, and Chinese leaders of expatriate press services and other refugee organizations.

Westerners released from Chinese prisons were usually deported to Hong Kong, where their appearance was noted in the English-language newspaper, the *South China Morning Post*. Upon reading such a report I would telephone the consular or religious leader to seek an introduction, or ask a friend to do so on my behalf. In the case of Chinese, most of those I interviewed had been living in Hong Kong for some time (though one or two had just arrived), and they would be introduced to me by members of the refugee-intellectual groups mentioned above, who in some cases were already having interviews with me in relation to their own thought reform. Over time, as my work became known, others would take the initiative in suggesting people I might wish to interview. While there could be conflicts and difficulties, I came to feel a certain degree of comfort in those arrangements and in the work I was doing.

My evolving method was thus derived from the circumstances of the research. They required that I modify my training and experience. Even during my earlier psychiatric residency I had the sense that technical aspects of the doctor-patient relationship (including distancing and neutrality) had been emphasized at the expense of the human encounter, the interaction of two people with needs and aspirations. Now I gave still greater emphasis to that interaction and sought to combine it with disciplined research probing. I tried to balance my passion for research information with a recognition that I was working with vulnerable people who should not be pushed too far. Some of them—especially Westerners just days out of prison—seemed still to be "confessing," still telling their story to someone in authority. But as they realized that they were no longer under external coercion, the "confession" could give way to increasingly autonomous exploration. In a way we were both out there in strange geographic and spiritual territory, and we had something to offer each other.

What they had to offer me was clear—their experience with thought reform. What I had to offer them was less obvious but also important. They had been put through a traumatic procedure that could leave them confused about what had been done to them; most were in need of some kind of healing, and many sought to explore with me their emotions while making confessions and undergoing reeducation. I was well aware that I was not and should not be their formal therapist. Most, in fact, had little concept of psychological therapy as such. But I quickly sensed the importance of bringing a healing spirit to the encounter. No one went through thought reform without retaining a certain amount of anxiety and confusion, which in some could be almost immobilizing in their intensity. In responding to their questions and their emotional state, I was (as I later learned) applying the neo-Freudian psychoanalyst Harry Stack Sullivan's principle of "reciprocal motivation," of both sides getting something out of the interview. My being a physician was helpful in all this. A physician was a person you could talk to, from whom you expected an atmosphere of healing, and I had that requirement of myself.

I became increasingly aware that I was working not in a medical or a psychiatric office but "out there" in history, in an environment whose currents were created by a harsh, revolutionary project. I was interested in how people's earlier lives could make them more or less vulnerable to the pressures of thought reform. But I was most concerned with how the process operated, and what it did, in one way or another, to virtually everyone. I did not believe that the passions and confusions stirred up by thought reform could be represented by psychiatric categories (neurosis, psychosis, character disorder), and that was the beginning of a general disinclination to apply such categories to people responding to larger forces and in that way overclinicalize the world. I was trying to make use of my background as a clinician to identify psychological experiences of people caught up in historical storms. This was consistent with a longstanding interest in the study of history, and curiosity about its impact on individuals, that went back to my high school and college years. I've come to feel a little bit like Freud, who once said that psychoanalysis was his indirect path to his major intellectual interest, the study of ancient cultures. For me, modified psychoanalytic psychology has been a path to my essential intellectual preoccupation, that of the collective human behavior we call history, and especially the destructive behavior in recent history.

Now I could talk to people who had been subjected to an explosive historical moment: fifty Westerners, with whom I averaged fifteen to twenty hours of interview time (in English, as it was then the lingua franca for Westerners in China); and fifteen Chinese, averaging thirty to forty interview hours (including time required for translation). That came to more than a thousand hours of interviewing former participants in thought reform, supplemented by hundreds of additional hours talking to everyone I could find who had broader knowledge of the history and origins of thought reform, whether they were Chinese or Westerners, academics or diplomats, journalists or missionaries, businessmen or administrators, or expatriates of one kind or another who happened to be in Hong Kong. I decided against tape-recording any of these interviews because it seemed inadvisable in the highly suspicious Hong Kong environment, especially in the case of those emerging from a hypercontrolled thought reform experience. Instead I took extensive, one might say furious, notes, which a wonderful British secretary named Mrs. Partridge learned to decipher and type up for me. Whatever my confusions, I went about the work with an impassioned thoroughness.

I quickly realized that interviews would mean little without extensive exploration of their immediate and wider context. So I read everything I could about thought reform in China (much of it from press translations made available by the American consulate); about the Chinese Communist revolution and modern China (with emphasis on youth, rebellion, and change); about Chinese culture and civilization and the overall experience of Westerners (especially missionaries) in China; about the history and culture of Hong Kong; and about methods of confession extraction and other forms of psychological coercion in the Soviet Union (especially during the purge trials of the thirties). I found myself a regular visitor to English-language Hong Kong bookstores and had very active accounts with booksellers in England and the United States. I got a beginning sense, which I could build on later, of the extent to which thought reform, while drawing on Soviet Communist practice, derived mostly from Chinese cultural tradition, including the Confucianism at the center of that tradition.

All of this background probing resulted in the "mosaic principle" that became an important part of my method in this and subsequent research. The mosaic had at its center the interviews, which were the pragmatic core of the work. The invaluable background information—current, historical, and cultural—created the remainder of the mosaic, without which the interview material would be isolated and the entire research less comprehensible.

The financial support I was able to obtain for the research emerged both from the Hong Kong environment and from my prior military work with POWs. The group to which I sent that first application (soon after that walk through Kowloon) was called the Committee for a Free Asia, its name subsequently changed to the Asia Foundation. I knew the Hong Kong representative of that foundation, a retired university professor much interested in my work, and he rather quickly arranged for support while making clear that it was to be temporary and that I should arrange for longer-term backing elsewhere. It all seemed respectable enough as the foundation included on its board of directors an array of university presidents, prominent writers, and businessmen. Only much later did I learn that the group was sponsored by the CIA as part of its widespread policy of countering Communist intellectual and cultural influence. Though no one tried to influence the work in any way, I couldn't help but feel a bit tainted by the backing, as must have been the case with many scholars with a similar experience.

The more substantial research support revolved around David McKenzie Rioch, who was to become a very important person for me during those early professional years. A neurologist and psychiatrist and a leading figure at the Washington School of Psychiatry, he had been a disciple of Harry Stack Sullivan, considered by many the greatest of American-born psychoanalysts. Rioch was at the time the civilian director of neuropsychiatry of the Army Medical Service Graduate School at Walter Reed Army Medical Center, and he used his position to further advance research of various kinds in psychiatry and social science. Burly and externally crusty, Rioch was an unusually kind man who took much pleasure in helping young people he considered to have promise. I had met him only briefly during a trip he made to Korea as a consultant, and was referred to him by mutual friends.

Though I was highly unsure of myself as a psychiatric researcher, I could write to him with some confidence about the importance of thought reform and my beginning knowledge of it. Rioch was highly responsive, and a few weeks later wrote to tell me that a grant of ten thousand dollars (a respectable sum in those days) could be made for a year's work including salary and research expenses, and suggested that nine months of it be spent in Hong Kong and three months analyzing the data in Washington. He proposed that the grant be made to the Washington School of Psychiatry, where I would be appointed as a member of the faculty for that year. The grant began in October 1954 and covered my time in Hong Kong until leaving in late June of 1955. Rioch never became an intellectual mentor to me but he had deep sympathy for my work and was a wise and generous advisor and sponsor. He also conveyed to me important insights emphasized by Sullivan and the neo-Freudian school of psychoanalysis that he helped form. These included a focus on group pressure and communication patterns in groups, as well as on "interpersonal relations" (as opposed to individual psychology alone)—all of which had much relevance for my work. Rioch also brought his own observations on the enormous influence that extreme environments could have on individual behavior. And through his high professional standing, he did much to bring my project into the mainstream of American psychiatry. In Hong Kong, however, I was mostly on my own.

Over time, I developed a rhythm in the work. I would drive about the colony in our 1948 Standard, a small British car that served us well but had a bit of trouble chugging its way up to the highest point in Hong Kong, called "the Peak." I would drive to the order house of a priest, conduct an intensive interview for two hours or so, and on my way back would find a convenient place for a swim in a nearby bay. I was hearing about painful forms of experience, but I was exhilarated by the work I was doing, living out the sense of adventure I seemed to crave. Lacking a mentor and well aware of my professional inexperience, I at times had the thought that someone more seasoned should be doing this work. But it was I who was there, learning much about a vast and remarkable project of mind manipulation, and also about the limitations of such a project. However fumblingly, I was creating a method, a way of evolving into a historically minded psychiatrist.

Challenges and Bad Dreams

Both my method and identity could be challenged. A middle-aged French physician I interviewed five days after his arrival in Hong Kong following three and a half years of physically abusive thought reform in a Chinese prison fired a series of questions at me: How old was I? (I was twenty-eight.) How long had I been in Hong Kong doing the work? And finally, the question really on his mind: "Are you standing on the people's side or on the imperialists' side?" He then further explained that this was important because "from the imperialistic side we are not criminals and reeducation is a kind of compulsion" but "from the people's side it [reeducation] is to die and be born again." I was to hear no better statement of the moral dichotomy with which participants could view thought reform.

The question broke through the protective mental scaffolding I had constructed. In all other discussions with people put through the process, especially Westerners from prisons, I was comfortable in our mutual assumption that something wrong and bad had been done to them. But this French physician was saying that in part of his mind he believed that his prison experience, however brutal, provided him with something close to a religious conversion, a spiritual rebirth. And even when representing the other part of his mind, which condemned the process as coercive and unjust, he did so in the language of thought reform, within which the "imperialistic" view is the profoundly immoral European and American perspective, in contrast with the "people's" view, which is revolutionary, virtuous, and represents not only the Chinese people but people everywhere. It was clear to me that he was still immersed in his thought reform experience and deeply confused about where he stood in connection with it. I wanted to answer in a way that was honest and at the same time avoid saying anything that would prevent this interesting man I had just met from cooperating in the research. So I said that I was part of the noncommunist world, but I was trying to gain an understanding of all aspects and views of thought reform. This satisfied him sufficiently for him to pour out his story, during the course of which he came to a much more critical view of his experience. He never emerged completely from that initial confusion, however, and our interviews helped sensitize me to varied and paradoxical responses.

There was also a more general challenge I faced in taking in the newness and the extremity of what I saw and heard. As a European or American man or woman told me about life in a Chinese prison, I had to convert those words about what were for me unfamiliar experiences into visual images of my own. The person before me became a helpless prisoner surrounded by hostile Chinese cellmates in a small room that was part of an old building, or was in a slightly larger room and subjected, while manacled, to the endless accusations of an interrogator who could completely control the administration of physical and psychological pain. This was an overall process of *translating words into visual images* that became central to my work. In the case of Chinese, I would imagine the person I was interviewing in a large classroom at a busy university, undergoing fierce criticism and "struggle" from fellow students. Or in a special "revolutionary university," which I saw as a nondescript building with cavernous halls in which students were subjected day and night to the emotionally suffocating and hyper-rationalistic currents of the institution's only activity, that of thought reform.

The man responding somewhat haphazardly to these challenges was far from a mature researcher. BJ reminds me that at the time my dark hair was cut short, fifties-style, and my face looked quite young and unformed. In a memoir of her own she placed me among New York Jewish intellectuals who seemed to come out of the womb with their horn-rimmed glasses. I remember myself as a tall and thin young man who swung back and forth between diffident reserve and assertive flows of words and ideas. I had a way to go before one could see in my face anything on the order of steady confidence.

Nor was I free of anxiety quite specific to the study I was doing. A dream I had at the time reflected my fears in a manner so bald as to be almost farcical.

> A fleet of small ships sailed from the Mainland carrying hundreds of Chinese Communist soldiers, who landed near our cottage [we were then living in what was called the "New Territories," adjacent to Mainland China] and took me prisoner (I think they let BJ alone), carried me back to China, and subjected me to a powerful version of thought reform. I seemed to cave in—or in any case did very badly.

The dream reflected a feeling of vulnerability at being so close to the Mainland, my sense of the power of the Chinese and their reformers, overall anxiety about taking on the work and about my life in general. But BJ and I could laugh at the dream's comic-opera absurdity. In it I seemed to be mocking my own fears.

In carrying out the project I was beginning a lifelong pattern of alternation between, on the one hand, movement and travel and hunger for worldly experience, and on the other, sedentary, methodical work on a particular problem, often in isolation. The first tendency has been a quest for new images, for transcendence of the ordinary and some form of originality. The other tendency has been my orderly, even compulsive "work habit" (in Erikson's term). That side of my character has been present since childhood, when I thrived on the consistent structure of classes in school and the planned activities of summer camps. Over the years I have been happiest when immersed in a long project, usually work on a book, and have tended to refuse shorter enterprises (articles, prefaces, commentaries) as diversions from that longer struggle. During those sixteen months in Hong Kong I settled into the identity of a research psychiatrist out in the world, immersed in ethical as well as psychological issues. My work habit came to include the fieldwork of exhaustive interview dialogues, reading in many directions, and constant recording of impressions about the work and the world. It was the work habit of a writer no less than a psychiatrist, and I was aware of doing something "out there" in order to bring it "back here."

The Bishop Who Wanted My Soul

Certain people I interviewed required me to modify my method considerably to make it responsive to them and to what they could tell me. For instance, I greatly extended the parameters of dialogue in my work with a neatly goateed seventy-year-old Belgian Catholic bishop whom I interviewed in a Hong Kong hospital where he was recovering from both physical wounds and psychological trauma resulting from the brutal treatment he had undergone during three years of imprisonment. Bishop Barker was articulate in describing his ordeal and upbeat in his demeanor, asserting that during forty years of missionary work in the Chinese interior he had, in effect, realized his boyhood ambition of becoming not only a priest but a doctor, soldier, and religious martyr. While his theology was simplistic (a struggle between God and the demons) he was keenly interpretive (emphasizing psychological parallels between Communist and Catholic practice), and poised and worldly in our exchange.

In pursuit of a spiritual agenda of his own, Bishop Barker soon turned things around by questioning me about my Jewishness. When I went to see him the next day, he told me, with a sly smile, that he had a present for me. He handed me a book by a Jewish psychiatrist whose experience with the Nazis led him to convert to Catholicism. I was astonished and awed by the sleight of hand (sleight of soul?) on the part of this man producing such a gift (which he had apparently located in the possession of another member of his order) from his hospital bed. (The book was called *The Pillar of Fire*, and I later corresponded with its German-born author, Karl Stern.) When our many hours of interviewing were more or less completed I told him that BJ helped me with some of the work, brought her to the hospital to meet him, and they became fast friends.

During our interviews I felt that Bishop Barker and I were more or less bartering our wares. He welcomed my psychological interpretations and generally therapeutic approach as helpful in his recovery, and in return he offered me advice on how to make the most of religious impulses of patients (direct Catholics to their religious confessions, Protestants to prayers associated with readings of the New Testament, and Jews to meditations on the Old Testament).*

My last meetings with Bishop Barker occurred three years later during a research follow-up trip to Europe and took place at the Catholic shrine at Lourdes, the only place our schedules allowed us to meet. We continued our dialogue, which in this case meant my questioning him about his work and feelings over the course of the three years, his detailed and highly sensitive replies, and then, at his insistence, his conducting of a small Mass for BJ and me in an isolated crypt far removed from the touristic paraphernalia of the larger shrine. (BJ had rushed to Lourdes to rejoin me and meet again with Bishop Barker and he had delayed his departure in order to be able to see her.) We were both moved by the aesthetic elegance of his performance, and struck by how far he had come from his humiliation in a Chinese prison.

The Believable False Confession

Another priest made me painfully aware of the mind's capacity under duress to spin out falsehood and then come to believe in that falsehood. I had read about false confessions made during the Soviet purge trials, but now I was encountering a firsthand description of a striking sequence of convoluted confession and belief that raised larger questions about the nature of belief and believability, which took one far beyond thought reform itself. Father Luca was an Italian missionary in his late thirties with whom I also spent many hours in a Hong Kong hospital. But rather than being interested in my soul, he was profoundly bewildered about what had happened to him in the Chinese prison from which he had been released just a few days before our first interview. A half century later I can still see his gaunt figure sitting opposite me, the restlessness and deep confusion revealed in his darting eyes and shifting thoughts and associations. He poured out his story of four discernible stages of confession and belief over the course of his extremely abusive three and a half years of imprisonment.

---

*When back in the United States I did for some years continue to treat patients. But from those first days in Hong Kong, I poured most of my professional energies into my research. And I came to realize that even a small number of patients, given the intense focus each required, drew considerably upon those energies. So while I took on various consultations related to my research, I gradually stopped doing therapy.

During his first days of incarceration he described himself as "determined not to admit to anything that wasn't true," and when observing fellow prisoners' "struggles" against one in their midst in the name of "help," he thought to himself that "to help means to maltreat people." But over the next month of relentless interrogation and sleep deprivation, including beatings and forms of torture involved with handcuffs and chains, he found his situation unbearable, became preoccupied with finding a way to satisfy his tormentors, and was willing to "say almost anything they wanted me to say." He produced a confession that included active participation in an espionage organization, with the operation of a nonexistent radio station. At that point he was so psychologically fragmented that he had little idea of what he believed and of reality in general ("To some extent I visualized this spy organization. . . . I imagined rather clearly a street with a house, a front room, and behind the front room a radio sender . . . like half dreaming . . . or writing a novel"). But his chief interrogator subsequently noticed that much of the confession was incoherent and contradictory, and ordered Father Luca to "think over" all of it and make a new confession based only upon "the truth."

After some respite from the brutality, Luca recovered his faculties sufficiently to produce a new, accurate document in which there was no espionage organization or radio center or spy activity of any kind. But then his cellmates, charged with helping him to record the confession, refused to allow him to submit this accurate version. Advanced as they were in their own "reform," they told him that if it were true and he had done nothing wrong he would "certainly not have been arrested." With both his wild confession and true account rejected, and experiencing life-threatening physical and psychological abuse, Luca became desperate for a solution. He found one, together with his cellmates and interrogators, that involved actual behavior interpreted as criminality: a conversation with a fellow priest about the advancing Communist armies became "passing military information to imperialists." Now grounded in actual events, the confession became (in Luca's words) "almost real," acceptable to prison authorities, and a basis for Luca's release and expulsion from China.

I knew that Luca, as a liberal priest, was especially susceptible to the Chinese (and often Western) historical argument that missionaries were inseparable from imperialistic armies; and also that the Communists were particularly intent on dishonoring by labeling as spies those who, like him, had found much favor with Chinese people. But I was nonetheless struck by this display of how relentless manipulators could not only extract elaborate falsehoods from their victim but in the process press that victim into creating falsehoods that were credible. At the same time I was somewhat relieved by the transience of the victim's belief in such falsehoods, and by the extent to which the manipulators could be entrapped by the very falsehoods they had produced through their extreme pressures.

I have never stopped pondering this illustration of the mind's simultaneous vulnerability and resilience. I thought of Kafka and the logical, guilt-suffused pseudoreality in which his characters are caught up; and about Borges and his powerfully imagined labyrinths existing separately from the world. But finally I returned to Camus, who once said, "We confess in order to avoid telling what we know." Luca and others had to avoid telling what they knew (the truth of what they had actually done or not done in China) in order to produce the distorted confession document that would affirm their guilt and conform to the thought reform narrative; whatever revisions they made, their continuing confession served to avoid that truth.

The Converted Jesuit

Some of the most remarkable hours I spent during my work on thought reform occurred not in Hong Kong but in northern France, at a small Catholic secondary school where I interviewed a Jesuit priest during the follow-up trip through Europe I made in 1958. As I sat with him in a modest room, part of an intensely Catholic environment in the bucolic French countryside, listening to his effusive praise for his Communist reformers and vigorous criticism of his immediate Catholic colleagues, I wondered whether I myself was hallucinating. Simon told me that his imprisonment "was one of the best periods of my life," and that "I had more freedom of speech in jail than I have right here."

It turned out that Simon was a man dependent on guidance and leadership from others and in that way was highly vulnerable to environmental influences. His unyielding conscience made him strongly susceptible to feelings of guilt, and to swinging from fierce resistance to uncritical embrace of the Communist worldview. Like many missionaries, he was also deeply affected by his desire to remain in China and deepen his connection with the Chinese people.

Crucial throughout was his strong personal inclination toward totalism, toward issuing what he called a "blank check" to a belief system. Only his commitment to Catholicism prevented him from remaining in China and joining the Communist movement: other than that "I accepted all their points of view—political and economic, everything." When I asked him how he managed to hold such views in his strongly anticommunist Catholic environment, he told me that he had an understanding with his superiors according to which he could believe anything he wished but was not to express his procommunist views publicly or make them known in any way to the outside world—an arrangement with which he was not entirely happy but which everyone found workable. His Jesuit colleagues seemed quite willing to play a waiting game, with the assumption that Simon's profound religious convictions and Jesuit loyalties would ultimately prevail.

As I heard all this I imagined him as the centerpiece of a vast tug-of-war: pulling from one side were his accusatory jailers, his interrogators, and fellow prisoners, all drawing strength from the amorphous but powerful entity of the Chinese Communist revolution and its fierce exposure of the dubious role of missionaries in China. Pulling from the other side were his immediate Jesuit colleagues and members of his and other orders, all of them drawing strength from the older and equally amorphous and powerful entity of the Catholic Church, which had the advantage of dominating both his past life and his immediate surroundings.

Was I rooting for one of them? I have no great love for religious hierarchies, including the Catholic one. But over the course of my work I had developed a particular dislike for the thought reform process, especially the prison variety, and did not want to see it produce and maintain so impressive a conversion. I also did not want to see contradicted my general impression that Westerners could emerge from the process deeply confused but tended to revert either to their pre-thought-reform identity or to a modified identity influenced by thought reform but recognizing its coercive nature. Actually I had little doubt that his Jesuit colleagues' patience would pay off. But Father Simon's conversion, however impermanent it might turn out to be, stunningly escalated my sense of the emotional power of thought reform.

The Chinese Source

To carry out my study of thought reform, I had to immerse myself in the culture that created and practiced it. Here my Japanese experience was of only limited value. Chinese culture had been undergoing profound upheavals over the course of the twentieth century, having to do with cultural and military encounters with the West and with its own struggles against cultural tradition. And I was doing my work in a Hong Kong environment that was fluid, confusing, and inundated with suspicion. Chinese who came there had experienced thought reform in educational institutions where they were not subjected to the brutal torture Westerners had undergone in prisons. There was a similar emphasis on criticism and self-criticism, continuous confession—and above all, on sustained reeducation. Yet so different were the cultural and historical backgrounds Chinese brought to thought reform, and the institutions where the process occurred, that I often felt I was conducting two distinct research studies.

In the combination of exhortation and coercion, the exhortation could be much more powerful, given the actual corruption of the Nationalist regime the Communists replaced, and the impressive, even heroic, early achievements of the Communist revolution. But unlike Westerners, Chinese who fled from the Mainland could not view Hong Kong as a temporary place of recovery from which to return to a more permanent structure of home and family or religious group. In contrast, most of them had no place to go; they had to struggle simultaneously with the conflicts induced by thought reform and the complexities of British hegemony and Communist influence in a Chinese cultural area that felt inhospitable and unsafe. I needed Chinese guides, and found them in two men, Ma Meng and Lu Baotong, who were steeped in their cultural tradition but also had backgrounds in contemporary social science, including study in the United States. Now I was touching the heart of the Chinese revolutionary process.

I took to the complexities of Hong Kong and to work with Chinese in general. Compared to Japanese students and intellectuals I had known, they expressed their ideas and feelings more freely. I could experience the much-heralded Chinese focus on human relationships, part of the extraordinary attraction that China has long held for Westerners. That focus begins early for young children in connection with the intricacies of family life and the strong expectation that they become sensitive to appropriate attitudes in the family hierarchy, sensitivity that extends into adult life and one's relationships in the world at large. One Western anthropologist declared that Chinese culture had "developed personal relationships to the level of an exquisite and superb art." Once, when I talked to Ma Meng about the emphasis of the Washington School of Psychiatry, with which I had become affiliated, on "interpersonal relations," he responded by asking: "What else is there?" Particularly in my work with Chinese, I felt myself always simultaneously immersed in thought reform itself, in traditional Chinese culture—which was both a target and a source of thought reform—and in the twentieth-century Chinese legacy of antitraditional historical movements that did so much to prepare the way for the reform process.

Chinese Generations

For my work with Chinese, generational struggles were, psychologically speaking, the crux of the matter. I had been interested in such struggles as they involved Japanese youth, and had begun to see their broad significance for questioning authority in general in a changing society. In the case of Chinese, the orchestrators of thought reform recognized that traditional society was anchored in filial piety, and therefore put the overturning of parental authority at the center of the thought reform agenda. Indeed, I read of ancient parables sacralizing the practice of filial piety, some of which went so far as to describe the killing of a young child so that there would be more food available for one's elderly parent; or the cutting off of a piece of one's own flesh and boiling it in order to feed a sick parent. But from the early years of the twentieth century, Chinese student and literary movements fiercely attacked these Confucian principles. In the celebrated 1918 story of Lu Xun, "Diary of a Madman," filial piety becomes a literal form of cannibalism of the young, and traditional society in general is condemned as "over 4,000 years of a man-eating world."

I came to see generational conflict as a central dynamic for historical change everywhere. At about that time I read José Ortega y Gasset, who claimed that "the concept of the generation is the most important one in the whole of history," pointing out that the twenty-year-old, the forty-year-old, and the sixty-year-old create three different mentalities at the same historical moment, which causes "an internal lack of equilibrium," through which "history moves, changes, wheels and flows." I was able to deepen this perspective from readings of Freud, Camus, and Margaret Mead, and later wrote about it in connection with Japanese and Americans as well.

The Chinese Communists considered themselves the inheritors of the twentieth-century assault on filial piety, and constructed much of their thought reform project around that assault. Their grandiose goal was *to convert every filial son or daughter into a filial Communist*. So all thought reform programs in universities and revolutionary colleges culminated in each participant's fierce denunciation of his or her father, as a person and above all as a representative of the evils of the "old regime" (the Kuomintang, a revolutionary movement that became corrupt and autocratic under Chiang Kai-shek, whose armies were eventually defeated by the Communists in a protracted civil war) and the reactionary traditional culture. In this way the Communists were manipulating feelings of guilt on many levels, and were demanding an obedience no less extreme or sacred than that of the filial son who killed his own child or cut off his own flesh and fed it to a sick parent.

Yet the very Confucianism under such severe attack was, paradoxically, the source of much of the approach and techniques of thought reform. Confucianism had its own focus on "self-cultivation," involving criticism, self-criticism, and aspects of confession and reeducation. So much so that early Russian advisors to the Communist movement accused it of being "too much influenced by Confucian ethics." And although the Soviets undoubtedly transmitted to the Chinese much of their physical and psychological practices of confession extraction, there was no Soviet program that gave as much sustained attention to the "self-cultivation" involved in Chinese "reeducation."

I was able to trace the history of the practice of thought reform not only through my reading but through a long and valuable interview with Zhang Guotao, a leading figure in the early Chinese Communist movement until his defection in 1938. An elderly, elegant man who chose his words carefully, Zhang spoke with the authority of an insider who had been involved in high-level planning. He told me of crude reform techniques used as early as the late 1920s with captured enemy soldiers and some among the general population, the idea being to bring as many people as possible into the Communist armies. For intellectuals, training centers were set up as early as the mid-thirties in border areas in order to absorb the large numbers of educated Chinese who were drawn to the Communist movement, then based in the Yenan area of northwest China. Early Leninist models of pressured political criticism and self-criticism were greatly modified in the direction of an introspective group study process. Zhang smiled as he explained that such a moral and psychological emphasis seemed to come naturally to the Chinese reformers. I thought of the anthropologist's comment about the culture's making of personal relationships "an exquisite and superb art." And I came to view the psychological manipulations of thought reform as a modern, totalistic expression of a particular cultural genius.

The Revolutionary University

"Revolutionary universities" were descendants of early Party institutions and became (as I then noted) "the real ideological core of the entire thought reform movement in China," where the process "was apparently worked out by trial and error over a period of many years." I spoke of the ingenious psychological pressures being applied in an "air-tight environment, with no opportunity for any emotional outlet beyond the program," and of the graduates of those centers as "the most important source we have for a basic understanding of the overall thought-reform process."

One of those graduates whom I interviewed for many hours and referred to as Hu had experienced sufficient conflict to cause him to leave Communist China and come to Hong Kong. But before that he had been caught up in thought reform to the degree that he produced a highly accusatory denunciation of his father, all of it expressed completely within the Communist idiom. As he put it, he had become "so accustomed to that pattern of words that you feel chained." Over time Hu believed in some Communist principles, disbelieved in others, and was beginning to feel resentful about being so controlled, "but I couldn't tell or make out what were the things I did or didn't believe in." He said that it was fear that made him write such a document about his father. Years later in Hong Kong he still experienced fearful dreams about a Communist cadre resembling those who did the reforming who appeared to him as not quite "a substantial person" but more or less a supernatural monster whose visibility consisted of "only his Communist uniform," a creature with absolute power over him because "he can do anything he wants to me and I can do nothing to him."

Of course those who defected were a small minority. Many more undoubtedly internalized the parameters of expression and belief under the new regime, and others were sufficiently caught up in Communist ideology to become cadres and leaders who guided and "reformed" subsequent generations. But Hu also taught me much about the ultimate uncertainty of the results of thought reform. As he explained, "If you put this final thought summary [including the denunciation of his father] before me now, I could write a new summary contradictory to it in each sentence." That reflection helps us understand both the psychological power of thought reform and what I found to be a decline, over the years, in its effectiveness. When revolutionary enthusiasm in China at large radically diminished, so did the exhortatory appeal of thought reform, and the process could be increasingly perceived as punitive and coercive. Indeed, the Chinese most clearly revealed both the collective impact and the ultimate limitations of thought reform when applying it to their own people.

The Totalistic Squeeze: Chinese Thought Reform and American McCarthyism

While listening in Hong Kong to accounts of Chinese mind manipulation, I was also hearing horror stories about McCarthyite accusations in the United States. I felt myself close to drowning in a sea of totalism. The narratives of thought reform I was exposed to every day, some of them brutal and all of them troubling, inevitably took a certain toll on me. David Riesman later wrote me that, from his own reaction to the manuscript of my book on thought reform, he was struck by how difficult it must have been for me "to listen to those stories of cruelty and confusion." Actually I was affected not only by the cruelty and suffering imposed, but also by the extent to which minds could be altered and truth blurred to the point of near extinction. With Westerners, those manipulations were epitomized by the false confession. With Chinese it was the extreme denunciation of one's father and the assault upon all feelings in one's family and one's life that were deemed antithetical to Communist virtue. In the world I was studying the criteria for truth could be little more than what manipulators chose them to be.

Similar tendencies were emerging at that time (1954 and early 1955) in connection with the American anticommunist phenomenon of McCarthyism. Joseph McCarthy, the senator from Wisconsin who wildly waved to his (mostly television) audiences sheets of paper ostensibly containing the names of Communists who had infiltrated the State Department or some other institution, gave the entity its name. But there were many other manifestations of it in the form of blacklists of writers and actors, false public accusations, hostile inquisitions before congressional committees threatening jail terms for contempt, and calls for the political purging of universities.

Americans who looked us up in Hong Kong had their own narratives of friends being fired from teaching jobs, and of becoming fearful about what they said or wrote or even about which magazines they subscribed to. Most McCarthyite slander contained the thought reform combination of (in the words of Father Luca) "big accusations from small facts." Significantly, much of the McCarthyite rhetoric related to China, including a sweeping accusation that Communist influence in American institutions, especially the State Department, had been responsible for "losing China." There were also demands for confessions of Communist connections, for "naming names" and betraying close friends, and pressured accusations that resulted in various kinds of guilt feelings. To be sure, McCarthyism contained no systematic thought reform process, and there were ultimately contending voices that could reassert personal and institutional freedoms. But McCarthyism included manipulations of truth and reality that paralleled those of thought reform. And now we were talking not about Communist China but about my own democratic country.

So sitting there in Hong Kong, I had the sense that the two worlds had gone mad. Each seemed to have completely lost its bearings and I, living in both of them, was hard put to hold on to my own. One had to look for sanity in strange places—for instance, in old British colonials. We had drinks one day, gin and tonics, of course, with two such former officials who had spent much time in India prior to their Hong Kong assignments. They at first seemed quite refreshing in their willingness to condemn, in the most rational terms, the excesses of both Chinese thought reform and American McCarthyism. Then they somehow turned to memories of their own, recalling an empire they recognized to be rapidly disappearing. With a tone of urgent nostalgia, one of them remarked: "Of course it's over, but it was remarkable that we could rule India with three hundred men." Yes, they had seemed the only sane people around—until they revealed their own madness.

3

Finding a Mentor

RETURNING TO AMERICA in late 1955 was a very complicated experience for BJ and me. We had lived in the Far East for three and a half years—in Japan and Korea while I was in the military, and then in Hong Kong for eighteen months (during which BJ spent much time as a correspondent in Vietnam). I had little doubt that I would seek an academic career, but that was not much on my mind. What was on my mind was writing up my work in Hong Kong on the most profound expressions of thought reform, as conducted on the Chinese Mainland, first in the form of a few articles and then a book. I remember how meticulous and anxious I was about arranging for mailing my precious records of the work, by registered boat mail, which I was told was highly reliable (airmail from Hong Kong would have been too expensive for such a volume of material) to the Walter Reed Army Medical Center graduate school in Silver Spring, Maryland, care of David Rioch. Intellectually and professionally, that set of packages was me. I was both fearful about what awaited me and excited about what I had done in my Hong Kong research. Now I wanted to convey that excitement in a book that would do justice to thought reform as a remarkable and troubling human project and convey the extraordinary experiences described to me by participants, as well as the very broad political and psychological significance of all that I had learned. I had painful doubts about whether I could write such a book, but I had the sense that I could not really move ahead with my life until I had done so.

Nor was I immune to the general problems of the expatriate's return. Later, in the course of my 1958 European research follow-up trip, I could observe in men like Father Luca and Father Simon struggles not only with residual thought reform conflicts but with their deep ambivalence about having to leave China and return "home." They were reflecting a long tradition of Westerners who had gone to China to convert the heathen to Christianity but in the process became so deeply drawn to the culture and people as to raise the question of who had converted whom. The conflict went back at least to the sixteenth century, to the great Jesuit missionary Matteo Ricci: he and his fellow Jesuits embraced Confucian teachings and, in their writings upon leaving China, disseminated often idealized versions of those teachings throughout the Western world. Luca, Simon, and Ricci too did not cease to be emissaries of the Church, but struggled to combine their missionary identity with the very powerful "Chineseness" they had absorbed.

I had not undergone the assaults experienced by the people I interviewed, nor had I immersed myself in any East Asian culture to the extent that they had in China. But I had accrued my own version of an East Asia–linked identity along with many of the conflicts of an expatriate. I remember how strange our own country seemed to BJ and me, how odd the lives of people were here, with their routines of working in their offices and shopping in supermarkets. I felt removed from their rhythms and keenly aware of their knowing nothing of our extraordinary experiences in remote places. And I was wary of adapting too quickly to my American environment lest I surrender a part of me, my East Asian self, so important to my evolving sense, however uncertain, of who I was and wanted to be. At the same time I wanted to reclaim my Americanness by enabling it to include and integrate what had happened to me during those three and a half years.

That recognition included my appointment to the Washington School of Psychiatry and the Walter Reed Army Medical Center graduate school, as arranged by David Rioch, and I remained in the Washington area for a year working on the thought reform material. After publishing a few articles I then received, with the active help of Fritz Redlich, then chairman of the Department of Psychiatry at Yale, a five-year dream grant for "research and research training" from the combined auspices of the Foundations' Fund for Research in Psychiatry and the Ford Foundation. That grant provided a salary for those years, along with support for completing my work on thought reform and obtaining further professional knowledge anywhere I thought appropriate. (I was to spend three and a half years during the late 1950s at Harvard, and then two years in Japan studying individual psychology and historical change in Japanese youth.) But despite benefiting so greatly from the remarkable beneficence of American society at a time of unusual availability of such grants, those early years in Asia, almost seven in all, created in me a consistent sense of being an observer of my own country from the world outside. And part of me has always wished to stay that way.

An important aspect of "coming home" was embrace of a mentor. I was not consciously looking for one, having navigated the work in Hong Kong and my beginning writings about it on my own. I learned a great deal from wide readings connected with the study, but knew that my intellectual relationship to psychoanalytic and psychiatric tradition was callow. At the same time I was wary of much of what was being made of those traditions as narrow and often stereotyped.

I have a vivid memory of the moment when I found what for me was a resolution to that paradox, and an exhilarating suggestion of mentorship. One evening in 1956, BJ and I were sitting on a couch in the living room of the small house we rented on M Street in Georgetown in Washington, D.C. I read quickly and excitedly through an essay by Erik Erikson that had just appeared in the *Journal of the American Psychoanalytic Association* called "The Problem of Ego Identity." Erikson described how young people struggled to sustain a sense of personal and historical continuity, which, under duress, could break down and lead to an "identity crisis," which led to forms of confusion that should not be considered symptoms of psychiatric illness. Solutions could be found in rearranging and expanding the components of one's identity in ways that enabled one to feel a greater sense of coherence. Erikson was providing an individual model, applied particularly to young adult life, that included both inner sameness and inevitable change. As I followed his argument, I experienced an overwhelming eureka feeling of "That's it!" "That's exactly right!"

Erikson spoke directly to my sense of what had been happening to the Chinese and Westerners I had interviewed in Hong Kong. I announced my discovery to BJ, who recognized something important was happening, but neither of us could know how important. What I did realize was that Erikson's concept of identity could be a conceptual anchor for me in the book I was beginning to write. The same was true, I would soon discover, of his concept of totalism as a tendency toward all-or-nothing emotional alignments, whether in young people struggling with identity, or in collective expressions of political extremism.

To be sure, I had energetically carried out the research and written several articles about it without benefit of Eriksonian theory. But now I found my work illuminated by a representative of a great intellectual tradition. For while Erikson was a psychoanalyst within the Freudian movement he was a highly idiosyncratic one who was enlarging and humanizing that movement. Moving beyond its focus on instinct and defense (mostly sexual impulses and their repression), he conveyed a more complex sense of human beings and their world, including their susceptibility to cultural and historical currents. Just reading his work diminished my feelings of intellectual loneliness, and gave me a sense of moving closer to a theoretical structure that could enrich future work and, in a way hardly clear, my life in general.

Erikson's work was not new to me—I had read and admired his earlier book, *Childhood and Society*, five years before as a psychiatric resident. That book said much about identity, but I had not associated it with my work in Hong Kong. I seemed to have to do more on my own before I was ready for mentorship. At my urging, Fritz Redlich wrote to Erikson about me by way of introduction, and in my first letter to him (July 19, 1956) I described thought reform as "an attempt to bring about a change in identity in the participant through techniques which resemble induced religious conversion or a coercive form of psychotherapy." I was deferential, suggesting a meeting or meetings not of equals but of teacher and student, of consultations "at your usual fee." But I was not without a bit of youthful bravado, referring to the three papers I had by then written and mentioning a number of prominent people in psychiatry and social science with whom I had already been in touch.

Erikson was interested and wrote back asking me to send my papers to him, while enclosing a recent reprint of his own. We arranged to meet on a

Saturday in late August at his home in Stockbridge, Massachusetts. Such a meeting had every possibility of awkward anticlimax, but instead it became part of a dizzying trajectory. Then in his mid-fifties, Erikson seemed to me a magnificent presence: tall and slightly heavyset, with a great shock of gray hair susceptible to any breeze, and an impish and curious smile. He spoke in soft tones that were ironic, self-deprecating, and humorous. And his easy back-and-forth banter conveyed a sense of our being old friends who had not seen one another for a long time and had much to talk about. He quickly suggested that we walk, explaining that Europeans like himself believe that good ideas only emerge when people are in motion together. Though I had never held such a belief—I had always assumed that good ideas came while sitting at one's desk in solitude or perhaps in quiet conversation—it seemed to make perfect sense at the time.

So we walked for much of that day, always at a good, steady pace. I later estimated that we walked around the town of Stockbridge about eight times. When I found myself tiring, I experienced a second wind from observing the vigor of this new companion who was twenty-five years older than I was. I did feel myself on some kind of European trek—like hiking through the Alps, or on a prolonged "ramble" of German youth, a two-man *Wandervogel*—though neither of us any longer qualified for youth-movement status. Ideas and images poured out of both of us, varying from jocular observations to structured conceptual principles, and as I think back on that walk a half century later I still experience a sense of excitement, of mind expansion, and (in the words of the Czech novelist Milan Kundera) a lightness of being.

From my recollections, and especially from the detailed notes I later made, our conversation had three loose—very loose—stages. The first could be called "Martin Luther and Chinese Thought Reform." Erikson asked me for endless details about young Chinese undergoing Communist "reeducation," which he quickly and repeatedly associated with the experience of Martin Luther (about whom he was writing a book) in training for the Catholic priesthood. He described the whole atmosphere of totalism surrounding Luther as we associated back and forth from the political practices of twentieth-century China to the religious practices of sixteenth-century Europe. From the beginning there was no question of my formally presenting cases to him or his doing "supervision" of my research. We just talked.

Now I could begin to understand why Erikson agreed to meet me. With his sensitive antennae he quickly realized that my work on thought reform could speak to his own imaginative immersion into Luther's struggles with totalism, obedience, and the internalization of individual conscience. Erikson was in fact soon to go off to Mexico, where he would write *Young Man Luther*, his psychological study of that brilliantly creative, ultimately destructive, and always extreme religious figure. I was thrilled that Erikson was drawn to my work. And I was aware of learning a great deal about interactions between individual people and history, especially about Erikson's psychohistorical model or "great man theory," in which the historical innovator's solutions to his own profound psychological conflicts provide a breakthrough for all people in his historical era and can reverberate through subsequent eras as well. That Luther–thought reform exchange, in completely spontaneous fashion, was an early axis for what became a twenty-five-year dialogue.

The second theme of our ambulatory conversation had to do with Erikson's deeply ambivalent reminiscences about Vienna and the early Freudian movement. He talked freely about those days, emphasizing on the one hand that "they educated me" (his formal schooling went only as far as the gymnasium, or advanced secondary school), and on the other that the atmosphere was so "unhealthy" that he would have found it necessary to leave even without the Nazi threat. That unhealthiness lay in the group's self-enclosure and suffocating dogma, leading Erikson to draw parallels with my observations on the environment of thought reform. As he talked, I imagined him walking through the streets of old Vienna, and then he and I strolling through them together, the city sometimes appearing bright and clear and at other times dark and threatening.

He told me he had very low standing in that Freudian community because of his youth and especially his lack of a medical education (he had come there as a teacher of young children and an artist), and that although he underwent analysis with Anna Freud, he had little contact with her father. He expressed great hurt in telling how Anna Freud had subsequently rejected him privately and criticized his work publicly as deviating from the desired traditional perspective. My feelings on hearing all this were complicated. I was moved to be taken with Erikson into that legendary early circle. But I shuddered at his descriptions of its coercive atmosphere, while feeling confirmed in my aversion to subsequent psychoanalytic totalism. At the same time I viewed Vienna as a revolutionary environment and shared much of Erikson's reverence for Freud's intellectual breakthrough—while before me stood a compelling, though all too rare, example of what that revolution could produce.

We eased gradually into the third and broadest theme of our conversation, that of the present work of each of us and of our relationships to psychoanalysis intellectually and as a "movement." As we went back and forth between our respective book projects, I came to see mine on thought reform and his on Luther as bound together by our early dialogue. When *Young Man Luther* appeared in 1958, I devoured it more intensely than any book I can remember: my repeated use of my copy has left it with endless slivers of crumbling paper inserted between pages to locate important passages, its long-undone binding barely held together by Scotch tape. (The only other book in my library that has remotely rivaled *Young Man Luther* in evidence of extreme use is Albert Camus's *The Rebel*.) What I found in this Erikson volume was a stunning expression of psychoanalytic imagination in describing how a great man must "solve for all . . . and not for himself alone" the individual-psychological conflicts he confronts. Luther thus projected his individual struggles with guilt, conscience, and religious authenticity into the flow of Western history.

Erikson told me that he no longer had much in common with most fellow psychoanalysts and even less with the movement, but at the same time he made clear to me, as he did in his writings, that he still identified himself as a "Freudian analyst." I was puzzled, and a bit troubled, by this contradiction, until I came to realize how much his own sense of adult identity had been formed by the early Freudian movement. That inner professional core, and a continuing tie to the movement, however tenuous, was necessary to him for carrying out his highly original work, even though the content of the work, with its stress on identity and the person in history, was antithetical to the still-pervasive classical Freudian psychoanalysis and to the ideas of most contemporary representatives of it.

Of course Erikson quickly sensed my own contradictions in these areas, which he approached only gingerly. When I told him that I planned to enter psychoanalytic training in Boston, he looked at me with a mischievous half smile and said something to the effect that it would be "interesting." After all, who was better equipped to understand my combination of hunger for participation of some kind in a great intellectual development and critical sensitivity toward its dogmatic excesses and its inclination toward creating highly controlled environments. In *Young Man Luther* Erikson explored the "monkhood, . . . monkishness, and . . . monkery" of psychoanalysis and raised questions about its ways of treating young candidates. While aware of his distance from the psychoanalytic mainstream, I was encouraged that the issue was being raised.

Erikson and I were separated from one another by his European origins and a generational divide of twenty-five years. Also, he had started out as a visual artist, and never lost that perspective. And there was his long-standing relationship to psychoanalysis. Whatever his conflicts, it was *his* movement, while I was an outsider entering its training with skepticism and trepidation. What was remarkable was the similarity in our sensibilities. We shared a feeling of personal paradox toward psychoanalysis—deep respect for its intellectual power and equally deep aversion to its tendencies toward totalism. Our continuing explorations together of that paradox became central to our personal bond.

We also shared a principle that could be called respect for the broad human repertoire of emotions and a wariness toward labeling them as psychiatric pathology, especially in regard to passions called forth by large historical movements and events (such as Luther's sixteenth-century Reformation in Western Europe and twentieth-century Chinese thought reform). When I talked then to most psychoanalysts, they seemed to reduce people and events to small, mostly predictable categories of their thought system. Erikson could do the opposite, use his psychoanalytic thought to make surprising observations, raise lively questions, and generally expand discourse and understanding. I could join in to experience a kind of personal expansion in the process.

And as important as anything else, we shared a sense of absurdity about much that went on in the world, which seemed to give us a certain distance from painful issues we contemplated. I felt an affinity between his sly humor and the subversive bird cartoons I was just beginning to draw, mostly for friends, which were mocking and self-mocking about anything and everything having to do with pomposity and claim to virtue. Erik loved the cartoons—later we would call ourselves "fellow artists," a considerable stretch in my case (the birds are stick figures who serve mainly as spokesmen), but accurate about Erik, who brought a painter's eye and concern with form to his psychological work.

Taking on Erikson as a mentor was not a calculated act (I never studied formally under him) so much as a response to a deep inner sense of affinity and possibility. But in doing so I could connect my work with his compelling version of psychoanalytic thought. At the same time I could strengthen the professional identity I was groping toward—one that could bring a freely expressed psychological imagination into history, into the world. And I had found a teacher who affirmed my sense that I had done important work on my own.

Margaret Mead's Cosmic Community

The thought reform work also took me to a new professional community, highly scattered geographically but with a certain intellectual coherence. That community included not only Erikson and David Riesman (who was soon to become another mentor) but other innovative people such as Margaret Mead, Gregory Bateson, Jerome Bruner, Fritz Redl (not to be confused with Redlich), Jerome Frank, Erving Goffman, and John Spiegel. They were psychiatrists, psychologists, anthropologists, and sociologists who, broadly speaking, shared a certain sensibility: all were influenced by psychoanalysis but critical of its dogma, interested in the individual person but always in connection with collective behavior, and were concerned not only with conflict but with human potential in the face of conflict. And they were advocates of progressive social and political change. They were idiosyncratic people whose ideas and attitudes were both refreshing and influential.

One could not quite call them a group—perhaps virtual community with heart is the best term—but there is no doubt that Margaret Mead was the hub. I'm not quite sure who introduced me to Margaret (perhaps David Riesman) but the power of her presence gave me the sense that she had always been there and always would be. Our first meeting took place in the late fifties, during a brief trip I was making from the Far East, at her office at the American Museum of Natural History on the Upper West Side of Manhattan. She asked me a series of questions about my work on thought reform and my life in Hong Kong and about my impressions of Japan and Japanese youth; and we talked about the possible significance of my work for psychology and the social sciences in regard to pressured influence as well as historical change.

Then she suddenly shifted into a different gear. She began to spin out a splendid array of people and writings she considered important for me. Her all-encompassing mind and squat body swung into high action as she darted about the room, picking up copies of papers here and there and tracking down addresses, telephone numbers, and references. She included thinkers and writers concerned with all phases of behavior, but especially with human influence and with fanaticism; with cultural psychology particularly involving China, Japan, and Russia; or simply because that work was done by someone she thought interesting and original. Margaret had looked me over and decided that I was okay, and I could perceive the great warmth under her imperious tone as she offered so much to this new acquaintance.

Feeling myself something on the order of a rocket being thrust into the atmosphere from the most powerful of launching pads, I returned to my hotel room in a kind of euphoric daze to try to take in Mead's generosity and her overall presence. As I collapsed on my bed, the telephone rang and once more I heard that (by now lovable) voice saying something like: "This is Margaret Mead. I forgot to mention that Jane Smith did an important study of Chinese families which is not yet published, but you can get it from her in manuscript. She spends fall and winter months in America and can usually be reached at her North Carolina home, where her phone number is . . ."

We became good friends. In addition to being one of the world's great intellectual coordinators and a person of vast knowledge and lively insights on so many things, Margaret had another trait that one might not expect from a person of her dynamism—she was a wonderful listener. At a conference where I made an early presentation of my work on thought reform, her response combined large conceptual comments (concerning Chinese, American, and Russian culture and the role of confession in social change, etc.) and nitty-gritty personal interactions (between interrogator and prisoner and between research subjects and myself). BJ similarly had extensive discussions with her about every kind of cultural and psychological issue in adoption, although she did not necessarily accept Margaret's sometimes idiosyncratic views. (Don't adopt a child until the age of four so that you can know what kind of a person he or she will be.)

But there were some moments, whether at a conference or in private conversation, when Margaret's irony and self-critical faculties would desert her and she would pronounce quite foolishly on a subject of which she had little knowledge. I came to realize that with Margaret, particularly if she felt under some duress, one had to be on the lookout for at least a modicum of what can best be called bullshit. But she would quickly recover from that state and relax into her more usual flow of knowledgeable and shrewd associations.

Margaret seemed to live in a field of force that could combat anything nature had to offer. I have an indelible memory of her at a large conference on aging held in Puerto Rico, probably in the mid-seventies, at which she and I were keynote speakers (though she a little more keynote than I). Our two talks were to open the conference and were to be held in a vast outdoor patio of a garish tourist hotel (which we all enjoyed), but the sky looked menacing and a storm was clearly imminent. Margaret by then carried her famous staff—as much a weapon as a walking stick—which she proceeded to point to the heavens as though to demand that they hold back to permit her oration. It seemed to work as she held forth in her usual style with a discourse on the constraints on aging in our culture as compared with the scores of cultures she brought into her argument. Then it became my turn to talk (on "protean" possibilities of aging). I had barely begun my opening remarks when the clouds broke with a torrential rainstorm, and my talk had to be canceled and rescheduled. I admit mythologizing Margaret a bit, but that is how I remember what happened.

When Margaret became ill with pancreatic cancer in the late seventies at the age of seventy-seven, neither I nor anyone around her nor she herself was ready for her to die. In a conversation I had with her she expressed an interest in the cryonics movement, the freezing of bodies to be reanimated when science produced a cure for the fatal disease involved, saying that "I would like to do that if I thought it was possible, in order to be able to take a look and see how things are in the future." I was aware that Margaret had a needy side, and depended greatly on people around her for support and love, but such was her special energy—her own vital space in the world—that she had seemed invulnerable and permanent. I learned a great deal from Margaret's work, especially how premodern societies could undergo rapid forms of change (as described in her book *New Lives for Old*), but even more about how much knowledge and support a young person could gain from a floating community of divergent people who shared a sense of the freedom of the mind.

The Snake Sheds Its Skin

On the basis of my thought reform work, I was also introduced to members of a European community of anticommunist intellectuals. One encounter turned out to be painful, even humiliating, but illuminating in the discovery of an *antimentor.* Arthur Koestler had been a hero to me. His great novel *Darkness at Noon* was something close to a sacred text for anyone who sought to understand how Communists extracted confessions, and what those making the confessions experienced. Published in 1940, *Darkness at Noon* was Koestler's response to the Soviet purge trials of the thirties, which had caused him to leave the Communist movement. The novel describes the experience of Nicholas Rubashov, a leading Soviet official who is accused of opposition to the Party; he is coercively interrogated, affirms his false confession as reflecting the Party's correct claim to ultimate historical truth, and is then executed. Reading the book at the time of my Hong Kong research, I was stunned by Koestler's psychological astuteness in depicting the totalistic regime's demand for ownership of individual minds, and the victim's belief in his false confession and allegiance to his persecutors. I devoured much of his other work, including his riveting autobiographical volumes, *Arrow in the Blue* and *The Invisible Writing*, as well as his contribution to the highly influential collection of essays by disillusioned former Communists, *The God That Failed.*

I was awed by the life he had led as Hungarian-born Jew who had been imprisoned by Spanish Fascists (who came close to executing him) and by the Nazis. He had lived in Vienna, Palestine, and then England, and had even fought in the French Foreign Legion. He was a man who had done and seen just about everything, and written brilliantly about all of it. A friend had arranged an introduction to him and our meeting in 1958 took the form of a dinner BJ and I had with him and his wife in Paris, where I was about to begin those three-year follow-up interviews with Western priests and businessmen who had been put through thought reform in Chinese prisons. At the time Koestler, at age fifty-three, was perhaps the most celebrated of all communist-turned-anticommunist intellectuals.

Eager to discuss with him our common interests, I quickly mentioned my study of Chinese thought reform, but must have gone on a bit about my admiration for his important work and its contribution to my understanding. I noticed that as I talked his face at first registered nothing at all and then impatience and disdain. When I had finished my little soliloquy, he raised his head and, in a quiet voice that sounded to me like a chorus of thousands, said: "With every book I write, I shed my skin, like a snake." So much for any possible dialogue about thought reform and *Darkness at Noon*.

Whatever Koestler's nastiness, I had partly set myself up for his response. At the age of thirty-two, modest as my experience in the world was, I should have known better than to approach this ultimate cosmopolitan with such fawning reverence. But I say that now after a half century of further seasoning and a certain amount of ruminating about what transpired at that dinner. It's hard to recall just what I felt at the time, but it was something on the order of humiliation to the point of being extinguished.

There was more. The dinner went on, and although I cannot recall what we actually *did* discuss, I remember all too well what we drank. Koestler introduced BJ and me to Pernod, a green drink stronger than it looks, and such was his authority over us and our general discomfort that we found ourselves drinking a great deal of it. The next day we were both not only hungover but ill; never have I better understood the experience of feeling "green around the gills." In fact, whenever I have subsequently thought of Arthur Koestler, I have found myself enveloped by a green nausea. I came to see him as a Svengali figure who toyed with us, withheld from me what I wanted, and then poisoned us. And I, the student and critic of mind manipulation, had allowed it all to happen.

Actually, after I had written a few books myself, I came to understand something of what Koestler meant by an author's shedding his skin after each published volume. By the time others sought to engage one about a book, one's mind could be focused on a new project. But that of course did not mean that one had to disdainfully reject any inquiry into the published volume. There was an element of the sadistic in Koestler's account of his shedding, which provided me with a usefully negative model of both dialogue and mentorship.

Ten years later I was asked by *The New York Times* to review a book of Koestler's, *The Ghost in the Machine*. I remember trying very hard to be objective. And I did still have considerable respect for Koestler's intellect. Koestler spoke of the "endemic form of paranoia" dominating human history, and invoked a current neurophysiological theory as an explanation: the source of human self-destruction lies in our residual reptilian and lower mammalian brain structures. We can resolve the issue and sustain human survival, he argued, only by discovering a chemical substance that could right the balance and then distributing it universally. I thought both the diagnosis and the therapy patently absurd. They were also antithetical to my evolving emphasis on psychological experience in historical change. My focus by then was on the principle of symbolization, in which all adult mental experience is recast and given meaning by our large human brain. The same symbolizing imagination that could create Shakespeare's plays and sonnets could also view the destruction of the Jews as necessary to Germany's spiritual health. From that standpoint the source of our self-destructive behavior would lie not in the lower and older brain structures but in our higher and newer ones such as the cerebral cortex, which is generally responsible for symbolization. I felt that Koestler was negating our very humanity, and ended my review with the declaration that "man remains our problem, whatever we put into him, and however shaky his future as a species." I was saying that, whatever its pitfalls, we were stuck with the human mind and could not avoid its dangers by means of a chemical magic bullet.

Was my review an act of revenge? Looking at it now, I find it reasonable enough. No writing is without bias, and mine was affected by my intellectual convictions. But what of the influence of that excruciating encounter ten years earlier? Perhaps I took a bit too much pleasure in saying that Koestler's "suggestion of a biochemical cure for man's deficiencies [was] so cursorily and simplistically stated as to make one wonder whether the author really believes in it." Perhaps the residual Pernod effect made its way into that sentence.

Looking back on our encounter, we were two Jewish intellectuals who had in common a concern with Communist mind manipulation but were otherwise in almost every way antithetical. I was the earnest young American with an Enlightenment-related conviction that hard-won knowledge could lead to human betterment. I was approaching almost worshipfully a man who made no such assumption and in fact, through extreme experience of near death and something close to world destruction, had become a jaded observer of murderous behavior and was offended by expressions of earnestness and hope because these placed a misguided faith in human nature. But he combined this cynicism with a lifelong search for the absolute, initially through politics and later, as suggested in *The Ghost in the Machine*, through chemistry. That is, Koestler never overcame the lure of totalism, the quest for an all-or-none collective, even evolutionary, solution. His personal psychology contributed greatly to that quest: inclinations toward extreme dominance and violence in human relationships, culminating in his double suicide with his wife, Cynthia, in 1983 when he was seventy-seven years old and fatally ill and she, fifty-five and in good health. I doubt now that there was any possibility of real conversation between us. Our impasse revealed the perils of either a fawning or sadistically disdainful approach to any human encounter.

The Hidden Mentor

I found more authentic mentorship, though completely at a distance, from another legendary European intellectual. I never met Albert Camus, but what he wrote so illuminated my own work that I came to experience him as a teacher and an intellectual and moral soul mate. I have a painful memory of sitting down at breakfast with BJ at the Continental Hotel in Cambridge, Massachusetts, on January 5, 1960, and reading on the first page of *The New York Times* that Camus had been killed in an automobile accident in the south of France. Before I could say anything I felt tears run down my cheeks, as though I had lost a close friend or a member of my family. I was surprised and even a little embarrassed by my reaction.

I had discovered Camus's masterpiece, *The Rebel*, soon after returning from Hong Kong. It was a brilliant philosophical dissection of totalism. I was reading a great deal then in everything that seemed related to my work but came to feel that Camus was one of the few people in the world who really understood the appeals and dangers of the totalistic forces I was struggling to grasp. He spoke of "crimes of logic" resulting from the revolutionary's "total rejection . . . absolute negation, of what exists," and the deification of that stance. "Total revolution ends by demanding . . . the control of the world."

Camus's critique of totalism sounded Eriksonian (Erikson spoke of the young Luther as resembling patients in whom he encountered "a to be or not to be which makes every matter of differences a matter of mutually exclusive essences . . . every error or oversight, eternal treason"). Camus had an added literary flourish: "Totality is, in effect, nothing other than the ancient dream of unity common to both believers and rebels, but projected horizontally onto an earth deprived of God." (It is possible that Erikson, with whom I discussed Camus on at least one occasion, was influenced by him in formulating views on totality and totalism.)

Like Koestler, Camus drew upon the Soviet experience to point out that brutal interrogation could produce within days "an illusory conviction," and that "the only psychological revolution known to our times since Freud's has been brought about by the NKVD [the commissariat responsible for social control] and the political police in general" to demonstrate "the physics of the soul." He goes on to point out that, with such a regime, "Every man is a criminal who is unaware of being so." He explains that this stems from having embraced an attitude of "all or nothing," a "demand [for] . . . totality." Camus went on to say that such totalists "put an abstract idea above human life, even if they call it history, to which they themselves have submitted in advance and to which they will decide quite arbitrarily, to submit everyone else as well." He seemed to capture perfectly the mind-set of Chinese Communist reformers—as did his further comment that "pure and unadulterated virtue [becomes] homicidal." And similarly, "How intoxicating to feel like God the Father and to hand out definitive testimonials of bad character and habits." Equally relevant was Camus's overall comment that "politics is not religion, or if it is, then it is nothing but the Inquisition."

How did Camus know all this? He had himself joined the Communist Party in his early twenties, but was expelled from it two years later because of his independent attitudes. He had been profoundly affected by the Soviet purge trials of the thirties, and by the murderous revelations of the Soviet Gulag during the fifties. In between he had fought in the French Resistance and witnessed the death of a number of close friends. Camus drew wisdom from his survivals and could explore the history of rebels turned totalists from the time of the French Revolution through Nazism and Soviet communism.

What especially moved me about Camus was his insistence on combining his fierce critique of absolutism with a commitment to continuous questioning of any status quo. Here Camus came to differ significantly with Koestler, who for a time was his friend. Rather than Koestler's own totalistic embrace of anticommunism as such (including that of Joe McCarthy, the CIA, and even potential military confrontation with the Soviet Union), Camus was always concerned with the means employed to oppose wrongs and the importance of rejecting any claim of one's own infallibility. *The Rebel* was, after all, Camus's subject, and the book is about the struggle to remain rebellious while avoiding the trap of totalism. Camus tells us from the beginning that a rebel is "a man who says no," who resists oppression and violence, always in a quest for justice. He must also resist abuses perpetrated in the name of rebellion. Like Camus, I considered myself a constant critic of the status quo—in his terms, a rebel—who was confronting a version of revolutionary totalism. For Camus a rebel was not only a man who says no but "also a man who says yes as soon as he begins to think for himself." When Camus spoke of a rebel's "complete and spontaneous loyalty to certain aspects of himself," I knew he had touched something in me, however difficult to identify.

I did not appreciate at the time the courage it had taken for Camus to write that book, the extent to which he was ostracized by prominent pro-Soviet members of the French intellectual circles he had inhabited, which included a painful ending of his friendship with Jean-Paul Sartre. I had admired a number of Sartre's essays, especially his classic piece on anti-Semitism, but was appalled by his view that the Soviets should not be reproached for their extreme abuses in the Gulag because they were on the right side of history—as opposed to Camus's insistence on full condemnation of such murderous behavior by anyone. I had no parallel problem with the American left when I published my book on thought reform. But during the heady days of the late sixties, students raised the question of whether I wished to retract some of my critical views toward the Chinese Communists. I would like to think that my unhesitating "no" had something Camus-like in it.

Camus had his blind spots, notably concerning the Algerian FLN's struggle against the French for independence. He tried to be evenhanded in condemning the excesses of French colonials and their use of torture, as well as the terrorism of the FLN. But as a Frenchman from Algeria, he simply could not accept the inevitable: an Algerian future without the French. Here I was with Sartre, and for that matter many other Frenchmen who were by no means on the left (notably Charles de Gaulle).

But Camus was also aware of the broader twentieth-century responsibilities of intellectuals. In his 1958 Nobel Prize speech, he spoke of the writer's creed to confront "twenty years of absolutely insane history." He saw the task of his generation as that of "fighting openly against the death-instinct at work in our history" and "keeping the world from destroying itself." I wrote to my friend Les Farber that, while the speech was hardly optimistic, I experienced "nothing but exhilaration" on reading it because here was a man who "really understood the way things are, and could describe them with . . . artfulness and profound psychological wisdom." He became part of my special pantheon of writers, an unlikely group that would include Erik Erikson, Leslie Farber, Susanne Langer, Ernst Cassirer, Samuel Beckett, Norman Mailer, Saul Bellow, Don DeLillo, Robert Lowell, and Theodore Roethke. All of them brought wisdom to my evolving, often confusing, sense of who and where I was in the world. But Camus holds a special place in my confrontations with totalism.

I have never stopped reading Camus, and two of his other books, *The Fall* and *The Plague*, have had special meaning for me: *The Fall*, which recounts in a series of monologues the moral decline of a self-described "judge-penitent" who can pass judgment on himself and everyone else, was important in terms of the use of endless confession to avoid essential truths. With *The Plague*, in which an epidemic devastates a French city, I was especially struck by the physician/hero's commitment to combating the forces of destruction with no certainty that his efforts will succeed. In my 2003 book about my own country, *Superpower Syndrome*, I conclude with Camus's call for "thought which recognizes limits," together with his pithy observation: "He who does not know everything cannot kill everyone."

Whose Work Is It?

As hungry as I was for mentorship, I found it just about as important to avoid certain kinds of influence. In the case of two people, both prominent psychoanalytic researchers and teachers, enthusiasm for my work took on what I could only view as possessive dimensions. The first of these encounters was with Abram Kardiner, then head of the Columbia University Psychoanalytic Institute, to whom I was introduced by David Rioch in early 1956 to explore the possibility of training with him. Kardiner had been analyzed by Freud, and was one of the pioneers of American psychoanalysis. He had created a somewhat rebellious offshoot at Columbia as the first psychoanalytic institute to become an integral part of a university. And I admired studies he had done on psychological trauma during World War II, on psychoanalysis and culture, and on psychological consequences of race in American society. I was at first moved by the excitement he expressed about my work and then stunned by the extent to which he suggested becoming involved in it. He said that I should enter his institute: "Bring your data and we'll look it over together, and after you've had a couple of years of your training, we'll see how we can make the best use of the data."

Whatever my confusions during those early years, I had always assumed that I would write up the work myself as well as I could (which was the assumption made by people around me such as Erik Erikson, David Rioch, and Margaret Mead). Now Kardiner was proposing that I delay writing up or doing anything else with the data for a couple of years until I was sufficiently trained in his institute, at which time he would collaborate with me and have considerable say about what should be done with the work in general. While I knew that I could learn a great deal from Kardiner (whom I met at about the same time I did Erikson), I was deeply troubled by the idea of anyone taking over the work I had struggled so hard to carry out. I did not want to surrender my autonomy as a researcher and writer. So I fled.

My second encounter with a would-be mentor was with David Rapaport, a close friend and psychological colleague of Erik Erikson at the Austen Riggs Center in Stockbridge, Massachusetts. Rapaport's encyclopedic knowledge of psychoanalytic theory enabled him to locate Erikson's work within that theory ("to tell me what I am saying," as Erikson put it to me). Rapaport was a brilliant and pugnacious Hungarian Jew whom I liked and who visited us in Cambridge on several occasions. Our problem also involved his way of being enthusiastic about my work. In our correspondence, he sent me a few of his reprints on psychoanalytic theory. I wrote back expressing my appreciation for them, but did not mention them further in connection with my preliminary work on my book on thought reform. He had wanted more, and in a reply said that he was "rather sorry about what you write to me concerning the reading you did [of his articles]. I will be candid: I hoped that it would dissuade you from writing now, and prompt you to study further and to make further investigations before you do so. But everyone travels on his own risk." I tried to explain myself in a note back, but our correspondence petered out, as did our friendship. I did compose a mock letter (which I found in my library papers) but only showed to BJ: "This is to inform you that your rabbinical style of work does not speak to my condition."

I later learned that Kardiner was notorious for drawing upon and sometimes taking over other people's data, and that Rapaport, though generally kind and supportive to young people, could become tyrannical when they took what he viewed as the wrong direction. While I felt hurt and threatened by the two experiences, I accepted Rapaport's declaration that everyone travels at his own risk.

That encounter with Rapaport helped clarify differences between Erikson and myself. It mattered to Erikson that Rapaport could locate him within psychoanalytic theory, but I was of a different generation, less involved in the arcane distinctions on which Rapaport thrived. Significantly, both Kardiner and Rapaport represented what could be called progressive modifications of psychoanalysis. But I believe that both had an exaggerated faith in the capacity of those innovations to provide a new version of psychoanalytic science, into which work like mine had to be subsumed. To me that seemed the wrong way to go about things. At issue here was the principle of focusing on direct experience and keeping one's

conceptual interpretations close to the data obtained. I wanted to figure out how best to understand my data, borrowing from psychoanalytic
work that helped me to do that, rather than making the work a vehicle
for any school of thought. Again there was that difficult balance between
influence required and influence avoided.

I had another experience of protecting my work that was more directly
political. The McCarran Committee (a McCarthyite offshoot) wanted to
use me and my work to further sensationalize "brainwashing" as a form
of Communist infamy, and to do so as part of the right-wing offensive
against liberals and others for having "lost China" and for being "soft
on communism" in general. When informed that I was to be called to
testify before it, my reaction was a combination of simple fear—of being
victimized and humiliated by political bullies—and a more complex form
of moral anxiety having to do with the work having social impact in directions I abhorred. I was to have that concern with all of my research, but
the general mystique surrounding "brainwashing" lent itself particularly
to crude political manipulations.

So I went to David Rioch as a friend and sponsor with considerable
leverage on the Washington scene, and he anticipated my request by suggesting that he intervene to prevent my testimony. He was able to do that,
not by questioning the motives of the Senate investigators (though these
certainly bore questioning) but by claiming that such public testimony
would interfere with the progress of my important ongoing research. I
wished to use my own writings, especially the book I was preparing, to
explain what thought reform was, its relationship to Communist China,
and its significance for the rest of us. I knew that I had little ultimate
control over what people did with the information I offered, but I wanted
to do all I could to avoid its being taken over by self-appointed political
mentors with their own agendas.

4

———

Finding a Voice—with Help from Friends

WRITING THE BOOK on thought reform was especially hard for me. I had to be concerned not only with those I interviewed but with the spectacle of the largest nation in the world turning in on itself and subjecting virtually all of its own people—along with a smattering of foreigners—to a "reform" process that was systematic, coercive, and of profound psychological consequence. My book had to be mainly about that remarkable process, about the nature of its impact as well as its failures.

A chapter toward the end of the book I considered especially important included eight psychological patterns I believed to be characteristic of totalistic environments everywhere, environments (whether religious, political, or both) in which procedures resembling thought reform are likely to occur. I came to view them as the "eight deadly sins" of totalism. They were: *milieu control*, that of virtually all communication in an environment; *mystical manipulation*, maneuvers from above by an obscure but ultimate authority under the guise of group spontaneity; *the demand for purity*, imposed pursuit of absolute good in order to defeat absolute evil; *the cult of confession*, obsession with continuous all-encompassing and ever-critical self-revelation; *the sacred science*, claim to doctrinal truth that is both divine and scientifically proven; *loading the language*, the reduction of all human problems to definitive-sounding phrases, to the thought-terminating cliché; *doctrine over person*, a primacy so absolute that any doubts about prevailing dogma must be considered a form of personal deficiency or psychological aberration; and *the dispensing of existence*, the sharp line drawn between those who have a right to exist and those who possess no such right. This last feature of ideological totalism for me summed up its larger evil. The "dispensing" in question could involve no more than positions offered or denied in society, or it could mean killing those considered to be tainted by the wrong background or wrong thoughts.

The chapter was a form of psychological analysis, but I realize now that it was also a statement of personal credo. It was my way of extending the work into a universal frame and at the same time taking an ethical stand toward totalism and its indicators. Only later did I realize how much of myself I had invested in the study. I had to complete the book both to justify the whole effort and to affirm my sense of being a psychohistorical researcher out in the world. I seemed to need help in doing that, and sent the manuscript to friends with whom I had already been having informal discussions about the work and its relevance. They included Erik Erikson, David Rioch, Kenneth Keniston, Leslie Farber, Fritz Redlich, and above all, David Riesman. I also sent portions of the manuscript to Benjamin Schwartz and John Fairbank, two highly knowledgeable authorities on modern China who had also been interested in the study.

Beyond their comments on different aspects of the book, these readers' responses provided me with a beginning sense of what it was like to lead the intellectual life, to combine affectionate friendship with a continuous exchange of ideas. But there was nothing neat or orderly in all this, and my anxiety about completing the book was reflected in my smoking habits at the time (a light smoker until its end stages when I began to approach a pack a day, and unable to give up the habit, despite the surgeon general's report on its dangers, until the manuscript was sent off to the publisher). Until that moment of completion I would not leave for the new research in Japan. My miscalculations about time led us to rent our small Cambridge house prematurely, which required us to stay a couple of months at a pond house in Wellfleet and a couple more at the old Continental Hotel in Cambridge. But during that period, when incorporating suggestions for the manuscript, I was also, almost inadvertently, redefining my intellectual community.

The Passionate Reader

My closest and most dedicated reader was David Riesman. He responded to the manuscript with his entire being, viscerally no less than intellectually, and conveyed to me a deep sense of the book's worth, and therefore of my own. He also helped me to understand my work as that of an American intellectual, whatever its Chinese content.

Riesman and I met in 1957, when he arrived in Cambridge to begin his celebrated Harvard course on American society. We quickly took to each other and he invited me to make commentaries in his course and to attend the weekly dinners at his home for the dozen or so young people (mostly graduate students) who served as his "section heads." I was closer in age to them than to him (I was thirty-one and he forty-eight), but Dave and I formed an unusual intellectual bond in our intense yet easy associations to each other's ideas, in our increasing pleasure in talking to one another.

Dave was all mind. He had no small talk. When an idea struck him his quintessentially serious face would flash a quirky little smile that could in turn give way to an all-consuming exuberance. Though he expressed no philosophy about walking (as Erikson had), he and I established a regular pattern of long late-afternoon treks along the paths of Fresh Pond Park at the edge of Cambridge, providing us with needed exercise and an opportunity for continuous talk. Also sharing the exercise was our beloved Weimaraner named Runcible (a nonsense word coined by the British poet Edward Lear), who was as prominent a gentle beast as one could imagine (height of a small pony, weight about eighty pounds, lively yellow eyes, a svelte gray, muscular body) but to Dave completely invisible. Totally immersed in our thoughts, Dave never once referred to the dog; and Runcible, ordinarily very friendly, took the hint and ignored Dave as well.

There were so many things we talked about on those walks—ranging from the globally threatening to the intellectually gossipy personal. But there was one overarching theme that Dave could uniquely explicate, that of American society: how it worked politically, religiously, racially; how it took shape originally and was recast from the triumphalism that followed upon World War II; how our ill-advised policy of unconditional surrender contributed to our problems with nuclear weapons; and how one might think about, and advocate, social change.

Dave always returned to an emphasis on the fragility of American society due to its absence of traditional roots, its vulnerability to breakdown and to extreme and violent behavior by reactionary groups always waiting in the wings. I found my mind moving back and forth between thought reform in China and social and psychological currents in my own country, including susceptibilities to totalism. With his multilevel observations and his strikingly idiosyncratic associations, Dave taught me more about the way America really worked—about its group conflicts and ever-present dangers—than one could expect to learn in a lifetime of ordinary study.

Although we talked quite a bit about my manuscript, Dave's most profound responses came in letters, two remarkable sets of them: the first four during the last half of July 1959, totaling sixteen single-spaced typewritten pages written over that two-week period; and the second round of seven letters written intermittently from late October of 1959 through mid-January of 1960. In an almost nineteenth-century fashion, certain matters seemed to require the letter as opposed to the spoken word. It is hard for me to imagine any more sublime combination of close and sympathetic reading, deep appreciation, sensitive personal support, enlarging associations and comparisons, critical suggestions, and overall generosity of spirit. In general, the letters were as much a continuation of our dialogue as they were comments on the book.

He raised the question of why the Chinese released Westerners from prisons "to tell such tales when they could quietly shoot them after getting their confessions"; he commented on the significance of logic in thought reform and the potential vulnerability of priests because of their training, especially Jesuits, to such logic; and he reflected on the inevitable discomfort of Chinese I interviewed with interpreters they did not know. In my replies I often had my own new thoughts, so that in response to an observation of his on the religious nature of thought reform I wrote: "The Chinese communists are on a kind of treadmill of their own; they just cannot stop reforming their population."

Of course, Dave extended his associations far beyond the work itself. He mentioned a "sad thought" to the effect that "the Korean War may occupy for Red China the same place that the Siberian intervention [of Western troops opposed to the revolution] occupies with the USSR." He asked whether I might want to study "people damaged by American thought reform," referring to his meeting with Owen Lattimore, the China specialist victimized by McCarthy, whom he found to be "a broken man." Mentioning the creative use of men like Nehru of their prison experience, he observed that this was true for some of those I interviewed who spoke of having benefited from their ordeal. Here he invoked William James's concept of "the moral equivalent of war," in contrast with what Dave called the "underlived" quality of most lives. And he noted, among the many reasons for ending the Cold War, the need "to restore our ability to criticize in the Iron Curtain countries without being considered, or being in fact part of, the CIA network."

No response to my work has provided greater affirmation—of a particular project, a sense of self, a hoped-for future.

Other Voices

Erikson had to be a key figure in these responses. What he said would enormously affect my own sense of the kind of psychological voice I had evolved. Characteristically, his reaction was delayed and cautious, but in a handwritten letter from Carmel, California, where he then lived (dated simply "December, 1959"), his expressions of approval were resonant and to me very moving: I had made "a quite major contribution to the psychology of ideology" (a way of relating the book to his work, since that was a strong interest of his), had ordered and "clearly thought out" a great mass of material, "found the right level of discourse and [kept] to it with simplicity and pungency," all of which "surpasses entirely what I've been able to visualize on the basis of our conversations." Interestingly, in the same letter Erik turned to issues of friendship, apologizing for having been "an unreliable friend" because of the complications of "disengaging myself from the therapeutic profession" (he was moving away from clinical practice in order to concentrate on teaching and writing), and offered his "hope that the future will be simpler and clearer."

Nothing was ever simple or fully clear with Erik, but I greatly appreciated his words and said so in a warm farewell note before leaving for Japan in February 1960, mentioning that the publisher would be sending him galley proofs for the last few chapters. On August 30, 1960, Erik sent me a cablegram that followed me from Tokyo to Hakone, an outlying resort town where I was attending a conference, which read: "Therapy chapter fine whole book great achievement greetings Erik." It took me a while to realize how generous an act it was for Erik to send the cable with the wonderfully cryptic message expressed in the cablese of the time. His response to the book made me feel like an "adult" among psychological writers concerned with the larger world, and more of an equal in our friendship as well. It occurs to me now that the moment of greatest intensity in any mentor–disciple relationship—my situation with Erikson at the time—can signal the beginning of its end.

That idea was suggested by the response of my friend Ken Keniston, the only contemporary of mine to whom I seemed to have entrusted the manuscript. A psychologist with one of the most wide-ranging minds I have encountered, Ken wrote two fine books on young Americans, *Alienated Youth* and *Young Rebels*, which depicted an important historical sequence. He and I considered working together on a comparative study of American and Japanese youth, and although this never materialized we got into the habit of writing empathic critiques of each other's work. We also had endless discussions about our struggles with mentors, mine with Erikson and his with the much more problematic Henry Murray, the Harvard psychologist who was a great pioneer in the field but who could be highly destructive toward people around him. Ken read my manuscript in the context of our dialogue on mentors.

Concerning Erikson he observed "how well the various aspects of identity theory help explain the material, and how delicately you manage to move from identity to its earlier and deeper roots" in ways that "equal and at times surpass your mentor. Maybe it is time to leave." Whatever his hyperbole, Keniston was perceptive about the imminence of my "leaving" Erikson, not in the sense of a personal break but of emerging from his influence. Though Ken was with me at Yale and was to play an important role in our early Wellfleet meetings on psychology and history, he and I, much to my regret, subsequently drifted apart. But during the years that we were close, our friendship provided the special mutual affirmation of peers who could share intense intellectual struggles, in our case concerning the mysteries of psychology and history, and of mentors and followers.

Leslie Farber differed from all other readers in his extreme psychoanalytic iconoclasm. He had pretty much lost all belief in theory, claiming that the Washington School under Harry Stack Sullivan (which Rioch also had been part of) had, in its quest for exact science, turned man into a machine, while the original Freudian school, with its instinctualism, turned him into a prehuman animal. So Farber in his work focused (admirably though perhaps too exclusively) on direct experience, a phenomenological approach that enabled him to remain wary of conceptual interpretation as such. He also immersed himself in literature and in the work of those concerned with literature. When I first went to see Les and complained to him about the unreadability of much psychoanalytic writing, his answer was "Read the literary critics," excellent advice in an era of Edmund Wilson, Lionel Trilling, and Alfred Kazin. As I think of it now, Les seemed to view himself as a critic, not of literature but of his fellow human beings, always with a mixture of skepticism and a certain sympathy for their foibles.

Les was seriously interested in many other things: religion (at one point he seemed to consider a conversion to Catholicism), sports, sex, popular culture, and film (his older brother, Manny Farber, whom he much admired, was a renowned against-the-grain film critic). Our conversations, often with the help of a drink or two, were irreverent, free-floating, and great fun. I can remember our comparing the virtues of the sports images we called forth in dropping off to sleep: and under his influence I added that of the inimitable Don Budge serving an ace on the tennis court to my earlier standard image of the great Jewish left-handed pitcher Sandy Koufax striking out the side. Les wrote sparingly, leaving a legacy of about twenty exquisitely honed essays, whether about therapists' own self-deceptions and sources of redemption, or the intricacies and modest achievements of quotidian existence. Each of these essays is capable of changing a reader's life.

Since he was a great debunker and had taught me so much, I both needed and feared Les's response to that first book. I knew he would be candid, sympathetic, and unsparing. Much to my relief he wrote me of his considerable admiration for the work, but with a qualification that was not a small one. He urged me to get rid of all of my references to Erikson's identity theory, which he thought only cluttered the book and did nothing for my argument, insisting, "You say everything you have to say without it." Much as I admired Les and respected his literary sense, I had little inclination to follow his suggestion. One could say that I remained true to that eureka moment of discovering the relevance of identity theory for the work, and I kept those references. Yet it is also possible that something in me resonated to Les's words in helping me to take my subsequent work in very different theoretical directions.

The reading that most affected my professional future was that of Fritz Redlich. My sending the manuscript to him was my way of demonstrating an outcome of the five-year dream grant for which he had been so instrumental, but I was surprised at the intensity of his enthusiasm for the final section of the book, which I called "Totalism and Its Alternatives." In that section I included a discussion of what I called "open personal change" contrasting with that promoted by thought reform, and suggested its relevance for psychotherapeutic work. I realize now that its critical discussion of absolutism and argument for noncoercive approaches to human beings in general tapped directly into Fritz's own lifelong struggles. A refugee from Nazi-controlled Vienna with strong survivor inclinations to combat totalism, Fritz was a leading figure among those committed to more progressive and open directions in American psychiatry and psychoanalysis, especially in teaching institutions.

He saw me as a kindred spirit and perhaps something more. Men like Fritz at Yale, and Erich Lindemann, whom I worked with at Harvard, could experience considerable conflict between their sense of themselves as intellectuals who could do original work in their profession, and the attraction to power that contributed to their becoming departmental chairmen with considerable authority sustained over time. In our conversations, Fritz frequently praised my "intellectual" and "creative" energies, which I believe represented for him the side of himself he had given up. It was also the side he perhaps most respected. He could see that I had no such taste for administrative power—not only because I became so immersed in my research but because I lacked the temperament to make the hard decisions about people's lives required of those wielding that kind of power.

In any case, almost immediately after reading that last section of my book, Fritz invited me to be Yale's candidate for one of three chairs in psychiatric research to be set up in various parts of the country by the same foundation that had awarded me my earlier grant. The application was likely to be successful, because the foundation and its consultants already had considerable involvement with my work, and even more so because of the great influence wielded by Fritz.

But that didn't mean that all went smoothly once I received the chair. In running the department Fritz could play one professor against another or be manipulative in various ways (in what came to be called his "Viennese style") and at times asked me to take on duties that would have undermined the research the chair was meant to enable. Nor did I make things easy for Fritz, insisting on living abroad, in both England and Japan, under the terms of the chair, and later moving to New York City and commuting to Yale for part of the work week. Fritz and I had a number of discussions about these matters, one of them on November 22, 1963, that terrible day on which President John F. Kennedy was shot. We abruptly ended our discussion and rushed to the parking area so that we could turn on the radio in his car and listen to the dreadful news that followed. Fritz and I went through much together, and sharing that experience was part of our bond.

Toward the end of his life I took pleasure in helping Fritz return to his intellectual self in connection with an admirable undertaking. He began to discuss with me the idea of his doing a study of the Nazi era. In our talks I encouraged him to pursue a manageable project, make use of his professional knowledge and cultural background, and pursue the particular interest he expressed in Hitler. He came up with the idea of doing a detailed study of Hitler's medical and psychological history. He carried out the work in his mid and late eighties, culminating in his fine book, *Hitler: A Study of a Destructive Prophet*. So at the end Fritz could return to the part of himself he most respected. I expressed my affection for Fritz in dedicating a book of essays to him as the person "who made it all possible."

Thought Reform and the Psychology of Totalism (the kind of ungainly title likely to be used for a first book) was well received, with reviews appearing in some major newspapers, magazines, and academic journals—not creating a big splash but its impact building over time. There was a laudatory response in the *New York Times Book Review*, which was the occasion for another cablegram to Tokyo. This one came from my father and read something like: "New York Times says your book is an excellent study." That recognition from the *Times* and my father's loving exuberance merged in my happily churning mind, and BJ and I had drinks together with Tokyo writer friends.

But I still had large questions about who I was and what I knew. I was a young psychiatrist, not a wildly unconventional person, but one who had begun to do some odd things in the world. If the Hong Kong work was (in BJ's Darwinian banter) my voyage of the *Beagle*, what did I do with the "specimens" I had acquired when the ship reached port? I had lived six months in Korea, a year in Japan in the military, then seventeen months in Hong Kong and two additional years in Japan as a civilian. East Asia had become my research area, a kind of specialty. But I was neither a Sinologist nor a Japanologist. I had learned some spoken Japanese, which served me well but by no means eliminated my need for an interpreter in my research. And for all I had learned about China, I had no knowledge at all of its language and dialects. I was deeply interested in psychology and history, but nobody had yet mentioned the word *psychohistory*.* I had a sense I could do unusual work but at the same time considerable inner uncertainty about my relationship to my profession and to the world. I was profoundly affected by the Freudian revolution but out of

---

*Except for Isaac Asimov whose fictional psychohistory was a predictive, mathematical science.

sync with Freudian institutions even with neo-Freudian modifications. I wasn't behaving like other psychiatrists—seeing patients, running wards, or investigating causes of individual neurosis.

Rather than focus on individual psychological health, I was wandering about the more obscure territory of shared and collective behavior, extending out to vast movements. I remember at one point, still in the late nineteen fifties, raising precisely this question in my analysis, asking myself what kind of special knowledge, if any, I had acquired. What I came up with was a special grasp of the interaction of individual psychology with larger ideological and historical forces, especially when the interaction of the two resulted in patterns of totalism, mind manipulation, and potential violence. That was probably true, but as a way of defining myself seemed not only abstract but tenuous in its intellectual connections. I felt myself to be both adventurous and unmoored.

To remedy the situation I considered the possibility of obtaining a graduate degree in Japanese studies. I knew that would be a major enterprise, involving years of study and a lifelong struggle with the Japanese language. I went to see Edwin Reischauer, the Japanologist, to seek his advice on the matter. We had a rather odd conversation. I expressed to him both my interest and my misgivings, and said something to the effect that it would be "embarrassing" if I embarked on such a project and then withdrew from it or failed to complete it. His answer, in the form of a question, was almost Talmudic: "Embarrassing to whom?" Reischauer was, like Fairbank, a kingpin at Harvard, in his case a pioneer in developing and extending Japanese studies in the United States. He was simultaneously encouraging me to take the degree and suggesting that, should it not work out, that would not be the end of the world.

I was struggling with the question of how much to immerse myself in Asian studies, with how to evolve a core professional self that would maintain a balance between my experience in the Far East and my historically minded psychological research in general. I wanted to avoid any misstep that might endanger the whole fragile enterprise. My feared sense of inner embarrassment had to do with being seen as inauthentic by both Asian specialists and proper psychiatrists—though ultimately by myself. My decision not to seek the degree was a way of protecting the openness of my uneasy identity forays.

I reported the conversation to BJ and "Embarrassing to whom?" became another of our mantras—the question one of us asked whenever the word *embarrassing* would come up, and always in a mocking or self-mocking fashion. Don DeLillo had a wonderfully absurd approach to that kind of problem in his novel *White Noise*, in which the narrator, Jack Gladney, becomes the dominant figure in the field of "Hitler studies" he himself created. But he felt himself living "on the edge of a landscape of vast shame" because he could neither speak nor read German.

Over time, as I proceeded with subsequent projects, I became less uncomfortable about these identity conflicts. I increasingly connected my personal experience with my evolving concepts about the complexities of the self, and especially our capacity for putting together divergent elements of identity or what I sometimes called "identity fragments." I was full of those fragments. In professional terms I was a psychoanalytically oriented psychiatrist with idiosyncratic interests. I was also a researcher: on Japan, on Hong Kong and China, on individual psychology and historical change, on the experience and consequences of totalism, on the influence of ideology on individuals and groups. I was not (in 1961) yet a university teacher but was heading for an academic career and had received research grants along that path. All that was in addition to such basic identity components as a husband, a father, an American, a Jew, a man, and a human being. And in terms that encompassed both the personal and professional, I was something of an expatriate or alien, and even more of a maverick. Yet gradually, imperceptibly, and rather erratically, these fragments began to connect and even, at least some of the time, to cohere.

5

_____

Further Struggles with Totalism

Thought Reform and the Apocalyptic

It took me a while to recognize the apocalyptic dimension of thought reform, the principle of destroying (or anticipating the destruction of) the existing world in order to bring about magnificent world renewal. Early on, I saw its resemblance to a religious revival movement, with the experience of transcendence and of mystical higher purpose it combined with its relentless political and personal "logic." But China's Cultural Revolution of the mid and late sixties went further. It concretely played out a narrative of world destruction and purified re-creation. Since the Cultural Revolution was an extension of thought reform to the point of caricature, I immediately sought to learn all I could about it. My study of it prefigured my later preoccupation with matters apocalyptic, including my study of Aum Shinrikyo, published in 1999, which I called _Destroying the World to Save It_, and my examination of America's own version of apocalypticism in _Superpower Syndrome_, published in 2003.

At the time I did my work on the Cultural Revolution, BJ and I were involved in extensive world travel. In 1966–67 I followed closely from New Haven, New York, Cape Cod, and then London and Tokyo, and finally Hong Kong, the strange events occurring in China: vast legions of young fanatics, called Red Guards and Revolutionary Rebels, on cru-

79

sades of purification and making startling attacks on Party officials that included extreme public humiliation and considerable violence. They had been called forth by Mao Zedong, rendered a deity, creating vast photographic tableaux of the by now despotic leader addressing his worshipful minions, reminiscent of Leni Riefenstahl's depiction of Hitler at Nuremberg in her film *Triumph of the Will*. During two weeks in Hong Kong I was able to interview a number of observers of these events, including former members of the Red Guard who had defected, and also to obtain many firsthand documents. The participants were not only university students but "children of thirteen to eighteen with beautiful faces," as one observer told me. I later referred to them as "almost beatific" in their transcendent sense of virtue, "a strange young band of wandering zealots in search of evil and impurity." They themselves spoke of "breaking and smashing" and "inducing the catastrophe," and their targets included not only everything Western and anyone associated with the prior regime but Party bureaucrats and leaders deemed insufficiently pure in their revolutionary fervor. Typical was the manifesto of one group of middle-school students:

> We are the Red Guards of Chairman Mao and we effect the convulsion. We tear up and smash up old calendars, precious vases, U.S. and British records, superstitious lacquers and ancient paintings, and we put up the picture of Chairman Mao.

I had by then developed some ideas about death and death symbolism and looked upon the upheaval as emerging from Mao's sense of his own impending death as well as his fear of the death of the revolution. The extreme measures called forth—the smashing of objects and people considered un-Maoist or insufficiently Maoist, and the all-pervasive pictures of the great Chairman—were efforts at revitalizing and immortalizing both Mao and a fiercely purified revolution. Hence the title of the book I was to write, *Revolutionary Immortality*. But I was edging toward a stress on the apocalyptic as well. In commenting upon an observer's view that the ascetic dedication of the Maoist Red Guard resembled that found in Calvinism, I suggested that "while the Calvinists sought to 'establish the kingdom of God on earth,' the Maoists seek a kingdom of eternal revolution." The Cultural Revolution was thought reform gone berserk. At the time I was not aware of just how berserk, of how much killing and cruelty was called forth by this apocalyptic reeducation project.

The larger truth is that mind control kills. That became clear to me in following developments in China during the years after my original study. Chinese Communist leaders used to say that thought reform was a humane alternative to killing people—as in the case of captured enemy soldiers early on, and alleged counterrevolutionaries at all times. But a decade before the Cultural Revolution, during the 1958 campaign, the Great Leap Forward, *at least twenty million Chinese*—some observers believe *as many as forty or even fifty million—starved to death* because of the apocalyptic fantasies of Mao Zedong and those around him. Mao pressed thought reform programs on the Chinese population that emphasized not only mind over technology, but a more fanatical vision of mind as a substitute for technology. Thousands of "backyard furnaces" were constructed in place of large steel factories, resulting in a catastrophic combination of an extreme shortage of agricultural labor, false reports by cadres on crop losses, and inability to cope with a drought that occurred that year—all of which led to one of the worst famines in human history.

These apocalyptic impulses were behind the Chinese Communists' need to over-reform their population. They came into power as heroes, having survived their legendary "Long March" (a six-thousand-mile trek in 1934–35 to preserve the Communist forces) in achieving a brilliant military victory. They could emanate an aura of power and integrity, which drove the whole thought reform process. Through it, they imposed their standards of revolutionary behavior on their sprawling population. But they could not stop reforming. Even when it became counterproductive and a source of resentment, they kept reeducating their people, whether ritualistically or in explosive events like the Cultural Revolution. During recent decades, as China has moved away from the ideological phase of the revolution and plunged into capitalistic development, one has heard much less about thought reform. But whenever the regime has felt itself threatened—as in the case of the prodemocracy uprising of 1989 and the late-twentieth-century expansion of Falun Gong, an aggressive religious movement with cultic features—the regime has expressed the need to "reeducate" the offending individuals and groups. That regime retains sizable pockets of totalism mostly in the political sphere, incarcerating those who raise the mildest questions about democratic change. Thought reform seems mostly limited to these pockets, but one can hardly be certain that the apocalyptic impulses behind it have disappeared.

Thought Reform and Psychoanalytic Training

The work also sensitized me to milder expressions of totalism and near totalism. These could be more difficult to identify, and more controversial, occurring as they did in religious, political, and educational institutions in our own midst. Psychoanalytic training institutes were a case in point. Those institutes had already been criticized for such tendencies by members of the profession, about which Erik Erikson had alerted me further. In my case, the prior study of thought reform had to complicate my training experience at the Boston Psychoanalytic Institute.

Since I was already highly critical of psychoanalytic dogma and the Boston Institute was known to be among the most "traditional"—meaning dogmatic—of them all, one might well ask what I was doing there in the first place. The answer was the other side of my mixed feelings about psychoanalysis, my sense that my work ultimately stemmed from it and that psychiatry was increasingly bound up with psychoanalysis. Despite my reservations, I believed that I needed the training to get to the highest point of being a psychiatrist. And with or without the training, I saw myself as already entering a humane and imaginative Eriksonian version of that tradition.

I did not particularly seek out the Boston Institute as such, but I wanted to be in the Cambridge area for the "research training" provided for in my grant—involving people I was drawn to in connection with work on East Asia, in psychiatry, history, and social science. The European flavor of the Boston Institute had a certain appeal—the expatriate analysts in charge seemed to come directly from the horse's mouth, so to speak—but it also was associated with a strong sense of hierarchy. The institute did, however, have one importantly liberal policy, that of candidates choosing their own analysts rather than being assigned to them.

I chose Beate Rank, a pioneer in child analysis and former wife of Otto Rank, not because of her accomplishments or her name, but because of my impression of her when meeting her at a reception at her home. She was an elegant, bright, and vivacious woman in her late sixties, and I remember feeling that she would be responsive to my idiosyncratic life and that she would not hurt me. I was concerned that a more dogmatic person, especially a dogmatic male, might undermine what I most respected in myself, my unorthodox professional directions, by viewing them as psychologically deviant. That concern was not entirely unfounded, as orthodox analysts at the time could readily view attitudes and interests antithetical to their own as aberrant.

Beate Rank turned out to be the nurturing and supportive analyst I anticipated, but I did not experience my two years of work with her as transformative. She was a traditional analyst, which meant that we had sessions four or five times a week during which I lay on the couch and she said relatively little, though enough to be helpful in connection with family conflicts, such as those having to do with my sister's psychological needs. After some reluctance, she was sufficiently flexible to agree to my absence for the full two months BJ and I had taken to spending on Cape Cod during the summer. I do not know what she thought of my unusual professional trajectory—she never commented on it directly—but it was certainly not undermined in any way by the psychoanalysis and probably to some degree was strengthened by it. My own self-protective tendencies were geographical as well as psychological, as I had made an understanding with the institute that I would be in Cambridge for two years of analysis and classes and would then spend two years in Japan on my new research. Still at times I felt like an alien in the institute. I was intellectually at odds with the narrowly Freudian content of the seminars and the orthodoxy of most of the faculty. Everyone was friendly and soft-spoken, but I found the atmosphere to be highly authoritarian; others did also, but tended to be less sensitive to such things than I was.

My way of coming to terms with my dilemma was to include in my book *Thought Reform and the Psychology of Totalism* a discussion of troubling resemblances between psychoanalytic training and the thought reform process. I went about the critique in a very measured way (Riesman thought it was too mild). But I was aware that making such a comparison in a book on thought reform, especially for one who was himself in psychoanalytic training, was a considerable act of rebellion. I began by pointing out that psychoanalysis as a body of thought derives from intellectual currents—humanism, individualism, and free scientific inquiry—that have been historically antithetical to totalism. But I referred to the perils of the controlling organizational policies that can follow upon the revolutionary phase of any movement. While others had made criticisms along similar lines, my study of thought reform gave me a special perspective and a specific set of criteria for such a task. I noted that the institute became the complete arbiter of therapy, professional instruction, and acceptance into the profession, rendering the trainee a patient, a student, and a candidate. That structure could create an environment containing most or all of the eight characteristics of totalism I had described, from *milieu control* to the *dispensing of existence*.

I went on to question, from the standpoint of thought reform, three favorite concepts of psychoanalysis. The term *resistance*, for instance, is used very broadly to suggest inner opposition to therapy because of reluctance to make unconscious material conscious. Noting that thought reformers use the same word for whatever they viewed as insufficient embrace of their message, I asked whether what is called *resistance* to therapy might not be reasonable opposition to a therapist's ideas or approach.

Similarly, *transference*, or the patient's tendency to reexperience with the therapist earlier attitudes toward parents, when overused, could infantilize the patient and bestow a kind of omnipotence on the therapist; and the transference may extend to the entire psychoanalytic movement, just as a version of transference was expected by thought reformers to extend to the Communist Party and movement in general. Finally, the term *reality* is meant to suggest the "objective world," but such a judgment is bound to be highly subjective. As in the case of thought reformers (who could make a caricature of the term), the therapist's own ideological convictions (or those of the movement he or she was part of) could become basic criteria for "reality" and cure.

I realize now that I was extending my credo on totalism to my own relationship to my profession. I was also severing my connection with the psychoanalytic movement, and when I returned to the United States to assume the chair at Yale in the fall of 1962, after two and a half years in Japan, I made a decision not to continue with the training. By then I had immersed myself in work on Japanese youth and atomic bomb survivors, which had taken me still further from the psychoanalytic universe. I was now more clearly a researcher and had less need than ever to become a psychoanalyst.

From my present twenty-first-century standpoint, one has to wonder why it mattered so much whether I entered a psychoanalytic institute or left it. The psychoanalytic training scene is much more varied and eclectic now, and institutes have nothing like the power and even mystical aura they possessed in the past. My daughter Natasha was to train and thrive years later at the same institute I attended, and to encounter there a much more open environment than I had, including eclectic readings that questioned classical Freudian thought. But my own way of connecting and disconnecting with the institute had much to do with psychoanalysis as it was earlier, and with where my own intellectual life was heading. Yet I think it likely that my structural critique of the psychoanalytic institute could still have some relevance. Paradoxically, freeing myself from institutional Freudianism enabled me, not too much later, to experience Freud, as a man and as a thinker, much more fully.

Leitmotif

My thought reform study became a leitmotif for all of my work. Everything I've done since connects somehow with totalism and mind manipulation, and all too frequently with expressions of apocalypticism. This was of course my first study, and one never forgets the special impact of any first experience in a realm that matters, whether it's bound up with knowledge, threat, or love. All the more so when the experience initiates a way of working and living.

But there is also the reach of the subject's significance. There was no better window through which to view an unprecedented experiment in human manipulation on the part of a country constituting one-quarter of the world's population. Nor was there any process that could better reveal the power and danger of totalism, the threats to and possibilities for individual autonomy, and for mind-sets that better serve the human project. In my own experience I'm struck by the irony of how an encounter with a closed, manipulative process opened out my life.

Part Two

"Hiroshima Had Disappeared"

6

Getting to Hiroshima

The Thrilling Weapon

I can recall exactly where I was when I heard of Franklin Roosevelt's death in April 1945: riding on a subway train on Manhattan's East Side with a fellow medical student on our way to class. People in our train car talked excitedly to each other about it, pointing to screaming headlines in tabloid newspapers. I can remember feeling suddenly adrift and fearful at the loss of the only president I had ever known, a man who, during his thirteen-year reign, had come to represent for me more or less permanent leadership and guidance. But I do not remember where I was when I heard about the Hiroshima bombing.

What I do recall does not make me proud. I was pleased, even thrilled, that America possessed this powerful new weapon and had used it on a Japanese city, that it would bring about a quick victory and I would not have to go to war. I did not know what "atomic bomb" meant and viewed it as a vastly bigger version of the bombs we had been using, as "a kind of super-blockbuster," as one commentator put it.

My response was not unusual. It reflected a wartime mentality of blocking out the suffering and dying of "the enemy"—and in this case of the danger posed for the human future by a revolutionary new weapon. The most intense American expressions of joy came, not surprisingly, from troops who expected to be part of an invasion of Japan, whether already in the Pacific area or being readied for transfer to that area for the invasion. One of them later recalled: "We shot bullets into the air and danced between the tent rows, because this meant we were going to live, and not as cripples." And Norman Mailer, soon to be on his way to Japan, later told me that for three days he was "stunned and euphoric," that the weapon seemed "miraculous" in delivering him from what he thought of as an almost certain death. As he put it, "You couldn't say anything bad about the atomic bomb."

For soldiers, that attitude was understandable. But I was in no such danger, and there were a considerable number of Americans, including, I am sure, many nineteen-year-olds, who knew better. I sometimes think I've spent much of my life undoing that first unfeeling response.

My sentiments about the atomic bomb soon changed. I was troubled by radio and newspaper reports about a single bomb destroying a whole city, and then another, and disseminating poisonous radiation that threatened to kill just about everyone. There were sensitive voices that made clear that this was a completely new kind of destructive force, not to be understood as just another improved weapon. H. V. Kaltenborn, a leading radio voice, spoke of our own danger: "We must assume that with the passage of only a little time, an improved form of the new weapon we used today could be turned against us." Writers like Norman Cousins and Lewis Mumford, highly respected in my liberal circles, made clear that these new bombs could destroy all of human civilization and that building them was a form of madness. (I would get to know both men later on and was impressed by their commitment to opposing nuclear weapons until the end of their lives.) I found much less convincing the many American voices insisting that using the bomb was justified because of the Japanese surprise attack on Pearl Harbor and was even a humane act bringing about the end of the war.

Within weeks after Hiroshima and Nagasaki, I began to read about the warnings of scientists who had worked on the bomb. The names Leo Szilard and Eugene Rabinowitch became familiar to me, and when later in 1945 they and their colleagues created the *Bulletin of the Atomic Scientists*, a journal whose specific purpose was to articulate nuclear danger, I became an early reader and came to see the bomb as very bad and ominous. An antinuclear position seemed the only honorable one. In relation to nuclear weapons, I developed a Cold War stance of a plague on both your houses. When the Russians seized the initiative in advocating for disarmament, I could not quite take their rhetoric at face value. I attributed the failure of the 1946 Baruch plan for general nuclear disarmament and international control of atomic energy to intransigence on both sides, and was aware of America's desire to maintain nuclear dominance. I was horrified by the emergence of the hydrogen bomb in the late forties and early fifties, and then by the inquisition of Robert Oppenheimer in 1953 by the Atomic Energy Commission, which I understood to be punishment for opposing the new weapon.

Yet in all this I never made nuclear weapons a particular subject of study. Even in becoming a psychiatrist I did not stop to consider the extent to which the weapons affected human life in general, and our lives as Americans in particular. I knew that nuclear weapons were a dreadful new force in the world, but I had not thought much about their impact on the human psyche. I needed to find a way to open my imagination to the nature of this new force. This was when I met David Riesman at Harvard and began to think seriously about nuclear weapons.

The Antinuclear Circle

It is often assumed that scholars perform their work more or less neutrally—or "professionally"—and take on their moral advocacies as a result of what they discover. But I have come to an almost opposite view. What we choose to study as scholars is a reflection of our advocacies, our passions, spoken or otherwise. What we discover can intensify those advocacies, or perhaps in some cases diminish them, but it is not their source.

When I went to Japan in the first days of 1960 I had no intention of doing research in Hiroshima. I planned to conduct a two-year study of the interplay of psychology and history in Japanese youth, to be carried out in Tokyo and Kyoto, and that was pretty much what I did. But when I completed that study in early 1962, I decided that it would be a good idea to visit Hiroshima before returning to the United States and taking up my new position at Yale. The decision to go to that city was a fateful one for me, but it was by no means mere happenstance. For by then, mostly in the Riesman circle, I had been struggling imaginatively with nuclear weapons and their impact for almost five years.

Riesman was not only temperamentally and politically antinuclear but sociologically antinuclear as well. He spoke to me at length about ways in which the influence of the weapons penetrated our society and poisoned our institutions through the secrecy and paranoia they brought about, especially concerning draconian war projections in which hundreds of millions of people would be killed. I found myself thinking about their psychological impact upon strategists (You bomb New York, we bomb Moscow, then we stop); upon political leaders (We can use them but we can't use them); and upon ordinary people (It's terrible that the world will come to an end, but I've got to get to the office by nine).

It was not that Dave and I had discussed Hiroshima itself in any detail. From the standpoint of the late-fifties nuclear threat, Hiroshima and Nagasaki seemed already old hat, involving "tiny" weapons now dwarfed by their world-ending successors. Of course we were aware of the two atomic-bombed cities but we might well have shared the general resistance—even among antinuclear activists—to the details of what actually happened to people in them. Perhaps that is why I did not get to Hiroshima until ten years after first arriving in Japan and sixteen years after John Hersey's stunning rendering of the bomb in his influential volume, *Hiroshima*.

Dave and I talked about the absurdity of the shelter-building craze, as epitomized by what seemed at the time to be the society's major moral conundrum: "If during a nuclear crisis a neighbor should try to force his way into your shelter, where he would deprive your family members of needed oxygen, would you be justified in shooting him?" We thought that a society that focused on such a question was in deep trouble. Shelter building was always an important subject for us because we could connect it with collective denial, with aggressive weapons policies, and with American cultural attitudes having to do with fixing any problem and protecting one's family from the perils of the outside world.

I was inspired by Riesman's way of bringing critical intellectual thought to his passionate opposition to nuclear weapons. He became faculty advisor to an undergraduate antinuclear group known as Tocsin (perhaps the first American professor to work with such a group), and I remember his bringing me to a meeting of about twenty students and leading a lively discussion of many of the issues that he and I had been talking about.*

Our group called itself the Committee of Correspondence (after the coordinating committees of the American Revolution), and our newsletter expressed highly critical views of both American and Soviet attitudes toward the weapons in the Cold War. Dave wrote a good part of the newsletter during what was probably his most radical phase. But I can remember contributions from such people as H. Stuart Hughes, the Harvard professor of European history, who would run for Congress on a peace platform; I. F. Stone, whom I had met years before at the Harburgs; and Erich Fromm, the psychoanalyst who had been Riesman's therapist and became his close friend. Each of these people also contributed to my developing sense that one could think and live in ways that were against the grain.

I also became involved with the enterprise and wrote a couple of short psychological commentaries, one on shelter building, and the other on the fallacious assumptions of nuclear strategists. However modest, they were for me a way of bringing professional knowledge into the public debate on nuclear weapons. The Riesman circle did not create a political movement but was a pre-sixties moment of reasoned radicalism, centered on nuclear weapons and the Cold War, that had an indeterminate influence on American intellectual life and a very clear influence on my own.

It was quite natural for me to continue the dialogue from Japan. During my two years of work on Japanese youth in Tokyo and the culturally dazzling ancient capital, Kyoto (1960–62), Dave excerpted passages of my letters in the Committee of Correspondence newsletter, especially when concerned with nuclear weapons issues. I questioned the advocacy of some in our group for unilateral American disarmament because I thought that arrangements for mutual disarmament would be "more generally acceptable psychologically" to Americans, while at the same time expressing my concern about "the still important totalist elements in [Soviet] ideology." When Dave wrote to me of his anxiety concerning the Berlin crisis of 1961, I wrote back about the discomfort of many Japanese with the belligerence of both America and the Soviet Union,

---

*One of the undergraduates I met there was Todd Gitlin, who was to become a leading figure in the student rebellions of the sixties, and later a keen sociological observer of American society and a good friend.

and mentioned as representative a Japanese student's comment to me that "both sides should calm down." Through my correspondence with Dave from Japan I was trying to keep in touch with the rest of the world and its dangers, and especially with critical perspectives on those dangers.

In a letter of January 9, 1962, I enclosed an article titled "Reason, Rearmament, and Peace." It was written at the request of the editor of a small journal, *Asian Survey*, as a response to an earlier statement by a Japanese military spokesman advocating "rational rearmament" of his country and denigrating opposition to it as "sentimentalism." In the article I questioned his version of rationality and irrationality, emphasizing the unique historical importance of the Japanese peace movement, related as it was to Hiroshima and Nagasaki. At the same time I asked for evenhandedness in that peace movement, as opposed to its tendency at times to focus only on American, and not Soviet, belligerence. I had no idea then that this article, when translated into Japanese, was to serve as a valuable passport in the peace-minded Hiroshima community for the work I was to embark on there.

There was another event, an extremely painful one, that occurred at the time, which had to affect everything. My father telephoned me in Kyoto to tell me my mother had been hospitalized because of complications of her cancer of the uterine cervix, and her condition seemed to be worsening. She had undergone radical surgery more than a year before and had seemed to do well until this recurrence. I flew to New York but reached her after she had lost consciousness, just a day before she died. I had never seen either of my parents rendered so weak and helpless, and was experiencing my first profound loss. My father was shaken but was managing all right.

Soon after the funeral I flew back to BJ in Kyoto. I poured out memories of my mother: the sense of her unconditional love along with her fearfulness about actions or directions that were unfamiliar to her. She expected me to achieve much in life but was worried lest I do something too unconventional or risky. A friend once said to me that I followed my father's mind-set of taking plunges and expecting success, as opposed to my mother's holding back to prevent problems and disappointment. At the same time my mother's devotion did much to infuse me with sufficient strength to attempt the kind of projects she feared. She was also the bearer of culture in our family, read novels, and had a modest musical talent. I remember social gatherings at which, after a certain amount of persuasion from guests, she would sing such unhip songs as "Sylvia's Hair Is Like the Night." I had not seen much of her or my father during that period of living abroad. But I loved her dearly and felt lonely and a little empty after her death.

BJ and I went to Hiroshima two months later and I subsequently wondered how my mother's death might have affected my work there. It was not involved in our decision to visit the city; that had mainly to do with our prior immersion in nuclear weapons issues. But it could well have influenced my approach to Hiroshima survivors. My own experience of loss could have further sensitized me to the more extreme trauma and loss of those exposed to the atomic bomb.

The Five-Day Visit

BJ and I arrived in Hiroshima by train from Kyoto on April 2, 1962. On that early spring day, the city looked bright with lush foliage and sprightly new buildings everywhere (though we did not have to look far to find encampments of men and women, some with keloid scars, living in the streets). So much happened during that visit that in my memory it lasted ten days or two weeks, but my records make clear that it was just five days. During that time I was at a fever pitch, exploring everything I could, speaking to a wide variety of people from early morning into the evening hours. I did not see myself as embarking on a study but rather as immediately engaged by the city. People were for the most part eager to meet with me—not too many Americans had come to Hiroshima in search of every kind of detail concerning what had happened in that city.

I met with leaders of survivor groups, religious figures, doctors, university professors, and city officials, most of whom were themselves direct survivors of the bomb. I also spoke to Americans who lived in the city as missionaries or peace activists. I described it all in a very long letter I dictated to David Riesman a few days after returning to Kyoto. I seemed to want to tell him, but also record for myself, what I had observed and personally experienced in Hiroshima. Later I realized that the letter had another function: it enabled me to articulate my strong inclination to remain there and carry out a systematic research project. Eight years earlier in Hong Kong, I had to struggle hard to acknowledge to myself my great desire to stay in that city. This time, with Hiroshima, it was very different. I could quickly see myself staying and doing the work.

I associated the moment of my decision with the completion of an interview with a psychologist at Hiroshima University. After a few comments about the survivors, he spoke of their entering "a psychological-moral-historical sphere at the very center of mankind's dilemmas." What struck me most forcibly was that, seventeen years after such a tragic turning point in human history, no one had attempted a comprehensive psychological study of what had occurred in Hiroshima. There was official American research on physical aftereffects, mainly from radiation, but none that recorded systematically what went on in the minds of survivors, individually and collectively, throughout the city and beyond. I said that my experiences in Hong Kong and Japan, together with my moral concern, could serve me in studying and communicating something useful "about these ultimately unknowable and perhaps insoluble issues." What I considered unknowable and insoluble was the full human impact of those two bombs. I mentioned the difficulty I had finding language for what I saw and experienced in Hiroshima. And I said that BJ and I, after viewing the exhibits of the Atomic Bomb Museum, sat down in a nearby hotel lobby feeling "anxious and depressed," and "tried to grasp the meaning of what we had witnessed. We are still trying." I can say the same almost a half century later.

Dave wrote back that he and his wife, Evey, felt strongly that I was the appropriate person to go ahead with such a study. But I still needed the approval of Yale Medical School and specifically that of Fritz Redlich, head of the Department of Psychiatry. Our previous arrangements were that I would begin work in the department in the early spring of 1962, in connection with the research chair that I had been awarded. I was actually already occupying that chair, since we had arranged for me to be on salary from Yale for the last eight months or so for my work on Japanese youth. My memory has always been of a wonderful exchange of letters with Fritz, in which I told him of my strong desire to do a research study in Hiroshima, and by return mail he offered full support and inquired about my research needs. The memory is essentially accurate, except for one point. I made much less a request than a statement of what I intended to do. I wrote from Kyoto on April 17, ten days after returning from Hiroshima:

> We're now in the process of making a change in our plans, which I wanted to tell you about. I'm finishing up my interviews in Kyoto and Tokyo, but I've recently become interested in the situation in Hiroshima. During a recent brief trip down there, I discovered that no one has yet undertaken any psychological study of the effects of the atomic bomb, and decided I would do what will be at least some exploratory work on the subject. I'll be going there again shortly to make definite arrangements, but my present plan is to work in Hiroshima from early May through perhaps late August or September.

I went on to say a little more about how I would go about the study, about the work's larger significance, and about the uniqueness of my vantage point. Overall, I was very sanguine about Fritz's reaction, both because I knew him to be concerned about large human issues and also to be eager to connect his department with potential achievement. I mentioned the work's "moral as well as psychological dimensions" and its value for "the social psychiatric perspective we have so often discussed." Fritz responded quickly and warmly, and did everything to help me in the work. It is true that I made it a kind of fait accompli, but it was Fritz Redlich who enabled me to do that.

A Different Researcher

There was a parallel in converting an intense visit to Hiroshima into a research study with what I had done earlier in Hong Kong, a certain continuity for me as a psychiatrist eager to work on large events in the greater world. But I was now a different person. I was no longer that wet-behind-the-ears itinerant psychiatrist who had landed in Hong Kong a few months prior to his twenty-eighth birthday and had to make up in boldness what he lacked in experience. Arriving in Hiroshima just before turning thirty-six, I was a bit more seasoned. I had done two research studies, had written a book, and had a university appointment. While hardly without self-doubt, I now had a certain amount of inner confidence, and I knew that my academic standing could help my work in Hiroshima, whether with university teachers there, leaders of various groups, or ordinary survivors.

Most of all, I had a tested research method, which centered on individual interviews but included a mosaic of historical and cultural influences. I knew that I could apply it and emerge with a measure of insight into what I was studying—in this case, the effects of the atomic bomb. I did have a certain low-level anxiety, this time not about inexperience but about the problem itself. I realized that the atomic bomb ultimately defied my method or any other approach to studying it. A phenomenon that threatened to end the human race could hardly be fully grasped by even the most dedicated researcher. But I also believed that I could contribute to the general dialogue (often nondialogue) on precisely that phenomenon. Through my psychological interviews in particular, I was convinced that I could arrive at truths that could not be obtained by any other method.

There was a significant difference in the locales of my first two studies. Hong Kong in the mid-fifties was an anachronistic British colony in a Chinese cultural area whose main identity had to do with the interaction between China and the West. The people I interviewed did not really belong to the city but had come there as a place of refuge they planned or hoped to leave. Hiroshima, in contrast, had long existed as a medium-sized provincial capital, which would have been a highly stable place were it not for the bomb. An ancient "castle city," originally founded in 1589 on Japan's inland sea, Hiroshima has been in turn the capital of a major Japanese fief of the Terumoto clan, an early center of culture, and in the nineteenth and twentieth centuries a modest industrial metropolis. Its name literally translates as "broad island," suggesting the city's relationship to the sea and to the many branches of the Ota River that run through it.

Though focused on the darkness of the atomic bomb, I experienced Hiroshima as a compelling and attractive city. The upheavals after the war included an influx of former residents returning home from military or imperial service, and of outsiders from various parts of Japan who sought new opportunity in this depopulated place—some compared it to the "Wild West" in America. Although its identity became inseparable from the atomic bomb and there remained much chaos in people's lives, Hiroshima was still a well-defined metropolis with its specific historical continuity. Almost everyone I met was a permanent resident, and during my six months of living there I could feel more a part of a particular place than I did in eighteen months in Hong Kong.

In addition, I had become a father and thought more in family terms. Our son, Kenneth Jay (in Japanese diminutive *Ken-chan*), was born in Tokyo in 1961. We duly registered him as an American citizen at our embassy. He would later express regret at being ineligible to become president because of his birth abroad, but that in no way curbed his energies, apparent early, especially in relation to what was to become his talent for managing technology. BJ and I vividly remember celebrating his first birthday with a little gathering that included a few Hiroshima friends and members of the children's group, the Folded Crane Club, which BJ worked with. We were a family more or less anchored in a small house on the outskirts of a Japanese city, as opposed to the peripatetic couple BJ and I had been in our various domiciles in Hong Kong. From the time of Ken's birth, and four years later that of his sister Karen (who would come to be called Natasha), our children became an active force and a reminder of purpose in our work and our lives, an important part of our adventurous narrative.

While the British crown colony had been for me primarily a place to study thought reform, in Hiroshima I became connected to an urban community, however tangentially, and felt a certain responsibility toward its various social groups and their sensitivities. I had a clearer presence in the city than had been the case in Hong Kong and became something of a curiosity as word got around that this tall American scholar had come to Hiroshima to learn about people's experiences with the bomb.

I was also involved in a very different form of witness. In Hong Kong, though I had not used the word, I had been witness to a destructive form of mind manipulation, and sought to make my retelling accurate and demystifying. In Hiroshima my witness was specifically focused on the suffering of people exposed to a cruel weapon at the hands of my own countrymen, but I had to confront the weapon's broader threat to the human future. I was now ready to open my imagination to what had happened in that city.

7

The Visceral Immersion

M Y FIRST INTERVIEW was a harsh lesson in the difference between
gentlemanly discussions about the bomb and a visceral immersion into its full effects on specific human beings. I thought I had prepared myself for this interview by talking with many people about the bomb's overall impact. But I could not possibly be prepared for what I would hear.

The man I interviewed was a thirty-year-old shopkeeper's assistant who had been exposed to the bomb as a child of thirteen at 1,400 meters from the hypocenter (surface position directly beneath the center of the explosion), a location at which most people were killed. His story was one of grotesque deaths and self-lacerating survival. His mother saved him by helping him out of the debris, but she weakened and collapsed; after attempting to carry her, he had to abandon her because of the spreading flames and smoke, feeling that "if I stay, we both will die." He was to hear her calls for help ringing in his ears for the rest of his life. He soon learned that his father had been killed in the flames, and he observed first his grandmother and then his baby brother die before him after having experienced the dreaded "spots" (bleeding under the skin, an acute effect of radiation that frequently foreshadowed death). He described terrible scenes of confusion and mass dying; many people having the spots, or their hair falling out, and others simply becoming increasingly weak until they stopped breathing. He then lived the life of an orphan, shunted about to various temporary homes, always feeling profoundly lonely and looked down upon, and as an adult had difficulty holding a job or sustaining relationships. Over the years he had never been free of excruciating fear of delayed radiation effects and, observing so many others' deaths, thought, "Sooner or later I, too, will die."

After the interview I returned to the small Japanese inn where I was staying. I was alone, as BJ and our infant son Ken had not yet moved to Hiroshima. My way of coping with the interview's devastating effect on me was to dictate my impressions. I began as follows:

> May 14, 1962, 11:00 p.m. I am back at my inn, and I have just emerged from a hot relaxing bath, but I have by no means recovered from my first research interview in Hiroshima. The story that this young *hibakusha* told me was so grim and terrible that it seems less authentic drama than gruesome . . . melodrama—except that sitting across the table and hearing it told by the human being who experienced all those horrors rivets me to its reality.

In this less than fully coherent way I was trying to say that the sequence of victimization described to me was so sustained and unrelenting that it lacked the shifts, variations, and nuances we ordinarily associate with a personal narrative.

I also noted a paradox in my reaction:

> I had . . . sought out this reality: it is the subject of my research. But at the same time I felt myself so shocked by it that I wished to deny and reject it. I've often said that one of the troubles with people's attitude toward nuclear weapons is that they are simply unable to imagine the consequences of such weapons, but now I understand my own statement for the first time.

What I had come to hear I did not want to hear. I was not too different, after all, from everyone else.

I was intent on examining the various levels of my reactions:

A feeling of simple horror accompanied by considerable anxiety, causing me to, at times, hesitate and waver in directing the course of the interview and leaving me limp at the end of it; an analytic quest for understanding; . . . a sense of moral involvement—a feeling that I must do whatever I can, by means of this research or any other path, toward preventing the kind of thing that I was hearing described; and a sense of the great difficulty of doing justice to this material because of the extraordinary demands made upon one in every way; along with the feeling, both vague and pressing, that there must be a way of dealing with this subject to say something new about [its various] dimensions.

I was struggling, under duress, to hold on to my research function. My difficulty lay in the pain I experienced when translating survivors' words into mental images. During that first interview I "saw" him being pulled out of the debris by his mother and then leaving her to die after a failed effort to carry her out, saw his baby brother weakening and dying with his skin covered with spots, and saw around me an entire city dominated not only by death but by the most grotesque forms of dying. My imagination had to enter realms more extreme—more unacceptable—than any I had previously encountered.

After a few more similarly searing interviews with survivors, I found myself becoming anxious, uneasy, preoccupied with images of death, unable to sleep. I knew that the work was important and that the kind of interviews I was doing were the best way to get at people's experiences. But precisely those interviews were the problem, causing me to feel overwhelmed and vulnerable. I began to wonder whether I could really carry out the project.

Then, within just a few days, I found myself changing. Much of my anxiety lifted and I felt increasingly calm and able to focus more clearly on my interview protocol and on the psychological significance of what people were telling me. The change was a great relief for me—it became clear that I could continue the study. What I had experienced was an involuntary defense mechanism in reaction to trauma, which I came to call "psychic numbing" or diminished inclination or capacity to feel. In this case it was "selective professional numbing" of a kind necessary to anyone conducting this kind of project. It is something on the order of a surgeon who, even if compassionate, cannot afford to experience the emotions of a patient or family members when performing a delicate operation. I continued to be pained by what I heard but no longer immobilized. And I began to think a great deal about the balance between feeling and not feeling necessary to the work in Hiroshima, to my work in general, and to the work of anyone who deals with extreme suffering. Perhaps not surprisingly, I was to learn that survivors of any disaster were likely to struggle, much more formidably and over years, with that same balance.

I've often been told that I had shown great "courage" in carrying out such disturbing studies as the effects of the atomic bomb in Hiroshima and the behavior of Nazi doctors in the Holocaust. But I have a different view. I could stay and work in Hiroshima because I sensed that the study was right for me, for who I was; that I had arrived at an appropriate intersection of my evolving work with an important world event. I don't consider myself a particularly brave person in the face of threat, and I don't seek out dangerous situations requiring physical courage. But I had a strong commitment to the work in Hiroshima, and whatever the impediments and doubts, I did not want to abandon the effort.

My Method Evolves

Of course, there was something strange about an American coming to Hiroshima and asking people how they felt about the bomb his country had dropped. In my book I refer to my situation as Kafkaesque, but a more accurate statement would be that my work brought about a Kafkaesque situation for survivors and an uneasy association for me. Kafka's characters are exposed to dreamlike environments in which reality, though partly recognizable, is radically skewed in a menacing fashion. One is vaguely accused of a crime, or one finds oneself transformed into an insect—all in a setting that is both strange and partly familiar. For survivors I interviewed, the bomb created a death-dominated environment so extreme that many thought of it as supernatural, but it all took place in their familiar city, on its streets or in their workplace or home. Though they were mostly motivated to talk to me, an American coming to their city to ask them about their experience could suggest to them another layer of skewed reality. My problem was that, although opposition to the bomb was a strong aspect of my identity, I nonetheless had a shared nationality with the weapon. I could not—no American can—completely divest myself of all connection to those who had used the bomb in our collective name. What I felt was not mea culpa guilt but rather a more vague unease at having some kind of relationship to the menacing force I was studying. That unease was alleviated by the sense of collaborating with survivors in bringing out their stories.

The method I brought to Hiroshima—combining intense psychological interviews with a cultural and historical mosaic—had to evolve further in my work there in connection with its specific research environment. I retained my emphasis on dialogue, which meant exploring in detail the extreme experiences of survivors while being open to their questions to me about what I was doing in their city. I decided to interview two distinct groups of survivors (or *hibakusha*, as they were called). The first or "special group" consisted of those who had become public figures as prominent religious or political leaders or spokesmen for survivor groups; they could be highly articulate about not only their individual experience but shared tendencies in the city. My second group was chosen randomly (every five hundredth name) from a list of more than ninety thousand people kept by the Hiroshima University Research Institute for Nuclear Medicine and Biology. These were officially designated survivors because they had been within the city limits at the time of the bomb, had come into the city within fourteen days of the bombing and entered a designated area of about two thousand meters from the hypocenter, had been in physical contact with bomb victims through disposal of dead bodies, or had mothers who fit into any of the above categories and had been in utero at the time of the bomb. I wrote to Dave that I felt a bit strange in drawing upon a random sample in this way:

> I hope it does not sound too callous to think "scientifically" in this fashion about such a horrible event, the repetition of which threatens to wipe us all out; and there are times when I think it would

make more sense to just scream out in pain and tell the world the terrible things even a "little" bomb can do, rather than worry about such things as samples and balanced results. But I know that the work will have greatest validity and impact if I follow these precautions and [this] method, and they need not, of course, prevent me from eventually reporting my results in a human and readable fashion.

It turned out that the most profound psychological responses in the two groups were basically similar. But including them both enabled me to establish fundamental patterns in all Hiroshima survivors and to learn much about collective behavior among leaders and followers in groups that emerged after the bomb.

I was wisely advised by Shōji Watanabe, a social worker who assisted me, to pay a brief initial visit to the homes of people in the random group, most of whom would be in quite humble circumstances. This was a show of respect for them, especially coming from an American, and a way of easing their discomfort about being asked to meet with a psychiatrist or any figure of authority. I remember trudging through the streets of the city with Watanabe—a young man who lived out his religious principles by dedicating himself to the well-being of *hibakusha*—during the excruciatingly hot Hiroshima summer days, looking for the homes of people whose names we obtained from the list. Also with us was Kyōko Ishikure, my remarkable bilingual assistant throughout the Hiroshima work as well as the earlier research on Japanese youth. The task was complicated by the old Japanese method of numbering houses not according to where they were located but to when they were constructed. When we finally found a particular house, Watanabe would introduce me either to the survivor or a family member and I would explain in my limited Japanese that my purpose in doing the work was that of contributing to world peace by learning all I could about what people had experienced in connection with the bomb.

It was especially important to make that explanation because of the deeply ambivalent feelings of Hiroshima people toward American doctors who were studying the bomb's physical aftereffects as part of an official group carried over from the Occupation, the Atomic Bomb Casualty

Commission, or ABCC. The ABCC was an outgrowth of the Atomic Energy Commission, which funded it, and which was also responsible for the production and testing of nuclear weapons, a relationship well-known in Hiroshima. People submitted to examinations out of concern about their health, particularly about the possibility of radiation effects, but expressed considerable antagonism about being made into "guinea pigs" since the official policy of the ABCC was to provide no treatment. No wonder people suspected that American doctors were there for the purpose of preparing their own country for another nuclear war. And to make matters worse, most of the ABCC physicians came from Yale Medical School, where I had just received my appointment.

Distinguishing myself from the ABCC was helped by a translation of my article on the Japanese peace symbol, "Reason, Rearmament, and Peace" and its appearance, through the efforts of Hiroshima friends, in the widely distributed *Asahi* weekly. The word got around among both prominent and ordinary people in Hiroshima that I was a man concerned about the dangers of nuclear weapons. I could then come to be seen as resembling other American peace activists who had spent time in the city—people like Norman Cousins, Earle and Barbara Reynolds, and the missionary pacifist Mary McMillan—but differing from them in undertaking a detailed study of what had happened to people in Hiroshima.

I adopted a policy of tape-recording all interviews and having a bilingual transcript (with Romanized Japanese) prepared. But summaries I dictated soon after each of the interviews were just as important. They included impressions of the atmosphere of the interview and reflections on anything that seemed significant, surprising, or puzzling. These summaries became what I called my "Hiroshima research diary," which meant much to me even at the time because it provided the sequence of what I was learning and experiencing in Hiroshima. The summaries were my messages to myself on the state of the research and the researcher. As I pore through this research diary forty-five years later, I realize that it contains the essence of my encounter with Hiroshima and its people, much sadness and pain but also affectionate bonds in a common cause.

Early in the work I devised a simple protocol—a sequence of questions for each person I interviewed. I would first explain why I sought the meeting and the purpose of my work, then ask a few relatively neutral questions (date and place of birth, present job, education, etc.), and then ask about their experience with the bomb, which they knew to be the raison d'être for our meeting. I asked for great detail about place and conditions (indoor or outdoor), family involvement, others encountered, observations of all kinds, and subsequent struggles and fears. Then I went back to their pre-bomb experience and early lives in general, but usually returned to the atomic bomb and their added observations, altering the sequence according to the flow of each interview. In order to connect the interviews with the larger mosaic, I asked about Hiroshima's past and its post-bomb history, feelings toward America and other countries possessing nuclear weapons.

I tried to be aware of survivors' needs and avoid pressing them too far about such painful memories. But they were mostly eager to tell their stories in great detail; in this way, and in the encouragement and support I offered, the interviews could have a significant therapeutic component. I sought to have a minimum of two interviews with each person, as I found that there could be a rush of information and feeling in the second meeting about experiences that may have been mentioned more limitedly, or not at all, in the first. Through this overall approach my Hiroshima study became an exhaustive rendering of the human consequences of the bomb in that city. Rather than a statistical study removed from the human encounter, I was constructing something on the order of an experiential history of exposure to the atomic bomb.

By then I was more clear about the principles of my psychohistorical work, which still drew heavily upon Erikson but differed importantly from him in approach. I followed Erikson's model of immersing himself in the historical era he studied (as opposed to prior psychoanalytic tendencies to reduce history to individual psychopathology or collective manifestations of the Oedipus complex). But while Erikson focused on the interaction of the great man (or person) with prevailing historical currents (as in his studies of Luther and Gandhi), my own emphasis was on individual interviews with groups of people who had been significantly involved in a particular historical event. I was looking for common psychological responses, or what I called "shared themes." In the case of *hibakusha*, I knew that these shared themes could shed light on larger human struggles with nuclear weapons, with grasping what they are and what they do.

I realized that, in order to understand what people told me in the interviews, I had to explore Japanese cultural attitudes toward death: studies of Shinto funerals, folklore concerning the danger to the living of the newly dead (especially when they died through violence or other aberrant circumstances), the ancient "double grave system" (the body buried in one grave and the soul in another), and personal forms of Buddhist worship in which a family shrine (or *butsudan*) could enable one to converse with dead family members. I had to consider the history of the city of Hiroshima, especially its postwar experience of collective death and then partial rebirth in the dramatic appearance of cherry blossoms and other vegetation the following spring; and also the extremity of its depopulation by the bomb and repopulation largely from the outside.

And I explored with knowledgeable consultants the nuances of key Japanese words used by survivors. For instance, in describing how they coped with their ordeal, a number of survivors invoked the work *akirame*, usually translated as "resignation" and considered to represent a kind of passivity before the great forces of destiny. But survivors also associated the word with a form of active reassertion. They would sometimes quote the ancient Japanese (originally Chinese) saying "The state may collapse but the mountains and rivers remain," suggesting that the forces of nature, to which they were spiritually connected, would outlast the bomb's destructiveness. But I did not view *hibakusha* as representatives of an exotic culture so unique in its attributes as to be separate from all others. Rather I approached them as reflecting potentially universal responses that could be expressed only within the framework of their particular culture.

That universality of Japanese *hibakusha* responses was to be confirmed later by Americans exposed in various places to nuclear radiation: to plutonium waste at Hanford, Washington, in connection with the production of the Nagasaki bomb; to nuclear testing over decades at Rocky Flats, Colorado; and to ground zero at test sites in Nevada, through which GIs were marched shortly after nuclear explosions. In all of these cases, there were symptoms similar to those of Hiroshima survivors in connection with what I called the "invisible contamination" of delayed radiation effects.* In trying to explore all levels of behavior in Hiroshima, my immersion into the city's experience was as much that of an anthropologist as a psychiatrist.

I remember only one survivor who refused to see me because I was an American. Another said that she could not let an American enter her home but did come to see me at my office. But I had the impression that others were drawn to see me precisely *because* I was an American. There was a certain appeal to telling one's story to someone from the country responsible for the event, especially when the survivor had the impression that the American listener was sympathetic. We were transmuting the potential anger of Hiroshima survivors and the potential guilt of an American investigator into a shared effort at exposing and combating the destructiveness of the atomic bomb. The new bond replaced the Kafkaesque discomfort on both sides.

Beyond my being an American, there were currents of mistrust directed in general at people who got involved with Hiroshima, whether as leaders or observers of any kind. One survivor asked me whether in my work I was, like so many others, "selling the bomb." The phrase was widely used in Hiroshima to express suspicion that people (whether outsiders or survivors themselves) were making use of their city's tragedy for their own personal benefit, financial or otherwise. Another survivor asked me, "Do you, Dr. Lifton, feel that your heart is completely pure and beautiful?"— a question I could hardly answer in a simple affirmative. Those suspicious queries reflected the sense that the bomb had been so destructive in the suffering it caused that responses to it had to meet absolute—that is, impossible—standards of purity.

I took these questions seriously about my own relationship to Hiro-

---

*More generally, whether studying events involving Chinese, Japanese, German, or American culture, my inclination has been to connect experiences with the broader human psychological (or psychobiological) potential—with "human nature"—rather than to isolate them as culturally unique. I came to understand all collective human behavior as containing three interwoven components: the universal potential just mentioned; the cultural shaping, over many centuries, of that potential; and recent historical forces, which often challenged those cultural forms.

shima, and came to recognize that for all people involved with the city there were at least two levels of motivation: passionate dedication to the issue itself, including deep sympathy for survivors; and elements of self-interest having to do with personal achievement, recognition, and career. I came to accept this combination of motives in myself but the image of "selling the bomb" or "selling Hiroshima" stayed with me, and influenced my behavior when my book *Death in Life* received a monetary award.

From the beginning survivors spoke of their experience as "beyond words" or "impossible to describe." That sense is not limited to actual survivors—I had it as well—or for that matter to Hiroshima. But in that city I learned quickly how inadequate words are for our profound feelings—for what moves, threatens, or satisfies us most deeply—the principle of the inchoate nature of our most primal forms of experience. For people in Hiroshima there was the added element of an unprecedented dimension of death and suffering, a dimension for which the mind had no reference point. That is why John Hersey's 1946 book *Hiroshima* was criticized, however unfairly, by reviewers such as Mary McCarthy and Dwight Macdonald, for describing the struggles of individual people in ways that failed to convey the revolutionary nature of the new weapon. I tried to confront this problem by placing the words of survivors (which were the most authoritative descriptions) at the center of the work. I could then supplement the words and shared themes of survivors with a larger mosaic that included: the messages of leaders who emerged from among the survivors and people closely associated with them; the responses in literature, art, and film; and then a general psychological comparison of survivors of Hiroshima with those of Nazi death camps. This mosaic did not eliminate the problem of inchoateness—nothing could—but it did contribute to a more encompassing narrative that gave strong articulation to what survivors said and felt.

One Plane, One Bomb, One City

The words of some survivors had a particularly profound influence on my own relationship to nuclear weapons. I have especially in mind a man, in his early sixties when I interviewed him, who was, appropriately enough, a professor of history. He brought extraordinary intensity to the three interviews we had in August 1962, "as though the experience had taken place yesterday," as I noted at the time.

He described his approach to the bomb as that of an accurate historian, or what I would call a visceral historian. That is, he wished to record everything that took place "without pity" so that people would "know about it, not only with their minds but [would] feel it with their skin." His testimony was highly unusual in going back and forth between the painfully personal and the shockingly panoramic. The personal account included his wife's grotesque death from acute radiation effects and his self-condemnation because he was unable to feel any emotion when she died and because "I did not give her all the care I should have."

His panoramic observation had to do with nothing less than a city vanishing:

> I climbed Hijiyama hill [at the outskirts of the city] and looked down. I saw that Hiroshima had disappeared. . . . Of course, I saw many dreadful scenes after that—but that experience, looking down and finding nothing left of Hiroshima—was so shocking that I simply can't express what I felt. I could see Koi [a suburb at the opposite end of the city] and a few buildings standing . . . but Hiroshima didn't exist—that was mainly what I saw—Hiroshima just didn't exist.

His mind had great difficulty taking in what he observed: "I couldn't imagine a bomb which destroyed the whole city." And in listening to him, my mind struggled as well with what he told me. The image I formed was one of vast emptiness—of a large area with nothing in it but vague and desolate remains. That image connected what he was saying with pictures I had seen of Hiroshima made soon after the bomb. But as his description proceeded, my image included, at least fleetingly, the city that had been there prior to the emptiness, and in that way became a before-and-after image of a disappeared world. I was struggling to witness his witness, to respond to his declaration that "all of Hiroshima was destroyed by this one small bomb and this should be made known to the world."

He remained preoccupied with massive disappearance, nonexistence, nullity. He was convinced that the only way to commemorate the bomb was to clean out the area of the precise hypocenter so that it was "devoid of anything at all," and in that way could convey the message that "such a weapon has the power to make everything into nothing." He connected that perspective with the Old Testament story of Noah's ark, which for him, he said, was "more than a myth [because] except for a few humans and animals, it is a story of everything becoming nothing." And he also imagined a more contemporary narrative in which groups on earth continued to drop their atomic bombs on each other until threatened by creatures from other planets, and only then would they find a way to live in harmony with each other and protect themselves from this external danger. He was struggling to connect his experience of world destruction with an apocalyptic narrative in which a virtuous remnant would bring about resolution and renewal.

Only later did I recognize how much I have been influenced by this historian's sensibility of nuclear nothingness. In my writings and talks I would acknowledge that, while more people were killed in Tokyo during a single night of saturation bombing than by the atomic bomb in Hiroshima, "In Hiroshima it was one plane, one bomb, one city!" I began to talk about "imagery of extinction," of exterminating ourselves as a species with our own technology. I came to see such imagery as potentially present in everyone, derived as it was from the experiences of Hiroshima and Nagasaki. I knew that atomic bombs, however powerful, were finite in their impact, as compared to hydrogen bombs, which were capable of literally infinite annihilation. But my own imagery of world destruction derived nonetheless from my exposure to Hiroshima, and most particularly from the historian's message.

Over time in the antinuclear movement some of us raised objections to the concept of "nuclear war" and favored instead the term "nuclear end." We were rejecting the apocalyptic promise of renewal, saying that nuclear weapons were only half apocalyptic: the destroyed world might have no chance of reconstituting itself. Much discourse on nuclear weapons misleadingly invokes that apocalyptic renewal, in keeping with the human craving for a vision of continuing life after the deluge. But the idea of a nuclear end could be more widely recognized when physicists began to project the possibility of a "nuclear winter"—the blocking of the sun's rays by explosions of sufficient megatonnage to produce all-enveloping debris, and the lowering of the earth's temperature to an extent that plant, animal, and human life could no longer be sustained.

Hiroshima could be rebuilt, impressively so, because even after the bomb there were still people with some energy within it, and there was an outside world with much greater energy to participate in the rebuilding—neither of which would be true after a large-scale, hydrogen bomb holocaust. Yet Hiroshima—and especially the passionately visceral historian—provided me with images that convey our terrible nuclear truths: apocalypse without renewal, nuclear end, nuclear extinction. One plane, one bomb, one city.

Spiritual Annihilation

Among the most difficult words for me to grasp in Hiroshima were those of a few *hibakusha* who said that the emperor's surrender speech of August 15 was even more devastating to them than the bomb itself. How could that be? What could be more devastating than the horrors of the atomic bomb experience?

One example was a physicist at the university. He told me how, at the time of the bomb, "My body seemed all black, everything seemed dark, dark all over . . . then I thought, 'The world is ending'"; how he walked through the city looking for bodies of relatives and encountered huge numbers of corpses; and how his mind became insensitive to everything around him (like a "saturated" or overexposed photographic plate). Yet he could still mobilize energies in providing some help to others. His response to the emperor's surrender speech, however, was a trauma of a different order, especially for one who had been an unquestioning Japanese patriot and had lent his scientific knowledge to the military:

I felt the entire structure of my life crumble. I decided to quit the university. . . . This collapse of the foundation of my life was much more a psychological sentiment than anything else. . . . A loss of a sense of meaning in my life . . . a very personal feeling, a loss of a sense of anything I could rely on . . . a kind of despair.

An elderly widow described similar feelings in more simple terms:

Hearing his words . . . I didn't think about the war itself. . . . [W]hat
I understood well was that we were defeated. . . . I listened in tears.
It is impossible for me to put into words how painful it was. . . . I felt
terribly sorry for the Emperor . . . and this feeling remains with me
even now when I imagine how he felt then. . . . The A-bomb—we
didn't understand anything about it at the time . . . so I think the
Emperor's words were harder to bear.

And a prominent writer, who at the time of the bomb experienced a
sense of "the collapse of the earth which it was said would take place at
the end of the world," responded even more strongly to the emperor's
speech with a sense of "an indescribable emptiness . . . which almost made
me dizzy . . . as though I were in a mist where there were no other people
and my legs trembled. My body was so shaky I found it difficult to walk."
Others spoke of despondency and emptiness, or "state of collapse" or
"vacuum state." Of course what they had gone through at the time of the
bomb and the subsequent nine days contributed greatly to their reaction
to the emperor's speech. Yet that reaction was so extreme that for many it
seemed almost to eclipse the atomic bomb.

I knew at the time that the emperor had been a god figure, as politically
exploited by the leaders of the Meiji Restoration of the late nineteenth
century who had crafted a national religion from an ancient mythology.
I learned later (mostly from the work of the historian Carol Gluck) that
this construction of emperor worship had been a way of containing what
was called the "thunderboltism" of explosive pressures toward overturning the feudal system and bringing about radical social change. In that
way the Japanese expressed a version of political genius by resorting to
a sacred imperial restoration to achieve—and manage—the social revolution that created their modern state. The Meiji leaders could do this
by strengthening the symbol of the emperor in representing old cultural
patterns while they systematically imported principles from the West of
governance, education, and industry. But there was a cost: an aggressive
emperor-centered ideology was to have much to do with Japan's role in
World War II.

The novelist Kenzaburo Oe, in his 1994 Nobel Prize acceptance speech, described in the Japanese psyche a long-standing "split between two opposite poles of ambiguity"—ambiguity toward Western-inspired modernization and equal ambiguity toward traditional cultural forces focusing on the emperor. But by the time of World War II, emperor-centered ideology had become antithetical to evolving social realities, what I've called an ideology at the end of its tether, which inspired extreme behavior to negate perceptions of its anachronistic nature.

The emperor who spoke on the radio to the people of Hiroshima was a godly guru who was never previously viewed or heard by ordinary citizens. In that sense, World War II was a holy war in which one fought and killed, not for oneself but for the emperor, and each soldier was both a vassal and a "baby" of that deity. The country became a vast emperor cult embarked on a sacred venture in which defeat was not imaginable. To be sure, many Japanese had doubts about the emperor's claim on their person, and doubts about the possibility of victory in a hopelessly devastating war. But the *hibakusha* responses I quoted suggest the extent to which ordinary provincial citizens could still be immersed in that blindly totalistic worldview.

In reflecting further on people experiencing a sudden annihilation of the ideological and psychological structure of their existence, I wondered whether there were biblical equivalents and consulted my theologian friend Harvey Cox. He immediately referred me to the book of Lamentations in the Old Testament, whose first lines describe the pain of the destruction of Jerusalem and the deaths within that city:

> *How solitary lies the city,*
> *   so full of people!*
> *Once great among nations, now become a widow;*
> *Once queen among provinces, now put to forced labour!*
> *   Bitterly she weeps in the night,*
> *   Tears run down her cheeks. . . .*

Then later lines refer with seemingly greater horror to the destruction of the city's spiritual existence, as brought about by God's intervention:

He stripped his tabernacle as a vine is stripped,
And made the place of assembly a ruin.
In Zion the lord blotted out all memory,
    Of festal assembly and of Sabbaths;
King and priest alike he scorned.
In the grimness of his anger.
The Lord spurned his own altar
And laid a curse upon his sanctuary.

Both Hiroshima responses and biblical writings suggest that the destruction of one's physical world and the death of most people in it become inseparable from the annihilation of one's spiritual or symbolic universe. But for the human mind, functioning as it does on symbolization, spiritual annihilation is the ultimate assault.

The Nail in the Sneaker

Children loom large in my Hiroshima experience. *Hibakusha* conveyed to me intense images of helpless children, very young ones, badly burned, crying for their mothers, left to die because nobody was able to help them. Many schoolchildren were instantly killed or severely injured close to the hypocenter, where, on the morning of the bomb, large groups of them had been assigned to labor, either in factories or in building fire lanes, in preparation for anticipated "conventional" bombing. I heard many stories of parents searching desperately throughout the city for their missing children.

One of my most anguished interviews took place with a balding sixty-year-old man who spoke with unrelieved pain about the death of his twelve-year-old son. The boy was killed while working near the hypocenter, his body never found. The way the father told the story was that he had returned late from a business trip and had slept very little the previous night. So when his son, before leaving the house, asked him to remove a nail from his sneaker, the tired father placed a piece of leather above the tip of the nail and promised he would take out the whole nail when the boy returned later that afternoon. He went on to describe his futile search for the boy through the city, during which he encountered many dead and dying boys about his son's age. The father was left with a lifelong self-accusation that the nail he had failed to remove slowed the boy's attempted escape from the flames and caused his death.

Actually it is unlikely that the nail had anything to do with the boy's death. The father felt the need to reconstruct the story in that self-accusatory way because of parents' profound sense of responsibility, psychological and even biological, for the safety of their children; their surviving their child's death can be experienced as an unbearable generational reversal. I thought of the endless examples of such generational reversal caused by the bomb, of the breakdown of the ordinary relationship between age and death.

This father went on to declare, "No matter what wonderful things America has done for us, I will feel resentment toward America until the moment I die." As he spoke, I felt partly accused and at the same time enveloped by his angry grief, unresolved after seventeen years. I also contrasted what I was hearing with my own privileged family status, as just ten days before BJ and I had held our little party for our son's first birthday.

Large disasters, especially those that are clearly man-made, are most powerfully represented by the killing of children. Hiroshima had its own Anne Frank, a girl named Sadako Sasaki, who died at the age of twelve. Anne Frank, who left a poignant diary of her life in hiding, was killed by the Nazis in Bergen-Belsen (she actually died of typhus) at age sixteen because she was a Jew. Sadako Sasaki was exposed to the atomic bomb at the age of two, just 1,600 meters from the hypocenter, simply because her family lived near the center of Hiroshima, where the bomb was dropped. It was highly unusual, almost miraculous, to have survived seemingly unscathed so close to the hypocenter. And for the next ten years Sadako developed into an apparently healthy, vigorous, and athletic girl—until stricken with leukemia resulting from delayed radiation effects. Then her very real history entered into legend: Sadako was said to have struggled to maintain her life by folding paper cranes in origami fashion, in accordance with a Japanese folk belief that, since the crane lives a thousand years, folding a thousand paper cranes can cure one of illness. According to the most popular version of the evolving legend, she died still thirty-six short of that number, and her classmates then added the missing paper cranes so that a full thousand could be placed in her coffin. In any case, a national campaign was initiated for the construction of a monument to Sadako and all other children killed by the atomic bomb. Financial contributions, along with paper cranes, were received from all over Japan, and the monument now stands near the center of Hiroshima's peace park.

To be sure, both Anne's and Sadako's stories have often been senti-mentalized. Anne was not just a sweet teenager who believed that despite everything people were good; she experienced resentments and frictions having to do with the privations of hiding and with her aspiration to be a writer. Sadako too undoubtedly had her complexities and struggles beyond the different versions of her legend. Anne died in a camp where the Nazis killed Jews and others, Sadako in a hospital from leukemia caused by the atomic bomb. Both Anne and Sadako have been important to me because, like many others, I could feel in each an expression of the larger evil of the event, however different the experience of the two chil-dren. Certainly in Hiroshima the later increase in leukemia in children and adults came to symbolize the bomb's endless "invisible contamina-tion." In that sense Sadako's story represents A-bomb victims in general but, like Anne's, it particularly invokes the annihilation of the smallest and the weakest human beings, of those we adults are supposed to protect both out of love and our commitment to the flow of generations so cen-tral to our sense of the future.

BJ did much to enhance my sensitivity to Sadako and to the vulner-ability of children in general. Professionally and personally preoccupied with children, she wrote a good deal of children's fiction, as well as books about the fate of children in both Hiroshima and Vietnam, and later a biography of Janusz Korczak, a Holocaust martyr who went to his death in Treblinka seeking to protect the children in the orphanage he ran in Warsaw. BJ told Sadako's story in *Return to Hiroshima*, the book she did with the prominent Japanese photographer Eikoh Hosoe. She also became involved with the group that formed around that story, Orizuru No Kai, or the Folded Crane Club. The group of children was led by an extraordinary adult, Ichiro Kawamoto, a day laborer (meaning one who worked irregularly at menial jobs) I called a "zealot-saint," who immersed himself fiercely into antinuclear activities of every kind. The children's group visited hospitals to help, and sometimes serve as family for, A-bomb patients; assisted with peace movement activities and greeted international visitors to Hiroshima with leis of folded paper cranes; and corresponded with children all over the world about the atomic bomb.

The zealot-saint had himself been orphaned at the age of twelve and paid special attention to children who had lost parents to the A-bomb. Seventeen years old at the time of the bomb, he had been working in a factory outside Hiroshima and joined a rescue team that entered the city in a truck almost immediately. His image of ultimate horror was that of a policeman attempting to force open the mouth of a three-year-old boy to feed him a biscuit, explaining that the boy, crying for food, had been clinging to his dead mother, who now lay covered in blood beside him—a scene that had become so indelible to the zealot-saint that he choked up with sobs when telling me about it seventeen years later. It was his idea to build a monument to Sadako Sasaki and he did more than anyone else to bring it about. He made passionate pleas to officials, media representatives, peace groups, and parents; mobilized children to help him; and managed to mount a haphazard but ultimately effective national campaign. Along the way he embraced Protestant Christianity and aimed at developing traits resembling those of Gandhi and Jesus. BJ befriended him and his wife, and when we went to visit their very humble shack, their way of entertaining us was to show us pictures of A-bomb orphans and letters written to members of his group from various parts of the world. He was never easy to be with and never still, always making demands on others to join him in helping those who were suffering most. I came to see him as a man with a near-fanatical mission to combat the bomb's evil.

In earlier years he had tried to help the homeless orphans who wandered about the city and frequently congregated around the old Hiroshima station, where they formed a nucleus for black-market activities and every variety of antisocial behavior. Known as *furō-ji*, or homeless waifs, they conveyed a sense of the total breakdown of society. The zealot-saint himself, of course, qualified for the status of the homeless waifs he assisted. Those orphans were no longer around when I did my study, but all that I read and heard about them created a strong picture in my mind. I still imagine them congregating around the old Hiroshima station as lost children whose very existence was a condemnation of the adult world that had made them into what they were.

With that image I think of Ivan Karamazov's lyrical insistence that he can accept no creator or creation that permits the suffering of children. At the heart of our sense of human morality is our relationship to such suffering, what we do to bring it about or alleviate it. My sense of the ultimate moral transgression of the atomic bomb is bound up with its massively random killing, maiming, and orphaning of children. That is what the story of the nail in the sneaker is really about.

"Can You Stop It by Sitting?"

In Hiroshima I also learned something about protest. I was intrigued by one survivor, an elderly professor of philosophy and longtime antinuclear activist, Ichiro Moritaki, who became well-known in the city for his practice of sitting zazen-style in front of the atomic bomb cenotaph (the official monument placed at what is believed to be ground zero) whenever nuclear testing took place. Unlike some other prominent antinuclear leaders, his confrontation of nuclear danger made no distinction between the testing of Russia, China, or the United States. He would sit, alone or with others who joined him, when anyone tested the weapons anywhere.

He aroused certain conflicts in me about my own public behavior in Hiroshima. I admired what he was doing and would have liked to join him in his sitting protest, but I was strongly advised by my Hiroshima friends not to do so. They pointed out that although the philosopher-activist was generally well thought of, he had critics and political enemies who questioned both his motivations and his method; and that if I wished to have access to everybody in the city, I needed to refrain from such public activism. So I combined my open antinuclear advocacy with public restraint and continued to admire the philosopher-activist from a distance.

When I interviewed him toward the latter part of my time in Hiroshima, I found him to be a vigorous man in his late sixties, tall and trim, with a prominent shock of white hair, and a gentle—I called it "soft"—manner. He was ramrod straight, whether sitting or standing, and I noted him to be "clearly a man of the old school." In fact, he was so much of the old school that during World War II, he had been a professor of philosophy and ethics and taught his students "love of nation" and "dedication to victory." In other words, he played an active part in promulgating the emperor-centered right-wing militarism of the time. After the war, he brought similar ethical passion to "atoning for my mistakes" and, in fact, understood all of his work for peace as part of that atonement.

I had heard much about the superficial conversions of Japanese intellectuals from right-wing convictions to Marxism or some other ideology of the left, but there was nothing superficial about this philosopher-activist. His change was anchored in his bodily experience with the bomb. He had been severely injured and lost completely the sight in one eye. After months of recuperation, he began to devote himself to aiding young children orphaned by the bomb and helped to form an organization for that purpose. Those young children were for him the heart of the matter. Moved by their suffering, he explained: "Just talking with one girl—with her alone—you feel that we should stop the bomb."

Only later, when working with antiwar Vietnam veterans, did I develop a term for this kind of emotional pattern. I called it "animating guilt" or "an animating relationship to guilt." By that I meant a transformation of feelings of self-condemnation into a sense of responsibility toward combating the destructive forces one had been part of. In his case, those forces included the Japanese militarism he had supported and the atomic bomb that he had miraculously survived; he was left with feelings of guilt toward victims of both Japanese militarism and the atomic bomb. The idea of atonement, he emphasized, "gives me power." He described his sequence from the purely humane to the larger antinuclear terrain in this way: "My intention [at first] was simply trying to help A-bomb orphans, but by helping them I found myself in the midst of the A-bomb problem." Over the years, he became involved with every form of protest—leadership of antinuclear groups, mass meetings, marches, petitions, and manifestos—before settling on his approach of zazen sitting before the cenotaph with a Buddhist rosary in his hand. He told me that it seemed natural for him to do so, as he had been practicing Zen since his student days. He found that there was "something special about sitting in front of this cenotaph" because he did so "on behalf of the dead, 200,000 people."

On one occasion, while in the midst of his zazen protest, a little girl asked him, "Can you stop it by sitting?"—a question he never ceased to ponder. He found the beginning of an answer when an American reporter called him a "human reactor," and he extended that idea to a principle he carefully wrote out for me in English: "Chain reaction of spiritual atoms must defeat chain reaction of material atoms." This idea suggested a Japanese, and broadly East Asian, cultural principle of "spirit over matter," but his protest also had a pragmatic component. If not quite initiating a "chain reaction," that protest had reverberations in Hiroshima and beyond.

He mentioned a conversation he had with Bertrand Russell at an antinuclear conference in England. Russell asked whether he had any hate or resentment toward the United States and he answered that his primary feeling was "preventing it from happening again." He said that Russell seemed skeptical of such a "lofty sentiment," but he himself considered it "just a frank answer." He had indeed channeled most of his bomb-related emotions, including anger, into his antinuclear passion.

But the philosopher also expressed strong doubts to me about what he was doing—about the way he sat (in a disciplined zazen position rather than a more casual one), and more broadly about whether his form of protest was effective or whether it simply isolated him from others. Without abandoning his quest, he was insisting upon his own fallibility. He even asked my opinion about his and others' forms of protest: "Is it possible for someone like you, who comes to Hiroshima from the outside and lives here for five months to make any suggestion about how we should proceed?" I told him I could offer little advice since he understood the Hiroshima situation much better than I did. I thought at the time he was just being polite in asking the question, but he might also have been trying to engage me in Hiroshima activism and could possibly have been seeking connection with American antinuclear groups. My reticence stemmed from both a sense of humility toward him and my policy of keeping a low activist profile in Hiroshima. As appropriate as that policy might have been for my work, it made me feel uncomfortable, even guilty, because it prevented me from sharing protest actions with a man I respected.

But we did become friends. And on later visits to Hiroshima, when my research was behind me and I had become more of a peace activist, we could discuss our various strategies, hopes, successes, and failures. An opportunity for my own "atonement," if I can use his word, came in 1975 when I returned to the city for work on a film based on my book. By that time he had become an icon in Hiroshima, and deservedly so, as he still sat before the cenotaph whenever any nation tested nuclear weapons. One day I was told that he was sitting in protest and decided to go to see him at the cenotaph. Without much thought or hesitation, I sat down beside him. While I could do no better than an ordinary sitting position with no resemblance to zazen, we greeted each other warmly and shared a sense of antinuclear communion. A photographer was there covering his vigil, and his photograph of the two of us sitting together was published in the local newspaper. This time I was glad to be quite visible in Hiroshima, at least in that way.

The philosopher-activist had more things to tell me about the demands of protest. Early in our first talk he said to me: "The more you look into the A-bomb problem, the more you realize how much you don't know about it. I've experienced the bomb myself—and formed an organization—and still the problem becomes for me deeper." He was confirming, with the considerable authority he could command, the unmanageable reverberations of that first atomic bomb. But he also expressed an important principle he had learned, that of radically extending the community one served. He recalled his prior focus on "family, clan, and nation," declaring that the atomic bomb changed all that, requiring a "conception of mankind as some kind of community sharing the same destiny . . . the same community of life and death." To be sure, many people were saying similar things, and the principle of the human community had been important to my own work from its beginnings. But that emphasis, coming from this particular man, undoubtedly influenced my subsequent nuclear-related concepts of what I called "species consciousness" (awareness of protecting the human species) and "species self" (a self-concept inseparable from all other human selves in sharing with them the ultimate questions of life and death). I have met no one who has better lived out a sequence from a destructive self-enclosed community to a life-enhancing universal one.

He taught me something else, although I did not learn it all at once. It had to do with the principle of persistence and the need for many-sided approaches to protest action. In *Death in Life*, I praised his way of sitting silently in zazen position as "bringing to *hibakusha* expression a combination of silence, sense of mission, and obeisance to the dead." But I added that it was also "isolated, slightly anachronistic, and of little effect." I now disagree with that evaluation. The protest did connect with people, was historically appropriate, and had an impact that was not fully knowable but surely significant. This retrospective judgment is consistent with a principle that has become something of a mantra for me, especially in connection with protest: "Everything counts." And, I would add, nothing counts more than staying power.

8

Entrapment by the Bomb

I DISCOVERED QUICKLY THAT the atomic bomb could not only destroy bodies and cities but also have an all-enveloping impact on the mind. Anyone involved with the bomb could become entrapped by it, especially survivors but also people who sought to engage it in their imaginations.

Survivors were entrapped by their lifelong fear of radiation effects, even if, over time and with reassurances from Japanese and American doctors, this fear tended to diminish. But associated with radiation fear was a sense of taint, of being inwardly poisoned to the extent of carrying "bad genes" that could be lethal to the next generation. For such a taint to envelop much of the population of two entire cities is a remarkable phenomenon. It is partly reminiscent of the experience of Jews and mental patients in being ideologically designated by the Nazis as carriers of bad genes and therefore subject to coercive sterilization, castration, and mass murder. The taint experienced by *hibakusha* was imposed on them not by an ideology but by the characteristics of a revolutionary weapon. In that sense one can say that at a particular moment in time the inhabitants of Hiroshima and Nagasaki were turned into functional Jews. Nobody was going to forcibly sterilize, castrate, or kill them, but they could be seen by others and by themselves as biologically inferior and dangerous.

I heard of *hibakusha* who voluntarily had themselves sterilized, especially in situations where both marital partners were thought to have been exposed to significant amounts of radiation. One prominent politician, himself a survivor, went so far as to tell me, "We should set *hibakusha* aside and not mix them with the rest of the population." However unusual such an advocacy, it expressed a sense of *hibakusha* as a population with a terrible stigma that had been imposed from the outside. Hence when they speak of themselves as "guinea pigs," they refer not only to being subjected to medical research without treatment but, more fundamentally, to having had the world's first nuclear weapon and its imposed stigma "tried out" on them.

Yet survivors could also retain a sense of special knowledge. One man I interviewed kept telling me, "I know things that others don't know," referring to the overall horror of the experience but perhaps particularly to a sense of world destruction. That special knowledge could lead to expressions of survivor wisdom in opposing the bomb, as in the case of the philosopher-activist and many others. But it could also, more rarely, take on its own form of entrapment by becoming part of a little-talked-about underground theme in Hiroshima: that of the *wish* for world destruction. A hospital worker declared to me: "I feel that I had very bad luck in having experienced the bomb. And sometimes when I am particularly upset, I feel that the whole world should be blown up." Another survivor described how she and others who had lost their families sometimes "cursed the whole world" and would say "I hope A-bombs will be dropped again and that the whole world will suffer the same way I'm suffering now." These tended to be temporary images of revenge, in which the amorphous "enemy" becomes the whole world.

Such a self-enclosed or "hermetic apocalypse" (lacking even the promise of world renewal) was an expression of total entrapment by the bomb. It was not only omnicidal but included a kind of cosmic suicide as well. I had the impression that survivors could best extricate themselves from this and other forms of entrapment by some means of asserting vitality, whether through family life and children, occupational success, or taking part in activities or movements combating nuclear weapons. But remnants of imagined hermetic apocalypse undoubtedly remain.

A different kind of entrapment can be found in political leaders and nuclear strategists who have advocated use of the weapon, creating policies inseparable from nuclear madness. That is what Stanley Kubrick told us in his classic film, *Dr. Strangelove or: How I Learned to Stop Worrying and Love the Bomb,* in which a technical accident launches an American bomber squadron bent on dropping nuclear weapons on Soviet targets, which would in turn activate a "Doomsday Machine" and destroy all life on earth. The film ends in an orgiastic mushroom-cloud apocalypse, revealing with ferociously zany gallows humor what is at stake in the nuclear entrapment that encompasses us all.

Immersing myself as I have in descriptions of death and pain by Hiroshima survivors, and then in the whole landscape of nuclear threat, I have frequently felt my own form of entrapment by the weapons and by their threatened world destruction. I have tried to extricate myself from that entrapment by finding openings to the larger world of human possibility, by exposing the nature and effects of nuclearism and taking a stand against that spiritual perversion. The remedy is far from perfect, but it is the best I know.

Psychic Numbing

From the beginning of my work I was struck by survivors' startling accounts of their emotions being suddenly turned off. Again and again they would tell me that, while aware of grotesque dying all around them, they suddenly ceased to feel. This could happen within minutes or even seconds after the bomb fell, and could also occur more gradually over days or weeks. They used phrases like becoming "insensitive to human death," undergoing "a paralysis of my mind," or (as in the case of the physicist quoted earlier) the mind becoming unfeelingly "saturated" with horror. I called the acute reaction *psychic closing off* and the overall phenomenon *psychic numbing*.

Death-related numbing enveloped the entire city. Dr. Michihiko Hachiya, in his classic *Hiroshima Diary*, wrote of "broken and confused . . . automatons" who walked about in the "realm of dreams." And the shopkeeper's assistant told me of severely burned people who "had a special way of walking—very slowly," like "walking ghosts," and "didn't look like people of this world." Another man said that at the time "I was not really alive." That kind of experience evoked in me the image of "death in life" that became the title of my book.

Later I was to discover similar observations by Primo Levi, the great
literary witness to Auschwitz, when he spoke of

> non-men who march and labor in silence, the divine spark dead
> within them. . . . One hesitates to call them living: one hesitates to
> call their death death. . . . They crowd my memory with their face-
> less presences, and if I could enclose all the evil of our time in one
> image, I would choose this image which is familiar to me: an emaci-
> ated man, with head drooped and shoulders curved, on whose face
> and in whose eyes not a trace of thought is to be seen.

Levi's "non-men" (or *Muselmänner*, as they were called) were created by
the hands-on cruelty of the Nazis, while the "walking ghosts" of Hiroshima were produced by the more distant technological cruelty of an
American revolutionary weapon. Grotesquely imposed numbing, then,
became both a consequence and a symbol of twentieth-century evil.

In referring to my own "selective professional numbing" in response to
interviews, I was recognizing its psychological relationship to the much
more extreme reactions of the survivors themselves. I was later to identify
a similar process, a different version of selective professional numbing,
in the physicists involved in making the atomic bomb. At times—during Wellfleet meetings, for instance—some friends and colleagues have
objected to my using the same term for such extreme experiences in
survivors, my own struggles with feeling, and the experience of nuclear
physicists. But I believe that all three, different as they are, represent a
common psychological process.

Consider the case of scientists making the bomb, as described by the
brilliant physicist Richard Feynman:

> You see what happened to me—what happened to the rest of us,
> is we started for a good reason, then you're working very hard to
> accomplish something, and it's a pleasure, it's excitement. And you
> just stop thinking, you know, you stop.

Feynman and other scientists, of course, did go on thinking about the
scientific and technical problems they faced in making the weapon. What

they stopped thinking about—or perhaps never thought about—was what their bomb would do to the human beings who lived in the city on which it was to be dropped. So Feynman might more accurately have said, "You just stop *feeling*." One cannot afford to feel—to imagine—what will happen at the other end of the weapon. Technological distancing always enhances the numbing of weapons users, most extremely and potentially disastrously in the case of nuclear weapons. Also crucial, as Feynman tells us, is the full focus on the scientific and engineering requirements of the project, the deep pleasure of creating and making.

I never met Feynman but I did get to know four physicists involved in the Manhattan Project (the term used for the overall effort to create the first atomic bombs): Philip Morrison, George Kistiakowsky, Hans Bethe, and Herbert York. I found all of them to be appealing people who were to recognize the danger of the weapon they helped to create and become leading antinuclear spokesmen. They emphasized how all participants in the Manhattan Project understood themselves to be in a desperate race against the Nazis, who had the deeply troubling advantage of the much more advanced state of German nuclear physics. I've often thought that, had I been a physicist at the time, I might have eagerly offered my knowledge to the Manhattan Project.

Ironically, the numbing of physicists at the Manhattan Project was enhanced by the dedicated community created there. Morrison and Bethe, who were both very close to Robert Oppenheimer, the director of the Los Alamos laboratory, emphasized what an extraordinary leader he was. Known to be arrogant in the past, Oppenheimer was not only stunningly brilliant in his coordination of everyone's work but also a friend, advisor, confidant, and facilitator of living arrangements who was always generous, decent, and supportive. The utopian community he did so much to create in an isolated desert area contributed greatly to the general numbing—not toward the purpose of the community, since everybody knew they were producing an atomic bomb—but toward the genocidal nature of the product that remarkable group was creating. Bethe, a German refugee married to a Jewish woman, emphasized to me the sense people had of being on a moral crusade on behalf of the future of civilization. No wonder they could "stop thinking" (or feeling), as Feynman said, or that they would undergo what was later described as a "half-conscious closing of the mind." That all changed with what Bethe called the "awful impression" the scientists experienced from the photographs soon shown them of the destruction of Hiroshima. All four of these men were to devote much of their subsequent lives to warning the world about nuclear danger, but before that they had shared a form of numbing that enabled them to become central contributors to the cruelest of all weapons.

Hiroshima survivors' dramatic cessation of emotion, then, led me to a concept of much broader relevance. I could take in survivors' accounts of acute and extreme numbing only by myself undergoing a more limited version, and both of us were in our situation because of the numbing of American physicists and military men. The numbing of *hibakusha* reflected a shattering of the psychic forms of the self, as opposed to a much lesser interruption of psychic function on the part of both the physicists and myself.

I came to recognize intense expressions of psychic numbing as characteristic of severe trauma in general. It was to be found in the "thousand-mile stare" of American soldiers repatriated from North Korea and in the similar demeanor of Westerners whom I interviewed soon after their release from Chinese prisons, both groups having been subjected to brutal, life-threatening programs of thought reform. And psychic numbing was much at issue in the rap groups in which I participated with Vietnam veterans (which I'll describe later) when they spoke of "learning to feel." The term made its way into descriptions of post-traumatic stress disorder in various editions of the *Diagnostic and Statistical Manual of Mental Disorders*, published by the American Psychiatric Association. In addition, I carried out research interviews with schizophrenic and depressive patients, in which I could demonstrate sustained forms of psychic numbing as central to their condition. Beyond that, I came to recognize what I called the numbing of everyday life, the barriers we automatically establish against the large bombardment of stimuli to which each of us is constantly subjected, barriers of numbing necessary to get through the day.

Psychic numbing is part of the human repertoire. For many *hibakusha* it was a lifesaving defense mechanism, a reversible form of symbolic death in order to avoid a permanent physical or psychic death. But some of that inner death could continue, even over lifetimes, in patterns of depression, despair, and unresponsiveness to other people and to the world at large. In matters of public policy, blunted feeling can be dangerous in the extreme. I've come to see psychic numbing as surrounding nuclear weapons in general—on the part of political leaders, scientists and strategists, and the general public—as a profound threat to the human future. At one point I considered writing a book titled "The Age of Numbing," a volume that would have encompassed much of my work.

I am aware that what I call psychic numbing can seem closely related to such traditional psychoanalytic defense mechanisms as repression, isolation, and derealization. But I have become convinced of the necessity of a concept concerned solely with feeling and nonfeeling, with direct psychological experience or its impairment. I have been sufficiently identified with it that, when meeting Arthur Schlesinger, Jr., during the mid-1970s, he could say to me, "Oh, yes, you're the psychic numbing man"—a form of recognition that did not thrill me. But the lesson from Hiroshima was itself indelible.

Science and Witness

In Hiroshima I had to think a lot about science and scientists, especially about physicians and their claim to science. It came down to the relationship of science and suffering, and ultimately of science and witness. Two Americans, in particular, became polar figures in connection with this issue: Earle Reynolds, who had taught physical anthropology and biology at Antioch College and then spent three years with the ABCC in Hiroshima before becoming a peace activist and the ABCC's most outspoken American critic; and George Darling, the director of the ABCC and a professor of human ecology at Yale. A third man, a Japanese physician named Fumio Shigeto, presented an alternative to that polarity. All three had bearing on what I myself was up to.

Earle Reynolds had achieved considerable fame by sailing his yacht through the nuclear test area surrounding the Marshall Islands as a form of protest, and later doing the same in Soviet waters. One evening BJ and I found ourselves in a taxi, together with a Japanese assistant, driving along the Hiroshima waterfront in quest of the man and the yacht. My immediate impression was of "how small" they both seemed—the boat a "puny object with which to confront the . . . nuclear monster," and Reynolds, a slight figure who seemed to look not at me but beyond me, and whom I found to be "determined, single-minded, inflexible, humorless, and mostly correct in what he had to say about the dangers of nuclear weapons and the need to do something about them." His scathing series of accusations against the ABCC included its suppression of his own research on the harmful impact of radiation on the development of children; its general negation of radiation effects, including those on workers who entered the city just after the bomb; and its failure to study the extremely important psychological impact because "it did not really want to know the full story."

Reynolds attributed these distortions to the ABCC's vulnerability to the political pressures of the Atomic Energy Commission, its sponsor, which wanted to downplay radiation influences. My impression was that Reynolds might have been exaggerating a bit but that he was telling us something important. Reynolds found much sympathy for his views in Hiroshima but people there were often uneasy with him, whether because of his verbal assaults on the powers that be (including the ABCC), his constant quest for antinuclear publicity, or his single-minded, unyielding, impersonal demeanor.

I wrote to Dave Riesman that Hiroshima journalists combined a certain amount of admiration for Reynolds with a "wish he would do his peace work elsewhere, preferably in America." I said also that Reynolds came into the category of "peace fanatics" that Riesman and I had discussed in the past, adding admiringly that "only . . . such a peace fanatic could be capable of this man's truly heroic actions." I was caught between my aversion to fanaticism of any kind and my veneration for a man whose actions were profoundly appropriate to the extremity of the nuclear issue, however difficult his demeanor. I was quite clear about where I came out: "Whatever the complexities involved, I feel that the voyages he has made, and perhaps will make, are a real claim to greatness."

Soon after, I went to see Reynolds's arch-antagonist, George Darling, at his ABCC office. Darling was an elderly, somewhat heavyset, friendly man who greeted me warmly as a Yale colleague. He then gave me a long exposition on the purposes and achievements of the ABCC, its extensive research and focus on scientific results based on careful study of comparative populations, and the reassurance it could provide survivors concerning their exaggerated fears. I felt there was some truth in what he said—one did want accurate studies—and the importance of reassuring survivors was also emphasized to me by a number of Japanese physicians. But I was troubled by what I called his "unmistakable tone of minimizing the effects of the bomb," which included a claim that, other than the increase in leukemia, the ABCC had found virtually no significant differences between the exposed and unexposed populations studied. Yet Japanese physicians had begun to report increased rates in survivors of many additional forms of cancer, findings that would much later be confirmed, reluctantly it would seem, by ABCC researchers.

I wrote to Riesman that it was one thing to carry out the responsibility of reassuring survivors, "but what was lost sight of here was perhaps the even more important moral responsibility . . . of making known to the world as quickly and clearly as possible the full dangers of atomic weapons." And I raised the question of whether there was American inclination—"explicit policy or unconscious pressure to hold back or minimize positive (that is, harmful) findings." That suspicion was later to be confirmed by M. Susan Lindee in her scholarly study of the commission. She uncovered an in-house ABCC document making clear that treatment had to be refused because it would be seen as "an act of atonement." She also concluded: "The Japanese perception that the ABCC (or rather, the United States government) was not entirely forthcoming in releasing information about the biological effects of radiation was frequently accurate. The information was a state secret because it was tied to a weapon that shaped U.S. Cold War strategies."

Reynolds and Darling became bracketed in my mind, and each in a different way posed problems for me. I felt connected to Reynolds's passionate antinuclear sentiment but uneasy about the lack of humanity in our encounter. Darling was more urbane and friendly, in a way more familiar and easier to talk to (I was to learn later that, among ABCC leaders, he was considered relatively liberal and internationally minded), but I was appalled by his consistent tendency to minimize the impact of the bomb. Ultimately I felt greater sympathy for the scientist turned zealous activist than for the "reasonable" mainstream scientist turned bomb apologist. I concluded that Reynolds needed his fierce one-sidedness to muster the courage and ingenuity required for his daunting antinuclear project.

As for the ABCC, there have been compassionate scientists associated with it: Reynolds was himself a case in point, and there was Warner Wells, who edited and cotranslated Michihiko Hachiya's *Hiroshima Diary*, which became a classic rendering of the early atomic bomb impact. But as an institution the ABCC wavered between science in the service of compiling accurate medical information, and science in the service of suppressing atomic bomb truths. (Years later, when Edwin Reischauer was ambassador to Japan, I told him about my misgivings concerning the ABCC. I had the impression that he was already aware of the problem and had considerable influence in what was finally, if belatedly done: separating the institution from official American ties in favor of Japanese control and internationalization.)

Japanese doctors could take a third position. Dr. Fumio Shigeto was known and much loved in Hiroshima for his tireless medical work with *hibakusha*. Himself a survivor, Shigeto was first head of the Red Cross hospital and then of the Atomic Bomb Hospital, built especially for survivors. A quietly energetic man in his early fifties, he spoke to me with deep concern about the medical and psychological problems of his patients. He made the clinical observation that (in direct contrast to what Darling told me) he was encountering a striking increase in the incidence of lung cancer (four times that of the general population) and stomach cancer (twice that of the general population). Much later the overall increased incidence of these and other cancers would be confirmed by ABCC studies. He also spoke of the pervasive fear of survivors of fatal radiation effects and a feeling, particularly prominent in older ones, that they could never recover completely so why make any effort to do so. Yet when survivors raised questions about whether they should feel free to marry, he told me that he always advised them to go ahead unhesitatingly as there was no clear medical reason not to.

As I walked with Dr. Shigeto through his wards I thought that it was impossible to know just how much of each illness could be attributed to the A-bomb itself. And I was later to write that one needed a unitary approach in which one understood that physical radiation effects combined with severe experiences of pain and loss and fear to bring about what was broadly talked about in Hiroshima as "A-bomb disease," a catch-all for any symptoms believed to have been caused by the atomic bomb. That could include established cases of leukemia and other cancers, or more amorphous feelings of chronic fatigue (which could have an understandable psychological component)—all of which, I wrote, illustrated "the malignant influence of the atomic bomb on every level of human experience." Whatever his combination of conviction and diplomacy, Dr. Shigeto had no bad words for the ABCC, insisting that its research was very important. But it was clear to me that, though his own observations would be considered less "scientific," he had become much more quickly aware than ABCC doctors of the physical and psychological atomic bomb truths.

Inevitably I raised questions to myself about where my own work stood in relation to these issues. From the beginning I saw my approach as broadly scientific, a systematic effort to obtain reliable information with scrupulous attention to evidence. It was in that spirit that I drew upon a random sample of survivors selected from the official city list, and developed a protocol that enabled me to ask the same questions of all the people I interviewed. The purpose of my scientific project was that of making known the human consequences of the atomic bomb to the world in general. That contrasted with Darling's vulnerability to official American political pressures in reporting or underreporting scientific studies. While I shared his concern about irresponsible exaggerations that could exacerbate fears among *hibakusha*, I saw my responsibility as that of uncovering difficult psychological truths rather than reassuringly stressing negative findings.

I shared Reynolds's insistence on full revelation of the bomb's effects, but my approach in that environment was through committed scholarship rather than his bold antinuclear actions. I shared Dr. Shigeto's sensibility about the vast impact of the bomb and his concern about the lives of survivors. But in contrast to his indefatigable medical responsibility to those survivors, I saw my responsibility to them as working together to elaborate their experiences in ways that had not previously been attempted, to add a psychological dimension to their witness.

Commemorating

My work in Hiroshima taught me much about the deep necessity of survivors to commemorate their atomic bomb experience and the profound inadequacy of every means of doing so. A fulcrum for this painful contradiction was the ritual surrounding August 6. As I went about my work in mid and late July of 1962, I could feel the tension building throughout the city. Newspapers printed many stories recalling people's suffering from the bomb, describing the often contentious opinions about plans for that year's commemoration ceremonies. People around us became agitated. Kaoru Ogura, the generous and knowledgeable man who did most to help me function in the city, not himself a survivor but very close to the whole experience, told me that working with me at night was tiring and he would have to reduce his time with me.* His fiancée, Kyōko, an actual survivor who was assisting BJ, said she feared she might no longer be able to do so because of the strain she experienced. Both actually continued to provide invaluable help. But there was a palpable sense of collective anxiety, along with a certain amount of diffuse anger.

In Hiroshima there was something sacred about the August 6 commemoration. But as in the case of Jews and the Holocaust, it was a profoundly negative sacralization. What a burden for survivors to require of themselves the deepest awe to commemorate a version of hell. Public ritual, the ceremony held near the hypocenter, was nonetheless of great importance to *hibakusha* because it gave recognition to their suffering, "consoled" the dead, and affirmed their own pride in recovery and rebuilding. Yet that same ceremony, survivors told me, could be painful in the extreme, both because of the symbolic reactivation of their entire ordeal, and because everything done—the honoring of survivors, the speeches, the release of peace doves—seemed too much a public display,

---

*Ogura was close to Shinzo Hamai, one of Hiroshima's true heroes. As a young city official at the time of the bomb, Hamai had distinguished himself by his selfless dedication to helping people under those extreme early conditions. He later became Hiroshima's first elected mayor, holding that office from 1947 to 1955 and 1959 to 1967. He encouraged my work and during two interviews with me he impressively described his efforts to balance an insistence that Hiroshima's full story be told with a forward-looking emphasis on the city's rebirth.

somehow inauthentic, unworthy of the dead. I knew that these ceremonies attempted to express the traditional poles of collective mourning: obeisance to the dead with pledges to continue their interrupted work, on the one hand; and separation from them and reassertion of life, on the other. But in this case no public effort at mourning could cope with the city's cauldron of remembered suffering.

Nor was I immune to some of these emotions in connection with the events of commemoration. I remember vividly a little ceremony of the Folded Crane Club in which its members floated lanterns along one of Hiroshima's riverbanks, each bearing names of children killed by the bomb, while chanting lines from Hiroshima's A-bomb poet, Sankichi Tōge: "Give back my father, give back my mother, give our sons and daughters back." In the midst of the floating of the lanterns and the chanting of Tōge's lines, a teenage girl suddenly broke down and sobbed uncontrollably. The adult leader of the group ran over to console her, spotted BJ and me a few yards away, and explained that the girl's brother had died of leukemia four years earlier. His voice then rose in a mixture of anger and pathos as he declared, "Please let them know about these things in America!" I felt compelled to do that.

As I look back on my experience with Hiroshima survivors, I'm impressed with the degree to which most of them somehow recovered and resumed their lives. They struggled with the impediments and confusions surrounding public and private mourning, commemoration, and memorialization. They conversed privately and quietly with dead family members. They sensed that no public ceremony, no monument, could be adequate for an atomic-bombed city. But despite everything, they sustained their lives. While the dead are more present in Japanese culture than in our own, survivors' perception of a "debt to the dead" is universal. That debt to the dead can take many forms, one of the most powerful of which is the lifelong responsibility to tell and retell their story, which for *hibakusha* is their own story as well, the story of Hiroshima as a warning to the world. No wonder that I became aware of the strong presence of the dead in all of our interviews.

Imagining the Real

I left Hiroshima for Yale in late October of 1962, and arrived in New Haven, Connecticut, in the middle of the Cuban Missile Crisis. That crisis turned out to be the greatest threat of large-scale nuclear war the world has ever experienced. My own strange reaction to it taught me things I hadn't wanted to know.

Following the disastrous American-sponsored Bay of Pigs invasion of Cuba, the Soviet Union, under the leadership of Nikita Khrushchev and with the cooperation of Cuban leader Fidel Castro, decided to secretly install in that country ballistic missiles with nuclear warheads. The presence of the missiles was detected by American spy planes, and President John F. Kennedy gave an ominous speech in which he condemned the Soviet action and declared a naval blockade of Cuba. People everywhere talked of all-out nuclear war. There was a terrifying sequence in which American naval vessels were sent to intercept Russian ships carrying nuclear missiles to Cuba—until the Russian ships turned back. At the time ordinary people knew little about details or of the efforts of both leaders to avert nuclear catastrophe. I met with some of my new colleagues at Yale, who were as alarmed as I was, and we sent a telegram to President Kennedy, urging restraint and avoidance of nuclear confrontation.

Having just left Hiroshima, my mind was full of images of a destroyed city and of grotesque individual suffering. And yet my sense of the immediate nuclear threat was somewhat abstract. Moreover, I was in the middle of a jarring reentry into my own country. It was difficult for BJ and me to extricate ourselves from the force field of Hiroshima and from our immersion in Japan in general—we had been there for two and a half intense years—and to find ourselves suddenly in the midst of what felt like alien American life. We were immersed in the details of moving into a newly purchased home in Woodbridge, Connecticut, just outside New Haven, together with our energetic sixteen-month-old son. We knew few people in the area and I was joining a new department of psychiatry while still preoccupied with Hiroshima and with the safety of my extensive Hiroshima materials (sent by registered boat mail). Though enthusiastic about my new situation, I was struggling with a formidable transition.

And there was another problem, an agonizing one. Our dog Runcible, the third party in my late 1950s walks with Dave Riesman, and a beloved family pet for more than six years, suddenly became ill with torsion of the intestine and had to undergo emergency surgery. The hours following the operation coincided almost exactly with the Kennedy-Khrushchev confrontation. I remember a terrible haze of nuclear threat and urgent talks with friends about its danger—along with visits to the veterinary hospital and anxious telephone conversations with the veterinarian. My mind struggled with two competing sets of images: one, a vast but amorphous panorama of nuclear destruction; the other consisting of a beautiful, spirited animal lying lifeless on the operating table of the veterinary hospital. When I later asked myself which set of images had been the most vivid and painful, I had no doubt that it had been those of the dog. The death of a specific creature, not even a human, had greater impact than the more cosmic but inevitably obscure threat of extinction.

My recollections were undoubtedly influenced by outcomes: nuclear war was averted, while Runcible died. And there were also feelings of guilt BJ and I experienced in wondering whether we had obtained the best treatment for him, or made the right decision in not having taken him with us to Hiroshima (where we had heard that canine heartworm was widespread), and whether his medical condition was influenced by the stress he underwent in being separated from us and then reunited with us. In relation to nuclear threat, we had no such guilt. But I know that I did have anxiety about a nuclear war, about my own death and the death of my wife and child, and about planetary death. That nuclear anxiety, I am now convinced, was at least partially displaced onto the dog's death, a very painful but manageable event. The whole sequence of course reflects the mind's preoccupation with what is immediate and concrete, and the difficulty it has making contact with the infinity of nuclear destruction—our difficulty (again in Martin Buber's phrase) of "imagining the real."

9

Dr. Hiroshima

HIROSHIMA LEFT MORE of an imprint than I realized—nothing you could tell by looking at me, but having to do with my sense of who I was, with the way I related to other people, and with how they responded to me.

Consider this incident that occurred in the Yale Department of Psychiatry. Ever since my work in Hong Kong I felt myself to be different from psychiatric colleagues. But now there was a new and stronger dividing line: I was separated from them by a cataclysmic experience they found hard to grasp and I found hard to explain. At the same time I was expected to be one of them in a department we shared, to blend with them on the basis of the knowledge and traditions of our profession. It was made clear to me that I was to be a kind of wide-ranging "intellectual." Besides continuing my research and writing, I had two main tasks: to conduct Grand Rounds, which had nothing to do with patients or bedsides but were presentations by guest speakers who were doing interesting work; and to give a seminar course for psychiatric residents on what we called Social Psychiatry. For the Grand Rounds I could include not only people from within psychiatry but others I admired like Erik Erikson and David Riesman. In my seminars with residents I emphasized studies that dealt with large cultural and historical issues, including my own work on thought reform and especially on Hiroshima.

Every year there was a Christmas party at which psychiatric residents performed an original skit in which they poked fun at their teachers. At one such performance, given a little more than a year after I arrived in the department, there was an all-too-recognizable character called "Dr. Hiroshima." As I remember it, that character would be shown to be chatting together with other members of the department, and would relate any subject that arose to Hiroshima. So when another doctor spoke of a patient requiring a particular form of attention, he would say, "That reminds me of the situation in Hiroshima," or, "Let me tell you about my experience in Hiroshima." Finally, after a wildly confusing exchange, he screamed "Hiroshima! Hiroshima!" and collapsed to the ground (I cannot remember whether he collapsed from his own excitement or was clobbered by someone in the Punch-and-Judy puppeteering style).

The residents of course were living out an annual ritual, something on the order of a carnival in which, for one day, hierarchies were reversed and the lowliest could deride those in authority and boldly expose their vanities. But the residents had picked up on something about me in my relationship to Hiroshima—an intensity bordering on obsession. I was a bit like Coleridge's Ancient Mariner, a compulsive witness to horror who insisted that any stranger he met hear out his tale.

I did not know how to respond to the skit. Part of me understood that I should accept it as playful creativity on the part of residents and go along with its humor, as did other faculty members who were roasted in one way or another. But because I was not aware of my obsessiveness on the subject, I felt ambushed, a bit humiliated, and alienated from my students and colleagues. Did they consider me an absurd fanatic?

But they got me thinking, and over time I could temper my behavior with them, which permitted them in turn to be more receptive to what I did say about Hiroshima. But I was also intent on sustaining my witness to Hiroshima as part of my way of being an idiosyncratic psychiatrist. As we got used to one another, we could relax a bit, hear each other out, and accept our differences. I formed a few lasting friendships with faculty colleagues as well as with residents who participated in my seminars. Some of those residents were sufficiently responsive to explore for themselves the possibility of following the model of psychiatrist-in-the-world I seemed to represent, but tended to retreat from that idea when facing the prospect of earning a living in our profession. Others could join me in active dialogue about my Hiroshima findings. For my side I seemed to require a combination of rapprochement (we were fellow practitioners of the same profession) and separateness (it was important to hold on to differences). Many of my relationships with colleagues took on what I would call creative ambivalence. Dr. Hiroshima would tone himself down, but would still be very much there.

The Hiroshima Volume

In writing my book I knew I would both rely on the experience of survivors and extend my mosaic to convey the bomb's all-enveloping reverberations. I can still remember hours and days and years of poring over survivors' translated words, and organizing them into a shared narrative of what happened to them and to their city. I did much of that from a large semi-attic study in our Woodbridge house. It was the first of several monkishly luxurious studies in which I've had the good fortune to work. Its cloistered quality was created by the eaves and the Colonial windows but it spanned across almost half of a mid-nineteenth-century house large enough to have once been an inn. I was told that the study had previously been used by a prominent Yale geographer to house elaborate maps, globes, and models of various kinds. I loved its view of a small pond on our property, which attracted mallard ducks, occasionally a heron, and a bit later our young son happily and skillfully rowing his small craft. My work on the book proceeded as well in more improvised studies in rented houses on Cape Cod and, beginning in 1966, in my favorite study of all: a separately standing high-ceilinged old shack, the original building on our Cape Cod land, renovated in brisk browns and whites, with a sideways view of the Atlantic and enough space to squeeze in forty people around its oak tables and along the walls during the Wellfleet meetings. Writing about Hiroshima, I began what was to become a lifelong tendency of contemplating horror from an exquisite setting. In dictating these words I now sit in the same spot behind the oak tables, not far from the large fireplace, looking out at the twilight silhouettes of pine trees and the ocean in the distance.

Work on the book consumed me from early 1963 through 1967. But there were major interruptions, the most beautiful of which was the birth of our second child, Karen (later Natasha), in Yale–New Haven Hospital in 1965. I was much chagrined over not being permitted to be present at the birth (the hospital was still backward in that way) but I was soon greeted and overcome by her dark, piercing eyes, which seemed, from the beginning, to look knowingly at me and at the world in general. Those eyes would continue to take in everything as an observant child, a fine student, and a wise woman. It was no surprise that she was to become a sensitive psychoanalyst. However idiosyncratic BJ and I have been as parents, we have treasured and sought to nurture the life-affirming energies of our children.

The book grew into a long one, centered on the interviews but extending to every form of response to the weapon. I have sometimes thought that a more concise and simplified volume could have been much more widely read. *Death in Life* had respectable sales, which greatly increased after the award, and has been included in many college courses, but has never been anything on the order of a bestseller. In contrast, I have frequently thought of John Hersey's *Hiroshima*, which I greatly admire, a short book written for a popular audience and extremely widely read, frequently by high school students. But I knew that my work had to be more inclusive and complex to be a true reflection of what I had observed and experienced in Hiroshima.

Over the course of the writing I sought psychological concepts that would explain what survivors told me. Though Erikson's work, and my dialogues with him, remained extremely important to me, his identity theory no longer sufficed. I read Otto Rank, one of the few early psychoanalysts concerned with death and with what he called "immortality systems." And I went back to Freud, who also had much to say about death, even if couched in instinctual language and not well integrated with the rest of his theory. Overall I found the subject of death to be neglected in psychoanalytic and psychiatric work, and I tried to derive new principles following directly upon experiences described to me. My original plan was to include in the Hiroshima volume my expanding explorations of theory concerning death and immortality. But I came to realize that Hiroshima needed a book of its own, and that my broader explorations had to become a separate volume, which I called *The Broken Connection*.

That two-book solution seems a very obvious one in retrospect, but I could arrive at it only after accumulating vast amounts of manuscript and applying Camus's philosophy of limits to individual books.

Although *Death in Life* was mainly the Hiroshima story, telling that story required a certain amount of conceptual elaboration that could not wait for a new volume. For instance, near the beginning of the book I noted that "the most striking psychological feature of this immediate experience was the sense of a sudden and absolute shift from normal existence to an overwhelming encounter with death." I was saying among other things that an extreme environment could overwhelm any psyche, no matter what its prior makeup, something I had learned from my earlier work on thought reform but not in such a brutally absolute manner. That principle of an environment taking over the individual psyche ran counter to much psychoanalytic thinking of the time, which stressed early childhood experience as determining subsequent behavior. My title, "Death in Life," was an image I used to suggest that "life and death were out of phase with one another, no longer properly distinguishable." That was a manifestation of the extreme psychic numbing I described earlier. I was not aware that the nineteenth-century British poet Alfred, Lord Tennyson had used the phrase "death in life" in his poem "Tears, Idle Tears," to describe the painful memory of love for people now dead. Nor did I know that the British psychiatrist R. D. Laing had used the phrase in his book *The Divided Self*, which I had not yet read, to suggest the inner experience of people thought of as schizophrenic. Also relevant to my title was my observation of "the replacement of the natural order of living and dying with an unnatural order of death-dominated life." That in turn had to do with what I called "a permanent encounter with death."

I found that *hibakusha* struggled not only to stay alive but to remain part of the human chain, or of the "great chain of being." They were struggling to hold on to what I called a *sense* of immortality, of being part of the continuity of human life. The concept had to do with two fundamental human characteristics: as cultural animals we feel ourselves bound up with collective, ongoing existence; and as creatures who know that we die, we need to come to terms with that knowledge. While the sense of immortality could include considerable denial of death, I understood it to be a way of symbolizing our larger human connectedness. I described five modes of symbolic immortality: the biological or biosocial mode (living on in one's family or one's "people"), the religious mode (living on in an immortal soul or eternal spiritual principle), the creative mode (living on in one's influences on other human beings), the natural mode (living on in eternal nature), and a fifth mode, which differed from the others in being an intense psychic state or experience of transcendence, within which time and death disappear.

When survivors quoted to me that ancient saying "The state may collapse but the mountains and rivers remain," they were insisting on this sense of immortality as part of eternal nature. That saying was much on my mind during discussions I had with fellow antinuclear activists as we tried to imagine a postnuclear world. We realized that nature itself was vulnerable to the weapons. And we imagined, in addition to the grotesque universal suffering and dying, the destruction of all libraries and museums, the cessation of the flow of cultural experience. There would no longer be any indication that human beings had existed, any record of a great chain of being.

The concept of symbolic immortality was also an expression of what I could call my spiritual sensibility. I have never been able to believe in concrete religious ideas having to do with the existence of God, in a messiah or an immortal soul, or in the historical accuracy of biblical stories. Nor have I been an agnostic, holding out a possibility in my mind of the truth of those religious claims. In terms of dogma, I am clearly an atheist. Yet I have always felt close to certain kinds of religious people. I have shared with them not only strong ethical convictions but a kind of spiritual energy on behalf of those convictions. It is what the theologian Paul Tillich called "ultimate concern," a form of passionate motivation that can be secular no less than specifically religious. That was what my old friend and fellow activist Arnie Wolf, himself a Reform rabbi, meant when he once said to me: "You are more religious than I am!" My concept of the symbolization of immortality, then, emerged both from observations on Hiroshima survivors and the sensibility of a spiritually committed nonbeliever.

A Jesuit theologian friend of mine, John Dunne, wrote in an article in a festschrift volume for me, that, whenever he came upon my term "symbolic immortality," he had the impulse to cross out the "symbolic." If there were anyone for whom I would do that, it would certainly be John, but the truth is that the "symbolic" remains crucial to my perspective. The issue arose again when I was invited to give the Ingersoll Lecture on Immortality at Harvard Divinity School in 1985. I said in my talk that I had "the feeling that I have come in through the back door" and had been "surprised by the invitation, and wondered whether the school had run out of lecturers who, when talking about immortality, would mean the real thing." But then I added that I myself had the "real thing" in mind in that "symbolization is at the heart of human psychic function, and our only path to what we call reality." That is for me the larger point. A sense of immortality is a matter of the human psyche, not of any greater outside or supernatural force—a feeling of being part of a larger entity that will continue indefinitely into the future well beyond the demise of the self.

In that way I identified myself as departing both from what I called Freud's "rationalist, iconoclastic" view that all talk of immortality was simply denial of death, and from Carl Jung's "mythic-hygienic" view that the teaching of an afterlife is to be encouraged as (in his words) "consonant with the standpoint of psychic hygiene." Mine was a "formative-symbolizing" perspective in relationship to life continuity. Since as human beings we are not only biologically, but culturally and historically connected with past and future, the sense of immortality becomes an appropriate expression of that connectedness.

All this was my way of coming to terms with Hiroshima. Survivors there had experienced not only the most extreme kind of encounter with individual death but also what I called a "fear of psychohistorical extinction"—of being at the forefront of the end of everything. And yet in completing that volume I expressed a modicum of hope:

Hiroshima was an "end of the world" in all the ways I have described. And yet the world still exists. Precisely in this end-of-the-world quality lie both its threat and its potential wisdom. In every age man faces a pervasive theme which defies his engagement and yet must be engaged. In Freud's day it was sexuality and moralism. Now it is unlimited technological violence and absurd death. We do well to name the threat and to analyze its components. But our need is to go further, to create new psychic and social forms to enable us to reclaim not only our technologies, but our very imaginations, in the service of the continuity of life.

I was beginning to elaborate a set of concepts around the model of death and the continuity of life, and that principle of human continuity became a mantra in my work. So did Hiroshima itself in terms of the threat it represented. That city still looms for me as a prism through which I view the world. There is in me still quite a bit of the Ancient Mariner telling his tale.

Reviews and Responses—Goodman and Macdonald

Death in Life was reviewed widely in newspapers, national weekly news-magazines, and various intellectual and professional journals generally quite favorably. But there was one notable exception, an attack in the *New York Review of Books* by Paul Goodman, a Gestalt psychologist and prominent New York intellectual, who vehemently objected to my nuanced approach, which, he declared, provided "a practical philosophy of life for the American empire in conditions of high technology." Why did I not instead, he asked, "protest and strike"? In addition to my hurt and anger, I was aware that Goodman was rejecting, or failing to appreciate, the larger principle of the importance of taking a scholarly approach to highly destructive events. I shared his sense of horror and rage in connection with the atomic bombings, but I had set myself the task of exploring systematically the psychological consequences of the weapon.

My work on destructive historical events was based on a specific conviction: we had to go beyond mere outrage and disgust to seek a fuller grasp of what led to an atrocity, what it did to fellow human beings, and what significance it had for the world that remained. I was to extend that conviction to my work on Vietnam, Nazi doctors, and violent cults. What mattered in all this was not so much the tone of Goodman's review as his rejection of the principle of full intellectual probing of the most egregious behavior and its consequences. I discussed these issues with friends, and in a rejoinder I wrote to the *New York Review*. The person I turned to most was Dwight Macdonald, a writer and editor whom I had come to think of as an American Camus. Dwight had weathered a number of storms on the American left, and had become a fierce critic of anybody's totalism while remaining sympathetic to many of the rebellious expressions of the sixties. He encouraged what he called my "objective inquiry into a complex moral question [as opposed to Goodman's] subjective moralizing." The difference between the two, he went on, "may be that between propaganda and contemplation, between what ought to be so, hence, must be so, and what is so."

At the same time I resonated with part of the Goodman review. Had I not experienced pent-up impulses in Hiroshima to "protest and strike"? I would act more boldly upon those impulses, but not at the expense of discarding scholarship or, more generally, a rigorous and complex approach to truth.

The Award

In 1969 BJ and I were living, with our two children, in our house in Woodbridge, Connecticut, whose grounds included the small pond with mallard ducks mentioned earlier. But BJ and I, both essentially urban types, needed to get away now and then from that bucolic scene and spent frequent weekends in New York City. We would sometimes stay at the old One Fifth Avenue Hotel, long since converted into cooperative apartments. When checking into that hotel one Friday afternoon, the desk clerk handed me a telephone, saying that a call had just come in for me. It was from John J. Simon, my editor at Random House. In a tone that combined excitement, surprise, and laughter, he declared: "You won!" "Won what?" I asked. "The National Book Award," he replied. It's hard for me to recall now just how I felt upon hearing that. I think it was mainly disbelief—partly because John had been a somewhat quixotic editor whose words didn't always register clearly with me, and more basically because I didn't see myself as a person who could win that award.

Of course I knew I had been nominated some months before, along with four other authors, all of them distinguished, in a category then called "The Sciences." One of those was the Nobel laureate James D. Watson, whose book *The Double Helix* was the one I was sure would be chosen. So I pretty much dismissed the whole matter from my mind, which was why I was momentarily confused by John's words. But I recovered quickly from that confusion and experienced what I can only call a quiet form of deep excitement. I wanted both to contemplate and celebrate the news, so BJ and I put our suitcases in our room and went down to the bar, where we smiled at each other, talked about how fine and unexpected it was, and about how much our time in Hiroshima meant to us. We drank a toast to the city, to the survivors we knew there, and to the award.

I happily succumbed to the literary hoopla of the ceremony and the dinner that followed. We were picked up by the private limousine of Bennett Cerf, founder and then still doyen of Random House. I remember him as a small, wiry man who was very pleased that two of his authors, Norman Mailer and myself, had won the award, Mailer for his marvelous chronicle of the antiwar march on the Pentagon, *The Armies of the Night*. At the dinner I was assigned to Robert Silverman, then essentially running the company, whose active involvement in international human rights movements I admired. I was a one-night literary lion, and as William James said to his wife after being celebrated by publishers in New York City, "I enjoyed being a lion."

The ceremony took place at Town Hall in New York City, and I have a compelling photograph of honorees on the stage in which I am sitting next to Norman Mailer and Jerzy Kosinski (who won the award in fiction for his novel *Steps*), Mailer leaning forward with his hands on his knees in the manner of a wrestler about to pounce, Kosinski looking tentative and angelic (though this complicated Holocaust survivor was neither and would kill himself many years later), and I with my fingers touching my chin on the order of a bemused "thinker." The sponsors made the mistake of setting up a generous bar backstage, and I heard a few of them express concern that Mailer, notorious for his alcohol-related misbehavior on public occasions, would do something wild and nasty. But Mailer astonished everyone by acting like a choirboy, and in his acceptance speech spoke almost in clichés about the importance of awards and how they made writers feel appreciated. John Berryman (who won the award in poetry for *His Toy, His Dream, His Rest*) turned out to be the hard-drinking bad boy of the occasion, and stumbled about the stage precariously during his talk, devoting most of it to denouncing a reviewer who, twenty years earlier, had said that his poems "lacked nobility." I had no idea how seriously troubled a man Berryman was until his suicide three years later.

(Nor can I help being struck by the fact that, among six winners of the National Book Award that year, two of them were eventual suicides.)

My own talk was taken over by Dr. Hiroshima and was, in essence, an interpretive antinuclear statement. I said that the weapons "cause us to feel severed from both past and future," give rise to "an age of numbing," and "become grotesque technological deities for a debased religion of nuclearism." I spoke of the rationale of the nuclear arms race as "the logic of madness." But I stressed that "we need Hiroshima to give substance to our terror—however inadequately that city can represent what would happen now if thermonuclear weapons were to be used on human populations." I also announced that I would turn over one half of the monetary award to a special fund for Hiroshima survivors, and divide the other half equally between the Council for a Livable World and Physicians for Social Responsibility, groups that "insist that we pursue science to promote life, and medicine to promote healing."

The National Book Award did not fundamentally change my life but it did affect it. The award bestowed on me, at the age of forty-three, a certain standing in the intellectual world, which undoubtedly contributed to my confidence; but that was accompanied by an expectation, not always laudable, that my work would and should continue to gain public recognition. Perhaps awards are always double-edged.

Acting on Hiroshima—Finding Medical Colleagues

While working in Hiroshima in the summer of 1962, I came upon a small notice in an English-language Japanese newspaper of a special symposium in the *New England Journal of Medicine* having to do with doctors and nuclear weapons. It mentioned a series of articles by American physicians describing the devastating effects the weapons would have if one or more were dropped in the Boston area. This was a time of great international tension focused on the nuclear arms race, just a couple of months prior to the Cuban Missile Crisis. Physicists were prominent in the antinuclear movement, along with religious and political activists, but doctors had not previously been heard from. Now I found it stirring that fellow American doctors were confronting the issue in the most vivid fashion. The group called itself Physicians for Social Responsibility (PSR), and when back in the United States I involved myself closely with it. However far I had strayed from medical work, I could feel in PSR's crusade a powerful affirmation of a large healing tradition. I later wrote to Bernard Lown, a leader in the movement, that "I've never ceased to view [PSR] as a life-enhancing alternative to what Hiroshima represents."

During the late sixties and early seventies the Vietnam War dominated everybody's landscape, and PSR as an organization underwent a period of decline. But then in the late 1970s and early '80s, the physicians' antinuclear movement simply took off and I found myself in one of those rare moments when my own activism converged with a decisive historical current. Helen Caldicott, the charismatic pediatrician, was a crucial force in rejuvenating PSR, along with its original organizers (Bernard Lown, Jack Geiger, Victor Seidel, and Lester Grinspoon), and we soon began what we came to call our "bombing runs," replicating the method used in the original *New England Journal of Medicine* symposium. In each major city throughout the country there would be a dramatic projection of overall effects of a 1- or 5- or 10-megaton nuclear bomb exploded in its downtown area: the enormous casualties, the unending consequences of radiation, and above all the incapacitation of almost all medical facilities. As I would put it in my own talk, "This time we won't be able to patch you up and get you back on your feet, as much as we'd like to be able to do that. The trouble is that you'll be dead and we'll be dead, and the few doctors who survive are likely to be in bad shape and with almost no functional medical equipment." I also emphasized how people in Hiroshima experienced a "lifelong immersion in death," and my mantra of "one plane, one bomb, one city." Now that Hiroshima message became newly powerful. In the past, even when treated respectfully, I felt that people were essentially saying: "Yes, it's wonderful work. We're glad you did it. But don't bother us too much with your terrible tale." But with Americans becoming increasingly fearful of nuclear war, especially during the early Reagan years, they were more open to what happened in Hiroshima as potentially applicable to everyone.

In PSR councils I and others stressed the need to avoid a simple message of doom and offer one of hope, and tried to do so in my own talks by suggesting our capacity to overcome the collective psychic numbing and the illusions that accompany the spiritual disease of "nuclearism." I

was joined by other psychiatrists in disseminating our psychological message, notably my close friend John Mark and the West Coast physician-
activist Judith Lipton. People were ready to hear what we said because
we were articulating their barely suppressed anxieties, did so in a professional medical fashion, and made clear that there was a better course to
take. PSR thrived despite bruising conflicts between Helen Caldicott and
the "old boys' antinuclear network"—over such things as power, scientific
accuracy, and antinuclear celebrity. There was much to be said for both
sides, given their remarkable antinuclear work. Again I recognized the
double level of motivation in those of us who become strongly involved in
public movements: a very passionate and genuine dedication to the cause,
along with more self-serving impulses such as vanity, personal ambition,
and competitiveness. This is the human equation. At the same time doctors became more than they had been as we all joined in what resembled
a religious crusade against nuclear weapons. A shy, tongue-tied fledgling
physician could be transformed into a knowledgeable and eloquent advocate of a collective medical conscience. There was a good deal of affection
for one another, a kind of camaraderie in confronting and transcending
massive killing and dying. The shared intensity and excitement could
become erotic, and together with a ready sense of entitlement, resulted in
quite a few affairs among PSR members. Taking in nuclear peril seemed
to have its compensations.

Also in the early eighties, the doctors' movement took its crucial step
into history by globalizing itself, although we didn't call it that at the
time. Bernard Lown, a leading American cardiologist, was the key figure here, seizing upon his friendship with Eugene Chazov, an equally
prominent Russian cardiologist, to take steps to render the movement
worldwide. He threw his considerable energies into what we first called
a medical Pugwash project (after the scientists' movement that brought
together American and Soviet physicists) and was to emerge as the International Physicians for the Prevention of Nuclear War (IPPNW). Bernie
was a steamroller with a conscience. He and I had ties dating back to
our internships at the Jewish Hospital of Brooklyn and, more recently,
in PSR, which he helped organize and for which he served as first president. During that early stage, Bernie naturally concentrated on creating
a Soviet delegation, and indeed the American-Soviet collaboration was

at the heart of the international doctors' movement. But Bernie had the wisdom to focus as well on Japanese participation, especially from Hiroshima and Nagasaki, and asked—one might say assigned—his Brooklyn comrade to help, which I was able to do during a trip to Japan. Much of the crucial early organizing was done by Eric Chivian, a younger man who was later to emerge as a leading psychiatric environmentalist.*

Chazov and Lown seemed to have much in common, except that Chazov had an outwardly milder manner and was highly placed in his country's political as well as medical hierarchy. They were both chunky and authoritative, accustomed to telling people what to do. Over drinks during late hours at IPPNW meetings, some of us would joke about "the two commissars" and their virtual interchangeability, speculating that, were each to be sent to the other's society, he could manage pretty well. We also shared some gallows humor about Chazov's having treated a number of Soviet premiers, most of whom seemed to have died from heart disease, and wondered whether current Party leaders gave any thought to changing their cardiologist. But behind that gallows humor was our awareness that Chazov was conveying the IPPNW message to those Soviet leaders, especially to Mikhail Gorbachev, who emerged as general secretary of the communist party in 1985 and came to adopt an antinuclear perspective resembling that of IPPNW. In a few talks I had with Chazov, I was convinced of his antinuclear passion and that of doctors close to him, as opposed to its absence in the political apparatchiks always included in the Soviet delegations to keep an eye on the others.

There was a considerable paradox concerning American and Soviet participation. The Soviet delegation received official support from its government (though there were inner divisions and Chazov was taking risks), but its members had to be very careful about what they said publicly, and even privately. They could not on any level, for instance, say that nuclear energy was dangerous because it could give rise to the weapons, since the Soviet government strongly favored nuclear energy. On the other hand, as members of the American delegation, we received no support at all

---

*Through Chivian and his wife, Susanna, I could become a coeditor of a collection of papers presented at an early conference for a volume that became an IPPNW bible: *Last Aid: The Medical Dimensions of Nuclear War*. (The Chivians did most of the work but John Mack and I were asked to collaborate with them and lend our names to the project).

from our government—the Reagan administration strongly disapproved of us and kept its distance—but we could say anything we pleased. Most of us, in fact, made very clear privately that we strongly opposed nuclear energy, though we agreed that our organization could not take that public position. Doing so, we understood, would have doomed the cooperation with the Russian delegation on which the entire project depended.

We had another genre of gallows humor, this one shared with our Russian counterparts. At every meeting either an American or a Soviet doctor would, with mock formality, offer a version of the following toast: "I drink to the survival of each of you, of your leaders, and of all of your countrymen. Because if you survive, we survive, and if you die, we die." That lugubrious toast was what IPPNW was all about. At our meetings in various parts of the world we emphasized the universal vulnerability to nuclear destruction, and our mutual self-interest in taking constructive steps together toward avoiding ultimate catastrophe. I found myself emphasizing that, just as we had to bring death into our imagination in order to live a full life, so we had to imagine nuclear catastrophe in order to act to keep the world going. We were extending to the rest of the planet what we had originally done in America, the whole process deepened and strengthened by the intellectual and ethical involvement of physicians throughout the world.

IPPNW, like PSR, was a cautious and conservative movement, very focused on medical and scientific projections. Our radicalism lay in our collaborative confrontation of the world-destroying nature of nuclear weapons and in the equally collaborative suggestions for breaking out of the world's nuclear entrapment. Yet I don't think that we in IPPNW fully understood the international impact we were having. I was amazed when our group was awarded the 1985 Nobel Peace Prize, but thought it, along with Lown and Chazov's trip to Stockholm to receive it, exciting and appropriate.

The whole doctors' journey strongly affected my relationship to medicine and healing. During the early eighties I was also writing and speaking about my work with Nazi doctors, always emphasizing their reversal of healing and killing. So in my head, and sometimes my words, I kept contrasting Nazi doctors who killed and IPPNW doctors who healed. In a deep personal sense, the doctors' antinuclear movement was an antidote to Nazi doctors. Having always been removed from medical work as such, I now felt myself part of the medical profession—or at least of a particular segment of it—perhaps for the first time. Antinuclear camaraderie led to shared medical identity as nothing else had. Now my contradiction was that of a man who jokingly described himself as a "former doctor" experiencing new pride in actually being one.

On the Courthouse Steps with the Berrigans

It was also as a scholar-activist that Dan and Phil Berrigan contacted me to testify at trials on behalf of them and their associates. The Berrigans were part of a Catholic left much influenced by Dorothy Day and her Catholic Worker Movement, and both Dan and Phil spent years in jail for their acts of civil disobedience in protesting nuclear weapons and the Vietnam War. At different times they asked me to testify about Hiroshima and nuclear threat or the psychological aspects of the Vietnam War, and about the symbolic significance of their and their associates' acts of civil disobedience in damaging nuclear weapons components or pouring blood on Selective Service files. But in most situations the judge prohibited such testimony, insisting that the trial concerned itself more narrowly with such specific violations as "breaking and entering" government buildings or destroying government property, rather than with larger issues of nuclear weapons or war-making. If permitted at all, my testimony would usually be relegated to sentencing hearings after the defendants had been found guilty.

Dan, a poet and Jesuit intellectual, was always considered the more sensitive and vulnerable of the brothers, as compared to Phil, a former Marine viewed as a blue-collar priest, fearless in his unrelenting acts of protest. But I found both brothers to be tough-minded as well as tender and to resemble one another in acting on their conscience and doing so with a saintlike consistency that was awesome and somewhat disconcerting. A priest who had been close to Dan told me how difficult he could be for disciples because he demanded of them the extreme sacrifices he himself was making, and that these demands in turn were much related to the strong influence of Phil's still more tyrannical conscience. But there was no doubt about the spiritual power of the two brothers, individually and as a team.

The nuclear weapons trial in which I became most involved was that of the "Plowshares Eight" in King of Prussia, a small industrial town in southeastern Pennsylvania, in 1981. The two brothers and six others had, in September 1980, broke into a General Electric plant there, hammered the nose cones of nuclear warheads being assembled, and poured blood on secret files connected with the weaponry. The judge had no patience with the Berrigans' argument of combating the greater evil, and simply declared: "Nuclear weapons are not on trial here. You are." He also gave short shrift to testimony during the sentence hearing by myself and other defense witnesses including Howard Zinn and Richard Falk (the international lawyer and activist who was a good friend), and handed out vindictive sentences of three to ten years in prison. But during the course of the trial itself, the defendants arranged a public meeting on the courthouse steps at which Falk, the biologist George Wald, and I gave our planned trial testimony. We were a ragtag group, a few determined speakers and an audience of not more than forty people, everyone exposed to the bitter February eastern Pennsylvania winds. The Emile de Antonio documentary *In the King of Prussia* depicted a scene that was affecting but not without its melancholy. I was unheroically bundled up against the cold, spoke in an earnest fashion about Hiroshima, and said that the current phrase about nuclear survivors envying the dead was inaccurate because, if there were survivors, they themselves would be "as if dead" in the extremity of their numbed incapacity.

I could not help but contrast the lives of the Berrigan brothers with my own, especially in terms of risk. Astoundingly, Phil spent almost eleven years in prison and was accurately described by a eulogist as "that rare combination where word and deed were one." It was a high point in my life in the peace movement when Phil introduced me with affectionate and comradely words for a talk I gave in Baltimore. Dan also spent years in prison, had severe health problems, and in the De Antonio film said, "I don't do particularly well in jail. I hate the humiliation. And yet one goes forward." I cherish the memory of Dan joining a Wellfleet meeting in the late eighties where, ever the fiery prophet, he reinterpreted for us the book of Revelation as a handbook for militant protestors. I was at one with Phil and Dan at the trial, but after it they went to jail and I went home. I was uneasy about the contrast in a way similar to what I experienced in relation to the actions of Ichiro Moritaki, the steadfast Hiroshima figure who sat zazen before the cenotaph to protest anyone's nuclear testing. But I did come to terms with my differences from both Moritaki and the Berrigans. They had their calling and their métier as spiritual and political activists. I found mine in ethically based psychological scholarship and a more limited form of activism. The Berrigans could make me uncomfortable, as they did everyone, because their lives challenged one's claim to morality. But they also helped me to clarify, and at the same time intensify, my own way of acting on a world defiled by nuclear weapons.

Hiroshima's Costs

Opening one's mind to what happened to people in Hiroshima and becoming involved with the city has its costs. I think of my friend, the BBC filmmaker Robert Vas. Vas had painful life experiences well before his encounter with Hiroshima, and in his introductory letter to me in 1974 spoke of having "lived through two dictatorships: the Nazi and the Russian and [having] left [Hungary] after the collapse of the 1956 Uprising." He said that the idea of a film on Hiroshima came to him while reading *Death in Life*. I responded enthusiastically and he soon visited me in New York City to discuss the film. He had come directly from the National Archives in Washington, D.C., where he had spent many hours viewing early, raw Hiroshima footage. He told me repeatedly how shaken he had been by the experience, reminding me of my own reaction years before to my first probing interview with a Hiroshima survivor. Vas was a short, slightly stocky man with a kind of anxious energy—responsive to everything he encountered and quick to express his feelings. We liked each other and found much shared sensibility. We exchanged warm letters in which (according to his original designation) I was "Robert[1]" and he "Robert[2]."

The film was to appear for the thirtieth commemoration of the atomic bombing, and I spent the month of May 1975 in Hiroshima working with Vas on it. Despite my enthusiasm for the project, a certain underlying anxiety was revealed in a dream I had the night before leaving Tokyo for Hiroshima. I was a doctor examining an ill child, asking him about the swelling on his face, only to be angrily rebuked by the child's father, who declared my question unnecessary since the swelling was all too obvious. The dream suggested discomfort about the film's possible exploitation of survivors, and perhaps a larger "symbolic reactivation" of the pain of my own overall experience in Hiroshima. I reinterviewed survivors I had originally seen in 1962, so that with a number of people I had two extremely intense encounters with thirteen years of silence in between. That was, as I later wrote, "like stepping out of a time machine—young men projected into balding middle age, teenaged girls into settled house-wives and mothers."

Some of the survivors showed signs of Japan's economic boom: a laborer I had originally encountered in dire personal and economic cir-cumstances received me in a sitting room dominated by golf trophies won by his son, who owned the opulent house in which both now lived. I found that survivors now tried to connect more with a collective sense of rebuilding the city and that memories of the past had somewhat receded, but that the bomb was still a painful presence in their minds and in their bodily fears. BJ spent part of the time with us in Hiroshima serving as a consultant and brought to Vas survivors she had worked with in connec-tion with the book she had done with the Japanese photographer Eikoh Hosoe, *Return to Hiroshima*. Vas and I experienced what I believe was a genuine collaboration: I provided background knowledge and advice, along with on-camera interviews with survivors and commentary; and he, in making the film, illuminated much with the images he was creating. While in ordinary conversation he could be ambivalent, self-doubting, and conflicted, when working on the film he was confident, decisive, in full control.

A few months later we spent five days together in London going over the footage that was being shaped for the final product. He seemed more anxious than he had in Hiroshima, and the discomfort he and his wife experienced in British society was manifest. But Vas and I retained our personal harmony. I remember how, after a gemütlich dinner at his home, he played a series of tapes for me from his vast collection, taking special joy in "conducting" the string quartets of Béla Bartók, his countryman. I had never experienced Bartók so powerfully or seen Vas so happy. He told me that, had he not become a filmmaker, he would have wished to be a conductor, and that he found much similarity in the two professions in the way one brought creative order and control to the world around one.

The completed film was sensitive and powerful, and in my judgment true to the Hiroshima experience. I wondered whether it could have been more innovative, but was in no way clear about what form such innovation might have taken. (The problem was that raised by Dwight Macdonald in his writings—and also by many survivors in their talks with me—about the difficulty conveying the revolutionary nature of the weapon, whether through documentary realism or any other method.) Mainly I felt great satisfaction in having my Hiroshima work translated with such skill and compassion into another medium, and done in a way that could bring about a broader awareness of that city. The film was shown in England and throughout Europe on August 6, 1975, as originally planned. It received considerable notice and on the whole very favorable reviews.

But somehow nothing was happening in connection with the film in America. BBC had a regular distributor in this country, Time Life Films, and when BJ and I made inquiries to them the answer we got was that American public television did not seem interested. It turned out that the distributor was doing little, if any, distributing. When BJ and I arranged a preview showing at the Museum of Modern Art, the Time Life people initially agreed to it but called me the night before to tell me that it had to be canceled, saying that the preview would somehow interfere with distribution in this country. I became incensed, told the caller that we would in no way cancel the film, that we would take every legal action necessary, and that I would be in touch with various people at BBC and Time Life in connection with such an outrageous demand. I did call everyone I could in both organizations, Time Life finally backed down, and we had a successful preview showing.

We were told that Time Life had behaved similarly in connection with a film critical of nuclear power, so that either that issue or political discomfort about telling Hiroshima truths could have been the source of their attitude with our film. BJ and I did some of the work of the distributor by contacting people in American public television, within which the Eastern Educational Network took on the film and helped arrange for it to be shown throughout the country. We then had a similar struggle with Time Life over not putting the film in their catalogue to make it available on campuses and elsewhere. But at some point BBC, for whatever reasons, arranged to turn over the film to a differrent American distributor.

Vas wrote warm letters of encouragement throughout the struggle with Time Life Films, and an upbeat cablegram before the Museum of Modern

Art preview. But in other correspondence he mentioned "ups and downs" with BBC and with other groups concerning his films in general. He also reflected on the power of his Hiroshima experience and the impact on him of the *hibakusha:* "The trip was one of the most important events in my life; I begin to feel the weight only now. You were right: Japan pulls you back. And Hiroshima moves you more and more fundamentally." He went on to say that he had brought back with him "a piece of burned stone, from the [A-bomb] Dome building" and that "I have it before me on my writing table, never out of sight." Those and related thoughts were interspersed with our correspondence about American reviews, which we agreed were favorable but rarely thoughtful or profound.

After a year of being mostly out of touch, Vas wrote me about a new film he would be making on the abuse of psychiatry in the Soviet Union, saying that he had learned I was publicly involved in the issue and asked to interview me. I enthusiastically agreed, and both of us expressed pleasure at the prospect of being with one another again. But a couple of weeks later I received a letter from a BBC assistant telling me that Vas was "unwell at present and may be away for some time," and then that the film project had been "temporarily suspended." When I telephoned an acquaintance at BBC I learned that Vas had killed himself, although no one seemed to know the details.

I had always worried about Robert's psychological state, but had never heard him speak of suicide and had no sense of that as a possibility. I berated myself for not having picked up clues and for not having offered more understanding and support. I thought especially of his agitation when it was suggested by people at BBC that the film be shortened, and of my having agreed with that suggestion. Perhaps I had been blinded to his condition by the warmth of our friendship and by his energy and talent as a filmmaker. The shock and pain BJ and I experienced were accompanied by a kind of anger. How could he do this—to us and to everyone else? In an essay I dedicated to his memory I spoke of Vas as "a Hungarian Jew who had known too many persecutions and dislocations" and "an artist able to infuse his work with his own survivor sensibility [who] made a brilliant film on Hiroshima and a year later killed himself."

Over the years I have thought more about Robert's suicide. Born in 1931, he was a teenager during the Nazi occupation of Hungary. I do not know the details of his suffering or of murdered family members, but it is likely that he was left with the kind of reservoir of despair I have encountered in many Holocaust survivors, which made them especially vulnerable to new threats or losses. I thought of Primo Levi, who wrote about Auschwitz as wisely as any survivor ever has, but killed himself at the age of sixty-eight soon after the death of his mother, who was then in her nineties. Vas had managed a second survival, that of the Soviet occupation and failed Hungarian uprising of 1956. Like Levi he was able to bring considerable survivor wisdom to his work, including films about the Holocaust and about Soviet oppression and the life of Stalin. (He also made documentaries on the German-American conductor Bruno Walter, the German playwright Bertolt Brecht, and the American comedians Laurel and Hardy.)

The part played by his immersion in Hiroshima must remain uncertain. But I cannot help remembering his reflections on the "weight" of that city on him and his keeping "a piece of burned stone" from the A-bomb dome on his desk, "never out of sight." Hiroshima seemed to become for him another tortured survivor experience, in confronting both its death-dominated content and its impossible demands on artistic form. Making the film, then, could have been a trigger mechanism for someone who carried so much potential despair in him. While suicide leaves a terrible legacy with family members and friends, it can also be a form of self-assertion, a solution to an insoluble life, a paradoxical quest for a future.

I too have felt the weight of Hiroshima. Like Vas, I had to immerse myself in death-haunted details of what happened there in order to tell a version of its story. But I did not go there with his legacy of painful survivals. I did not carry Vas's heavy load of sustained and repeated terror. In working in Hiroshima I could, perhaps more than Vas, permit myself the protection of selective professional numbing. In my work in general, I became aware of what I called pacing myself, both actively plunging into, and in some degree holding back from, the devastating events I studied. And I have been able to draw upon currents of hope and renewal in the lives of many survivors in their mission of atomic bomb witness. Yet none of that means I emerged unscathed from Hiroshima. While I have not responded with deep pessimism or despair, it has left me with persistent images of great suffering and of world destruction. Over time I found ways to transform these feelings and images into interpretive narratives. Vas seemed to be doing that with his films, but could not overcome his inner accumulation of twentieth-century survivor pain, or prevent its reactivation by Hiroshima.

Scholarship and Activism—and a Caring Friend

Death in Life contributed to the antinuclear movement as a scholarly text. But by the time it was published (in 1968) I myself had plunged deeply into a more activist mode in opposing both nuclear weapons and the Vietnam War. I became one of the more visible participants in protest on the Yale faculty. It was a relatively early phase in what was to become an unending struggle to achieve balance between scholarship and activism. Then I received some advice from a dying friend that put the issue in stark perspective.

Mary Wright had come to Yale with her husband, Arthur, a year or two before I had. They had both been students of John Fairbank, and were asked to rejuvenate Asian studies at Yale, which they surely did, though both were to die too young. Arthur was a mild-mannered man and a renowned scholar of Chinese Buddhism. Mary, a historian of modern China whose work had more bearing on my own, had opposite qualities: she was fiery, blunt, and outspoken in her insistence that we look realistically at the achievements of the Chinese Communists. Mary and Arthur were very welcoming to BJ and myself, and soon became part of a faculty discussion group that BJ and I founded. Both Mary and Arthur read in manuscript and gave me advice on my second book on China, *Revolutionary Immortality*.

But in 1970 Mary developed a rapidly growing lung cancer. When her illness was at an advanced stage, she asked me to come to see her. I remember thinking at the time that she wished to talk to me, as someone whose work had much to do with death, about her own closeness to death.

That was in no way the case. I had underestimated Mary. When I sat down with her in her comfortable living room overlooking Long Island Sound, she seemed thin and weak but greeted me with her usual intensity. Never one for small talk, she quickly got to the point. She said something like: "I know how intensely committed you are to your political protest against the Vietnam War and against nuclear weapons. I agree with your position on all of these matters and I admire your actions. But I want to point out to you very strongly that if you had done nothing but protest, you could not have written *Death in Life*. And writing that book and others like it has much more importance for the world, and much more influence in the directions you desire, than does any political action you may take. I just wanted to tell you how I feel about this." We talked a little more about politics, work, books, and what lasts. It was clear that Mary did not want to discuss her illness at all. She was handling that quietly and stoically. It was hard for me to find the words with which to respond and thank her—I hope she understood the depth of my gratitude. I told her I would take her advice very seriously, and I have.

I was stunned by Mary's act. That soul-stirring encounter reverberated in me much more than any theoretical argument. I've always known that I am primarily a researcher and writer of books. But Mary gave new clarity to that realization. I would continue to be an activist, but would remember Mary's cautionary words, along with her generosity and courage. What came next made that conversation with Mary all the more important.

Part Three

_____

Vietnam and the Sixties

10

Responding to Slaughter

Saigon Truths

BJ and I have always said that we were against the Vietnam War before it began. It all goes back to a scene in a Saigon café in 1954. We had flown to South Vietnam from Hong Kong, she as a journalist writing about what was going on in Indochina, and I as just a traveler taking time off from my research on thought reform. We were talking to a group of French correspondents and administrators, most of them about to leave. Earlier that year the French had been defeated at Dien Bien Phu, and BJ had been in Hanoi with other journalists when the forces of Ho Chi Minh (who were then called the Viet Minh) marched triumphantly back into their old capital. The Frenchmen at our table said such things as "You'll see what will happen. This country is nothing but quicksand. You'll make the same mistake. What happened to us will happen to you."

I was taken aback by this European cynicism and did not know how to respond. I had no illusions about American virtue. I knew that the extremity of American fear of communism could lead to disastrous policies, but still hoped that the procolonial actions of the Truman and Eisenhower administrations were a temporary aberration. I had a lot to learn.

We revisited Vietnam thirteen years later, after my research on Japanese youth and on Hiroshima, as well as some years of work on *Death in Life*. During the early and mid-sixties the euphemism of American "advisors" in Vietnam had given way to repeated escalations. There were increasing reports of American missteps, confusions, and then atrocities. In the process Vietnam changed in American consciousness from a background rumble to a foreground obsession. The country as a whole had not yet turned against the war, but divisions were becoming increasingly bitter.

For me all that took place in Vietnam was inseparable from Hiroshima. Indeed, by the time we made that 1967 visit to Vietnam, there had not only been major escalations in the war but considerable talk of a possible American use of a nuclear weapon. Early student protestors had made a similar nuclear emphasis, as suggested by words used in the 1962 "Port Huron Statement" inaugurating Students for a Democratic Society: "Our work is guided by the sense that we may be the last generation in the experiment with living."

We were in Japan in early 1967 for follow-up interviews I was conducting with Japanese youth, and I thought that a visit to Vietnam could teach me a great deal about what America was doing in that country—or, as I put it to friends in a lame joke, "provide ammunition for my antiwar position." When we got there, BJ and I had our division of labor, undoubtedly reflecting our comparative courage. She went north in the direction of the fighting, seeking information about casualties in children for a book she was writing. I stayed in Saigon for discussions with Vietnamese intellectuals and resident Americans.

I had no trouble finding articulate people to talk to. Educated Vietnamese, who were supposed to be on our side, were eager to tell me about everything wrong with the American presence in Vietnam, as were non-official Americans such as journalists and civilian employees of the military. And as for official American spokesmen, one of them in the embassy spoke to me in what came close to Orwellian "Newspeak": endless stalemate was "victory," psychological and moral disintegration was "progress." I thought of the words of the French Cassandras we had met in the same city thirteen years before who told us that America would make "the same mistake" as the French. But it was even worse than that. Vietnamese went on to tell me how the American presence deepened rather than resolved their dilemmas, how it interfered with needed democratic change and divested them of their autonomy. "This is not [any longer] our country," was the way one of them put it to me. And about the communist Viet Minh, he added: "We are against their terror but we understand them, and consider many of them patriots."

An especially revealing moment occurred at a small dinner party at the home of a young Vietnamese doctor. After a pleasant meal and much discussion of Vietnamese and American problems, the host brought out a violin, played a little Beethoven, and then launched into twentieth-century rhythms that sounded like romantic marching tunes. "Those were a couple of songs I used to play when I was with the Viet Minh," he explained. It turned out that he had spent several years with them as a physician and had even on occasion treated General Vo Nguyen Giap, a mythic figure second only to Ho Chi Minh in the Vietnamese communist pantheon. He muttered something about having left the movement for family considerations, but what he clearly wanted to convey was its profound appeal as contrasted with the deadening political confusions of the official government in the South.

Among my American encounters, some of the most grotesque involved ostensible applications of psychology and social science. For instance, an embassy official told me that the problem with the Vietnamese was that they "needed a father figure," which, presumably, Americans were to provide. I noted that to be "a vulgarism impressive in its psychological, historical, and moral reach." And I talked with a political scientist, a man of high academic reputation but a supporter of the war with close governmental ties, who told me that he was there to conduct large-scale research on "attitudes"—in the case of villagers in response to the installation of television sets by his research team for experimental purposes. I thought of Graham Greene's lethally naïve "Quiet American"—but called him instead the "Numbed American." Listening to him intensified my strongly developing interest in misbehavior of professionals in serving destructive projects.

I was relieved to find BJ fully intact when she rejoined me in Saigon. (Just a few months after we left, the early 1968 "Tet Offensive" of the North Vietnamese and the Viet Minh revealed how dangerous things really were in Vietnam when they succeeded in penetrating supposedly secure American bases everywhere, providing dramatic evidence of the futility of our entire military intervention.) BJ had succeeded in getting not only useful material for her book but also evidence that, even in Vietnam, American humor was not dead. Concerned about safety, she had asked a black GI she met about the degree of danger in that area. His answer: "It's a little worse than 110th Street but not as bad as 155th Street."

My Lai and the "Atrocity-Producing Situation"

But it was the revelation of the My Lai Massacre that really got to me. In November 1969, while on an airplane from New York to Toronto (where I was to give a talk on psychohistory and do a radio broadcast on nuclear weapons), I picked up a *New York Times* and read about how in a small Vietnamese village American soldiers had slaughtered about five hundred civilians over the course of a single morning. Mixed with my anger and outrage was a feeling of shame—the slaughter was carried out by my own country—and a more personal sense of having failed to take stronger action in opposing the war.

Two years before, there had been a "Call to Resist Illegitimate Authority," the signers of which pledged themselves to aggressive forms of civil disobedience that could lead to considerable legal culpability, as it did in connection with the burning of draft cards. Thousands of Americans signed the call, including a number of people I knew, but I did not. I'm not entirely clear about the reasons for my failure to sign, but I do remember great concern about the possibility of spending time in prison. I partly had my family obligations in mind, but the simple truth of the matter was that I was not yet ready for the potential sacrifice that such civil disobedience could entail. The slaughter at My Lai made such reluctance seem cowardly, and I wanted to call on new energies to oppose such slaughter and compensate for that earlier failure.

Soon after returning from Toronto I rearranged the papers on my desk—relegating the extensive materials having to do with *The Broken Connection* to a rear table, and placing front and center my chaotic but growing body of notes, clippings, and articles on the Vietnam War. I was changing course, on my desk and in my mind. I was telling myself that any research and writing I now embarked on had to be directed toward exposing truths about the war in the service of opposition. The activist tail was wagging the scholar dog, even if that dog insisted on carefully probing psychological and historical evidence. I was groping for ways of expressing, in my work and in my life, deeper opposition to what America was doing and becoming.

The sequence involved for me consisted of first outrage, then research to deepen knowledge, and then protest in the form of writing and action. Learning more about My Lai led me to my concept of the "atrocity-producing situation." What I meant by that term was an environment so structured, both militarily and psychologically, that an average person— "no better or worse than you or me," as I was fond of putting it—upon entering it, could be capable of committing atrocities. In Vietnam the military structure included a counterinsurgency war in a far-off, alien environment, involving a nonwhite culture, in which it was often impossible to differentiate enemy combatants from civilians; and military policies such as "body counts," "free fire zones," and "search-and-destroy missions." For the men, psychological responses could combine fear and helplessness, angry grief in response to the deaths of buddies, and hunger for an enemy as a target for revenge.

A few months after the revelation of My Lai, I heard of a soldier who had been there, had refused to fire, and had spoken publicly about the massacre. I eagerly sought him out, knowing that he could deepen my interpretive grasp of what happened in that village and what was happening in the war in general. During eight hours of interviews over two days, he did not disappoint me. As we talked quietly in the anonymous but brightly lit and comfortable New York City hotel room I rented for our interviews (he could best meet me in New York and I had not yet moved there from New Haven), I could join him in the menacingly amorphous landscape he described: "You have the illusion of going great distances and traveling like hundreds of miles, and you end up in the same place. But you feel like it's not all real." And experience with him the confusion about "the enemy": "No matter how much effort you put into it . . . [y]ou can't lay your hands on him. And the fact is that he might be anywhere . . . as though you are hunting a specific deer and you don't know which one it is and there's a deer herd all over you."

He explained further that with the company experiencing heavy losses, the men yearned for revenge and began to imagine "wiping the whole place out—the Indian idea that the only good gook is a dead gook." Then came the climactic emotional moment of the massacre: the funeral ceremony the night before held for a man named Sergeant George Cox, an older soldier with extensive war experience who played a special part in the company as an advisor and leader, a kind of father figure to the men. Sergeant Cox had been blown to bits by a land mine. I could be there listening to the company commander's fervent eulogy in which he described the virtues of the fallen sergeant and the company's task of carrying out his unfinished work. Then came the connection between angry grief and military exhortation: "Here's our chance to get back at them. There are no innocent civilians in this area." Sergeant Cox's death and eulogy, the American My Lai survivor told me, were a breaking point.

Now the men were given "more or less permission to gun down everyone and everything, sort of like, you can do it." In that way his words took me inside the My Lai dynamic as one of a fierce survivor mission of slaughter. He emphasized that the men did their killing while kneeling in a combat position, "like some kind of firefight [combat exchange]." But "if you're actually thinking in terms of a massacre or murder . . . shooting a bunch of defenseless people, why crouch?" He answered his own question: "Because your judgment is all screwed up. They actually look like the enemy, or what you think is the enemy." He was saying, in effect, that the men momentarily experienced an illusion that, in gunning down babies and old men and women, they had finally engaged the enemy, had finally got him to stand up and fight. In its entire structure—its combination of unrestrained military policy, enraged grief, and exhortation and release—My Lai was the quintessential atrocity-producing situation.

Listening to the My Lai survivor, I became a spectator in the grotesque scene of that atrocity. In slaughtering civilians, the men were attempting to bear witness to the deaths of their buddies, but it was a false witness because their victims were in no way the cause of those deaths. In telling the story, the My Lai survivor was bearing authentic witness to the entire atrocity. So part of the tableau he created for me included him as neither kneeling nor crouching in combat style but instead standing and pointing the barrel of his gun to the ground. I later learned that he was heard muttering during the killing, "It's wrong, it's wrong." He extended his witness by providing details of the slaughter to a former member of his unit who had not been at My Lai but put together information about it to make it known to American journalists and the American public.

Still, the My Lai survivor did not escape feelings of guilt in relation to the event, both because he recognized in himself some of the murderous emotions of the other men, and because he had not interfered with their actions. (A helicopter pilot from outside the company did help stop the killing by threatening to turn his guns on his fellow Americans if they did not cease shooting, a threat that would have been much harder for the My Lai survivor to make while himself in the middle of things.) As he put it: "There's no way I can feel that I was separate from the whole thing, especially when I didn't do anything to stop it myself. You feel sort of responsible, a part of it." So he was uneasy when publicly lionized, on at least one occasion fleeing from a ceremony at which he was to be presented with an award: "They think I must be a martyred Jesus or else a communist subversive, one or the other. Right? No, wrong!"

Yet he had shown courage and restraint in overcoming an atrocity-producing situation and helping to expose it, and I believed it important to probe the psychological sources of that courage and restraint. After hours of interviewing, I came to recognize three significant influences that played a part. The first was his early Catholic training that instilled in him a sense of the sacredness of life and contributed to his sensitive conscience, which he retained despite his subsequent break with the church. A second factor was his tendency to be a loner, to engage in individual activities such as boating and fishing rather than team sports, making him less susceptible than others to group attitudes such as the racism and hatred for Vietnamese prevailing in his company. But it was the third influence that I found completely unexpected and a little disconcerting. The My Lai survivor enlisted in the Army at a time when he was entirely at loose ends in his life: he had no clear goals, was drinking heavily, and in the process of flunking out of college. In the Army he suddenly found himself, excelled at every training exercise, was rewarded by quick promotions, and was enthusiastic about making the military his career. But what he encountered in Vietnam, and particularly at My Lai, shockingly violated his military idealism, his sense of what a true soldier did and did not do. That military identification was clearly the strongest source of his defiance of the atrocity-producing situation.

That gave me pause because I had always tended to associate military identification with belligerent war-making. At the same time I was fascinated by a discovery that called into question my prior assumptions and required me to look further into the phenomenon of military idealism.

Military Doves

I learned much about the phenomenon from a visit I made toward the end of the Vietnam War to the Virginia Military Institute (VMI), the oldest state-supported military college in the country, and frequently called the "West Point of the South." I was asked to have informal exchange with students, give one public lecture, and then have a debate with the other weekend guest, Walt Rostow, perhaps the leading academic-turned-government spokesman for war-making and escalation in Vietnam. I was intrigued by the invitation but also a little nervous about how my strongly antiwar sentiments would play in that environment.

Moments after my arrival at the VMI campus in Lexington, I knew that everything would be fine. A cadet-guide greeted me with a stiff salute, introduced himself, and declared in a kind of military cadence: "*Sir*, you'll find that we are mostly *doves* here, *sir!*" Once I came down from my euphoric Alice-in-Wonderland feeling, I could confirm the accuracy of his assessment. The cadets in general responded to my efforts at combining hard-hitting opposition to the war with reasoned argument. Then came the main event, the debate with Rostow. As I strolled leisurely through the lushly flowered southern campus on my way to the chapel where the debate was to be held, two cadets ran up to me, gave their robotlike salutes, and one of them, an African-American, shouted his message: "*Sir*, we've been discussing both of you in the barracks and we wanted to tell you that we hope you'll *annihilate* him, *sir!*" I was no longer surprised by such militarized dovishness, but I had to smile at the violent imagery in its service.

Entering the sacred space of the large chapel, I was confronted by a huge, and hugely bloody, painting depicting, it was explained to me, the martyrdom of a heroic contingent of southern student volunteers wiped out by Union forces. Despite the backdrop, the debate seemed to go well. I was energized by the situation, while Rostow seemed tired and dispirited, unenthusiastic about defending a war already lost, somewhat weary of the whole enterprise. I felt myself an angry David holding his own with, if not slaying, a fatigued Goliath. Faculty members later explained to me that there was great disillusionment with the military among the students because of its part in the Vietnam War. A large number of them had decided simply to serve their required three years as military cadets and then apply their training as engineers to civilian pursuits.

A group of "antinuclear admirals" were to deepen my understanding of military idealism when, during the early eighties, they formed the influential Center for Defense Information. I had a particularly enlightening conversation with one of them. He was a very courteous, conservative southerner who drove me in his late-model luxury car from Washington, D.C., to a conference on nuclear weapons in Virginia, looking and acting like a true pillar of American society. I asked him how, as a professional military man, he had come to his antinuclear position. That was entirely the point, he told me. He'd come from a family steeped in military tradition and above all in principles of military honor. Ingrained in him especially were two basic principles: defending one's country rather than attacking others, and always being committed in one's military actions to causing minimal loss of life. Nuclear weapons, he explained, rendered both of these principles impossible to live up to.

The founder of the center, Gene LaRocque, had been horrified when serving in the Pentagon and discovering that many in high places advocated a preventive nuclear strike against the Soviet Union. And later, when captain of a ship carrying guided nuclear missiles, he became deeply troubled by his own situation: "I could fire those weapons at any time. I had no instructions that said I couldn't." His resignation from the military had been precipitated by the wasted lives of the Vietnam War: "I hate it when they say, 'He gave his life for his country.' . . . We steal the lives of these kids." Like the My Lai survivor, these antinuclear admirals could call upon their military honor to bear witness to military behavior violating that honor.

My Lai in Washington

The revelation of My Lai resulted in my being invited for a series of appearances in Washington in which I could bring my interpretive psychological position on the war to members of Congress and others. Perhaps the most important of these was my testimony in January 1970 before the Senate Committee on Veterans' Affairs, then headed by Senator Alan Cranston of California. I had met Cranston socially the previous summer and liked his soft-spoken progressive views, and his policy of combining in his hearings support for veterans' health and educational benefits with opposition to the war. He arranged for his staff to schedule my testimony about "the psychological predicament of the Vietnam veteran."

In both my written statement and spoken remarks I spoke sympathetically of the soldier-survivor's deep confusion and terror in a counterinsurgency war, of his "impulse toward revenge, toward overcoming his own emotional conflicts and giving meaning to his buddies' sacrifices by getting back at the enemy." I mentioned the collective experience of an "advanced state of psychic numbing" and of "general brutalization," along with an ultimate feeling that the war may have no justification. I combined my psychological observations with an antiwar position, insisting that "we cannot separate the larger historical contradictions surrounding the American involvement in Vietnam from the individual-psychological responses of our soldiers," and that "if we are really concerned about the psychological and spiritual health of America's young men—and indeed about our own as well—we will cease victimizing and brutalizing them in this war."

When I finished reading my statement I remember Cranston smiling uneasily and saying something like "Those are pretty strong words," suggesting that he didn't disagree with what I said but felt it to be a bit outspoken for his sense of senatorial decorum. There were a couple of Republican senators at the hearing who challenged my observations by raising the question of how representative the veterans I talked to were of Vietnam veterans in general. Others were to raise similar questions about my work on the war. I tried to answer candidly by saying that I had nothing on the order of a systematic sample but mentioned the work of the historian Murray Polner, who had interviewed more than two hundred Vietnam veterans of very diverse views and concluded that "not one of them—hawk, dove, or haunted—was entirely free of doubt about the nature of the war and the American role in it" or free of the "gnawing suspicion that 'It was all for nothing.'" The hearing hardly made a dramatic public impact. But a few newspaper accounts quoted from my testimony, and among the handful of letters I received I particularly valued one from an Army captain who, as a defense counsel for soldiers, told of frequently encountering precisely the kinds of reactions I had described.

I was also introduced to the phenomenon of the congressional conference as a forum created by legislative critics of existing policies, at which professionals from the outside were invited to provide intellectual backing for that opposition. It was important that such conferences occurred, and they did bring strong antiwar sentiments to a Washington atmosphere that was long on posturing and short on concrete approaches to ending the war. The conferences dealing with Vietnam were sponsored by antiwar legislators: senators such as J. William Fulbright, Edward Kennedy, and Eugene McCarthy; and congressmen like John Conyers, George Brown, and Robert Kastenmeier.

The best of those congressional conferences I attended was one on War and National Responsibility, held on February 20–21, 1970, whose boldly declared purpose was "to publicly examine the full implications of American activities in Vietnam including—but not limited to—My Lai, treatment of prisoners of war, bombing of civilian areas, use of herbicides and chemical gases, Operation Phoenix [assassination of designated communist leaders in villages], and programs such as 'pacification,' 'search and destroy,' and 'forcible resettlement of civilian population.'" Present were many prominent intellectuals who opposed the war, including Telford Taylor, who could invoke his experience as chief American counsel at the Nuremberg trials to question the legitimacy of the war, and the political scientist Hans Morgenthau, who could document its disastrous effect on America's international standing. I referred to the widespread sense among Americans that the war was "not only brutal but ultimately absurd," and referred to the young in particular as feeling "betrayed and victimized—by the war, by our political leaders, by the older generation, and by our society in general." And, emphasizing the danger of using nuclear weapons in Vietnam, I brought Hiroshima into the debate and urged that we examine further what the use of those weapons in that city did to human beings. With Taylor I stressed the importance of the Nuremberg trials (though I was eight years away from my study of Nazi doctors) and supported his insistence that "people be critical within their own professions." At that conference as in talks I was giving, I emphasized the dubious role of doctors especially in the war, trying to put forward my increasing preoccupation with how professionals in general were behaving—and how they should behave—in connection with their country's murderous actions.

I have a poignant memory of a Washington trip involving a less public encounter with Senator Fulbright at a small luncheon arranged by a medical friend of his who wanted to put him in touch with kindred spirits. Fulbright was warm, and responsive to my ideas about the war and to the possibility of my participating in various congressional events. But he also seemed a bit depressed, even despairing, as he bemoaned the continuing destructiveness of the war and, more personally, the relentless attacks he was experiencing from political leaders as well as constituents for his antiwar statements and actions. I realized, perhaps for the first time, how painful it can be for a prominent leader to buck the American political tide, especially in connection with a war. I felt a strong wave of compassion for him, and at the end of the lunch as we walked away from the dining room I surprised myself by putting my arm around his shoulders and saying: "Please remember, Senator Fulbright, that many people deeply appreciate what you are doing. We need you to be strong and we'll do anything we can to help." I don't know whether my words had any effect but he did nod appreciatively at me. Looking back I believe I was speaking to him not as a scholar, as a psychiatrist, or even as an activist, but simply as a fellow American who was moved by what one brave man was doing.

11

———

Existential Evil

Among many short pieces that I wrote on Vietnam, the most significant for me was a review essay in the *New York Times Book Review* on June 14, 1970, on two books on My Lai: *My Lai 4*, by Seymour Hersh, and *One Morning in the War*, by Richard Hammer. It was the most overtly polemical of my essays. I was still the psychologist but one with raw feelings. I spoke of our country as entering a realm of "existential evil" and carried my analysis of complicity upwards to generals, the secretary of defense, and the president himself. And I agreed with a GI quoted as saying that what happened at My Lai was "just like a Nazi-type thing."

But as unsparing as I was about my country, I insisted that it was capable of better: "When I talk to students about My Lai, some simply shrug and say, 'What can you expect?' From the war, they mean—but also, from America. I, for one, enraged as I am . . . still expect more . . . [and] think the young really expect more from America too, as they are showing in their vast effort they are leading to turn the country around, to demonstrate, above all to themselves, that there is more to America than My Lai."

In that essay, more than in any other before or since, I was able to find a far-reaching mainstream outlet for an angry and radical psychological statement on the war. I did write additional pieces for op-ed columns in the *Times*, the *Boston Globe*, and other newspapers, including one titled

"Have Americans Become Murderers?" which was published both in the *Baltimore Sun* and the *Yale Alumni News*. I kept a diary of the events of the "Moratorium" in Washington, D.C., in 1969, which I published as "Death Power" in *Esquire* magazine. I put these views forward in an inter-term lectureship at the University of Hawaii in January 1971, dedicating the series to Daniel Ellsberg, who had recently released the Pentagon Papers.

I had many exchanges with other antiwar activists. Fred Branfman wrote to me about his invaluable observations on the air war in Laos, on the technological distancing of pilots and aircrews from the consequences of their actions. Helicopter pilots were in the thick of combat and had psychological responses similar to those of soldiers on the ground. Medium bomber pilots could only see tiny distant figures on the ground, while heavy bomber pilots saw nothing below and flew and bombed completely by instruments; both required acts of imagination to experience the consequences of their actions. When he mentioned his psychological pain in doing the work, I sent him a book of bird cartoons, telling him that they helped keep me sane and "might do a bit of that for you also." I also wrote to an Air Force brigadier general, Irby B. Jarvis, Jr., on behalf of a young doctor, Bruce Ashley, who had refused Air Force orders to go to Vietnam and declared himself a conscientious objector. My plea, quite predictably, had no effect. But it was part of my effort to mobilize whatever energies I could for combating the existential evil.

Crimes of War

That evil was to be epitomized by what were called "crimes of war." The strongest public expressions against those crimes came from leaders of two general constituencies: the antiwar veterans and the Catholic left. The government came down particularly hard on these two groups, went to great pains to infiltrate and dishonor them, because it sensed their moral authority. Compared to professors like myself, whose national influence was, to say the least, limited, protesting veterans and priests could have powerful reverberations throughout American society. Veterans had the authority of personal military sacrifice and direct experience of the war; priests had the authority of religious conscience. The FBI conducted its own war on such veterans and priests, and I was able to participate in two of the trials mounted against them for "conspiracy" against the United States government.

Prior to the trials, I began to appear on platforms with antiwar veterans, one of them in December 1970 as part of the "National Veterans' Inquiry into U.S. War Crimes Policy." It turned out to be a warm-up for the celebrated "Winter Soldier hearings" held in Detroit a few months later, a powerful occasion for what could be called angry confessions of participation in war crimes. There was little mention of God or Christianity in these confessions, but I believe they had a religious quality, both in their condemnation of the evil of the war and in their implicit quest for redemption. While I did little more than point to the psychological forces of the behavior they described, I felt that I was facilitating—and in a sense affirming—their quest. In the process, the crimes described penetrated my own imagination ever more powerfully and thereby contributed to various levels of my "radicalization." They had something of the same impact on the whole society, as images of the event were widely disseminated, culminating in a powerful documentary film.

The veterans' trial with which I was most closely associated was that of the "Gainesville Eight," members of Vietnam Veterans Against the War (VVAW) accused of conspiracy to obstruct the 1972 Republican National Convention in Miami Beach, Florida. "We pled 'not guilty' to conspiracy, but guilty of war crimes in South East Asia," was the way that the defendants understood their trial. I spent several days with the accused men in Gainesville, interviewing a few of them in detail in order to be able to testify about their specific motives in protesting at the convention. But I was never to give my testimony, this time because the judge so charged the jury that they were able to acquit the accused men on all counts without requiring a defense. That was so because FBI informants infiltrating the VVAW—and especially one agent provocateur—were the ones responsible for planning and carrying out the militant actions of the "conspiracy." It turned out that the Nixon administration's preoccupation with these antiwar veterans was related to its Watergate crimes; in both cases the Nixon White House was engaging in illegal actions in seeking evidence of collusion between veterans and the Democratic National Committee in an alleged conspiracy to interrupt the Republican convention. I did not understand that at the time, but I did have a sense of being in the middle of a version of the administration's "dirty tricks."

In my involvement in a conspiracy trial of the Catholic left, I had a still more satisfying experience. The "Camden 28" was a group of Catholic priests and laymen (with one Lutheran minister) who had broken into a government office in that New Jersey city in August 1971 and removed and destroyed draft files, resulting in a trial that was much trumpeted by then FBI director J. Edgar Hoover and Attorney General John Mitchell. The defendants had been inspired by the Berrigan brothers and emphasized "the burning of children" and other American crimes in Vietnam. Their charge of conspiracy against the Selective Service program and destruction of government property could have resulted in prison sentences of more than forty years.

But in entering the courtroom in the spring of 1973 I was astounded by the friendly atmosphere I encountered. The judge treated the defendants with respect, permitted them to explain the reasons for their act of protest, and responded sympathetically to their argument for the relevance of my testimony. He encouraged me to speak at length about war crimes and their importance for motivating protest, and about struggles with conscience on the part of many Americans. I did this in tandem with a priest-defendant who questioned me sensitively, my testimony blending with that of other expert witnesses (notably Howard Zinn on civil disobedience in American history). I had the sense that the narrative I offered entered more directly into the judicial process than in any other case in which I participated.

The courtroom atmosphere was undoubtedly influenced by the shift in American sentiment against the war and by the Watergate scandal, but the judge himself, a man named Clarkson Fisher, played a very large part, and interviews he later gave suggested that the defendants had prodded his own Catholic conscience. Also affecting him and everyone else in the trial was another bizarre informant situation, in this case involving a Catholic layman and friend of several defendants who was a professional handyman and took the lead in planning and carrying out many of the mechanical details of the break-in. He then reported his friends to the FBI, but had a change of heart during the trial and decided to go over to the defendants' side and confessed everything about his role as an agent provocateur. (I would come to see this man as exemplifying the phenomenon of "doubling" that I was later to describe in connection with my work on Nazi doctors.) Again, the judge's charge to the jury encouraged its decision for complete acquittal.

I could share with the defendants a rare sense of triumph, and in my exuberance following my testimony I invited two of them, young priests, to join me and my family at a Passover Seder at our New York apartment, probably the only Seder that BJ and I ever organized. Still high from the trial, the two priests and I delighted in our improvised riffs on resistance and liberation, as encouraged by the progressive Passover Haggadah we were using. (That was a far cry from the Seders I had experienced as a young boy at my maternal grandparents' home, conducted rotely in a language I could not understand, whose only redeeming feature for me was the children's game of finding the hidden matzo and then receiving a few coins as a reward [Hanukkah gelt].) But as BJ and I fumbled over unfamiliar details of foods and recitations, our guests politely asked to take a look at the English Haggadah text, and proceeded to plunge seamlessly into the sequence of the ceremony. As priests, their organic feeling for ritual contrasted with my own awkward rendering of what was supposed to be part of my own tradition—so much so that our ten-year-old son Ken commented, "They seem to know the book better than you do, Dad."

The American Friends Service Committee—the Quakers—also seized upon American crimes of war in a way that drew me further into the issue and led to a specific product. Stewart Meacham, a leading spirit in their efforts, called a conference in late 1970 on American war crimes, which included Richard Fernandez, then head of Clergy and Laymen Concerned About Vietnam, and Francine du Plessix Gray, the writer and sympathetic chronicler of the Catholic left. Also present were Richard Falk and the historian Gabriel Kolko, both scholar activists. Somehow, Richard, Gabriel, and I came out of the meeting agreeing to create a volume, *Crimes of War.* That result stemmed from the Quakers' insidious talent for turning one's individual conscience into a kind of friendly bully. Their persuasive power derived greatly from their own example of conscience-driven dedication to confronting Vietnam truths. Their choice of the three of us as objects of their persuasive power had a certain cunning, as they recognized that we were in a position to bring reputable scholarship to radical opposition to the war. Actually they did us a favor in evoking (in Abraham Lincoln's term) our better angels, so that we ended up creating not only the volume but a sponsoring group called the Education/Action Conference on U.S. Crimes of War in Vietnam to be the recipient of the book's modest royalties. Our edited volume, *Crimes of War*, had a legal section (Falk's), a political one (Kolko's), and a psychological and ethical one (my own). In my section, I included writings of Daniel Berrigan, the playwright Arthur Miller, the military psychiatrist turned protestor Gordon Livingston, the German philosopher Karl Jaspers, the political theorist Hannah Arendt, the Auschwitz survivor-writer Tadeusz Borowski, Erik Erikson, Kurt Vonnegut, and Jean-Paul Sartre.

I realize now that I was bringing to this focus on crimes of war my own nondoctrinal religiosity. Crimes suggest evil, a term I found myself increasingly making use of. For me such evil is specifically human and in no way related to the supernatural, but there is something about my passion in combating it that found kinship with religious people, particularly members of the Catholic left and the Society of Friends. We shared not just a conviction to oppose mass killing but the kind of intense individual conscience that derives from a larger spiritual affiliation with (however amorphously) humankind.

Vets and Shrinks

In late November of 1970, I found myself sitting in a small dingy room in the lower Manhattan headquarters of the New York chapter of Vietnam Veterans Against the War, together with Jan Crumb, cofounder and national president of the organization; two other VVAW leaders; and Chaim Shatan, a psychoanalyst and fellow activist who was about my age. The meeting had come about through a letter Jan wrote to me in which he sought to engage me in "two perhaps separate projects which we are trying to bring together as one"—providing help for "the severe psychological problems of many Vietnam veterans because of their experiences," and at the same time combating "the military policy of the war which results in war crimes and veterans' nightmares." He wrote to me because he had read my Cranston committee testimony and was familiar with my antiwar position and my earlier Hiroshima book. Then in his late twenties, Jan had turned his back on a military career and resigned from West Point to become an antiwar voice.

His letter could not have been more welcome, as I was being asked to combine professional knowledge with antiwar advocacy. A soft-spoken man with fire underneath, Jan told us how veterans intensely "rapped" with one another about the war, their lives, and their conflicts with American society, and often felt that they would like to have people around with greater psychological knowledge. He told me how Vietnam veterans in general felt badly treated by their society in having been sent to fight a dubious war, looked on suspiciously upon their return, and offered fewer educational and medical benefits than in the case of veterans of other wars. He stressed that antiwar veterans in particular felt deeply alienated from their society. He made clear that they did not want to go to the Veterans Administration for help or dialogue, as they considered it part of the war-making establishment. When I suggested that we form "rap groups" of veterans with psychological professionals, I was doing little more than responding to what the veterans had more or less in mind. It occurred to me that psychiatrists like Hy Shatan and myself were also experiencing war-related alienation from American society, so that the rap groups, which functioned outside ordinary social channels, were a product of this shared alienation. Though I had no way of knowing it then, I was also embarking on the most significant of my Vietnam War–related efforts, and the one that had greatest impact on me personally.

Mostly through Hy Shatan's efforts, we enlisted a panel of about fifteen psychiatrists, psychoanalysts, psychologists, and social workers to participate in the groups, about half of whom were to remain active in them over a period of two and a half years. I had met Hy in connection with work we shared on American war crimes and found him to be a superb colleague who combined enormous dedication with sharp insights about antiwar veterans (and would later play a central role in the successful effort to include a concept of post-traumatic stress disorder in the

1980 edition of the *Diagnostic and Statistical Manual of Mental Disorders* [*DSM* III]). We held to the name "rap groups" as a way of avoiding the term "group therapy." We were groping toward a perspective that could avoid a medical or clinical model while exploring personal struggles in the larger context of the Vietnam War, and of American society. For want of a better word, we referred at first to our psychological contingent as "professionals," but the veterans quickly simplified matters by calling us "shrinks."

So it was a joint effort of "vets and shrinks," which quite naturally took on an egalitarian flavor, everyone on a first-name basis, with the feelings and motivations of shrinks as well as vets always at issue. Our shrink contingent met a couple of times at my home to discuss what we were doing and experiencing. A few expressed discomfort with the informality of the rap groups and advocated more traditional principles of group therapy with clear distinction between patient and therapist. Most of us were on the side of breaking down those barriers and viewing our project as a social experiment. (I later came to see the rap groups as very much a sixties enterprise taking place in the early seventies.) The traditionalists either adapted to the unorthodox tendencies of the group or else tended to leave the project. The groups were to remain active for almost three years, meeting at first in the VVAW office and then later in a room in a small Catholic seminary. Members of the groups preferred these humble settings to the more luxurious offices of individual shrinks, which were tried once or twice but resisted because of a perceived clinicalization of the enterprise.

Our weekly meetings were scheduled for two hours but frequently ran much longer and could be hard to end. For some weeks the men poured out accounts of their war experiences, of participating in or witnessing, or hearing from others about, grotesque killing and dying. I was awed by the extremity of what the men described—unending menace and violence, devastating loss, and transgressions of all kinds including the mutilation of corpses. As in earlier work I found myself entering a bizarre realm I had never myself experienced. My strong inclination was to listen and learn before saying anything, to refrain from interpretations until I had myself taken in more of the strange world the veterans brought to us. Now I believe that the vets had a need not only to confront their own experiences but to establish a baseline with the shrinks, to make clear to us some fundamental truths about Vietnam in order to be able to work together.

Then, after some weeks, the vets began to insist upon dealing with immediate psychological struggles, which were considerable, having to do with relationships to those around them, with their changing sense of masculinity, and with their conflicts with the society to which they returned. When descriptions of Vietnam were not connected to their present lives, they would be critical of one another for "telling war stories." They spent a lot of time confronting macho emotions, epitomized by what they called "the John Wayne thing," which were frequently related to joining the military and then to violent inclinations both in and out of uniform. I was impressed by their astuteness in exploring the broader social significance of blind patriotism in connection with warmaking. They could then bring that more general critique of American society to their actual Vietnam experience.

I recall one such moment when about twenty of us, two of whom were shrinks, were sitting haphazardly but attentively in a ramshackle VVAW room and an angry, articulate vet recalled a particular scene in Vietnam. There had been an air strike on a North Vietnamese unit and his company came upon an ugly scene of dismembered corpses, and proceeded to mutilate the bodies still further and then engage in a wild victory dance. The vet remembered asking himself: "What am I doing here? We don't take any land. We don't give it back. We just mutilate bodies. What the fuck are we doing here?" He was describing a version of what I came to call the "counterfeit universe" of Vietnam, in which moral criteria were inverted and the price of survival was to internalize the all-pervasive corruption of the environment. He went on to tell how he rejected awards he was to receive for participating in it: "They gave me a Bronze Star . . . and they put me up for a Silver Star. But I said you can shove it up your ass. . . . I threw all the others away. The only thing I kept was the Purple Heart because I still think I was wounded." He was rejecting not just the medals but the assumptions of military glory that lay behind them.

Later in the rap group sessions the men were discussing how one might prefer to die in Vietnam, and a slight, shy vet who had said almost nothing for weeks suddenly held everyone's attention as he blurted out a story:

I heard of one helicopter pilot in Nam who was carrying a shithouse [portable toilet] on his helicopter. He crashed and was killed, and was buried under the whole shithouse and all the shit. I thought that if I was going to die in Vietnam, that's the way I would like to die.

Stories like those required no interpretation.

Vets were tender toward each other and responsive to each other's words. But there was one session in particular—this time in the seminary—in which there was a quick contagion of feelings of guilt that was both painful and valuable. It began with a vet's description of uneasy dreams, in which he would be riding in a friend's truck or a subway train and would suddenly find himself in a military vehicle, or back in Vietnam, where he would again be fighting and would sometimes die. Other vets and the two shrinks present commented on his fear of the military and of the unfinished business he had with it, encouraging him to recognize those feelings, even if troubling. In response, a veteran who had previously expressed resentment at any emphasis on feelings of guilt spoke agonizingly of "mistakes" he made in Vietnam as a platoon leader, resulting in a terrible ambush and grotesque deaths of some of his men: "Their faces . . . screwed up . . . all fucked up." And he added, "I don't know why it all happened—there was this damned fool war—and maybe I just wasn't old enough to have responsibility for so many men." He then darted out of the room, explaining later (to another vet who followed him to make sure he was all right) that he just needed to sit quietly for a while. Almost immediately, the vet who had been struggling with his dreams spoke in tremulous tones: "I'm shaking all over . . . because what he said hit me hard. . . . Before . . . we talked about guilt . . . but I didn't feel too much. But now I really feel remorse. I feel very badly about what I did in Vietnam—and it's a terrible feeling."

Other vets were supportive, emphasizing the importance of coming to terms with experiences and emotions. The group tried to maintain a balance between individual responsibility for what one did, and recognition of the extraordinary pressures of the atrocity-producing situation, which was in turn the responsibility of American society for creating. They insisted that the larger society confront this responsibility, just as they were attempting to confront their own. I agreed with them, and became aware of the courage and astuteness of many of these veterans in struggling to achieve this kind of moral equilibrium.

On other occasions, social criticism could become inseparable from painful guilt feelings, as in the case of a vet who told of killing a Viet Cong soldier with a knife, and then added in soft tones: "I felt sorry. I don't know why I felt sorry. John Wayne never felt sorry." He was rejecting "the John Wayne thing" and its glorification of macho detachment in killing. For the vets and for me as well, there was no better antidote than the great Country Joe and the Fish song, "I-Feel-Like-I'm-Fixin'-to-Die Rag," with its bitterly lyrical gallows humor poetry about sending men, in complete ignorance, to die in Vietnam. One former grunt said that until he heard that song he felt it necessary to be "reasonable about the war" but "when I heard the 'Fixin'-to Die Rag' I really just let it all hang out and say that it was really crazy. . . . It's really what I feel."

I myself played the song repeatedly, and saw in it the deep oppositional power of focused absurdity. I later compared Country Joe's words with the opposite sentiment of Alfred Tennyson's "Charge of the Light Brigade": "Theirs not to make reply, / Theirs not to reason why, / Theirs but to do and die." Needless to say, the "Fixin'-to-Die Rag" became my favorite rock song. And some years later, after publication of *Home from the War*, I was thrilled to receive a note from Country Joe himself, affirming our ethical camaraderie. I confess that I displayed Country Joe's note shamelessly to my two children as a happily shared connection with an element of American popular culture.

These experiences made clear to me how much social and historical forces could influence immediate behavior. Veterans closely explored the impact of the war on them and their susceptibility to social attitudes concerning war and peace in general. Those dimensions can be lost sight of because of the intense focus in psychotherapy on individual psychology. But under extreme conditions, as prevailed in Vietnam, it became impossible to ignore those larger currents and their effect on everyone's feelings and actions.

I was learning a lot, but that did not mean I was immune to my own awkward mistakes. During one animated session, vets began to discuss the two shrinks in the group. One of the vets noted the disparity between my status as a prominent psychiatrist at Yale and as an ordinary guy named

Bob in the group. Though made a little uneasy, he and the others seemed to accept that disparity but were more troubled by something said a few moments later by another vet: "What about Bob Lifton—taking all those notes? Is he really in the group?" In further exchange a few of the vets made it clear that they knew and approved of my intention to write a book on the project, since making known Vietnam veterans' experiences was one of the purposes of our work together. What they objected to was my becoming so immersed in note-taking that I was not fully "present" in the group. The second shrink, Florence Pincus, another fine colleague, praised the veteran for his courage in confronting me, adding that she had thought the same thing but lacked the courage to say so. I felt a bit stunned and very foolish, realizing immediately that the criticism was fair. I collected myself a bit and tried to add some levity by saying that veterans, lacking psychological training, had less to unlearn than shrinks. I admitted that the rebuke was justified, and from then on waited until each session was completed before writing down details of what had transpired. I came to feel that the incident had value: to the group in asserting its claim to the "presence" of everyone; and to me in making clear my responsibility to the immediate group as opposed to what I would write about it.

I learned something else that had great value for me in my psychological work in general. In relation to extreme experience, people have the capacity for rapid individual change. Responding first to a death encounter, and then to our intense group sessions, veterans underwent shifts not only in their feelings toward the war and toward their government and society, but also in their relationships with parents, wives, partners, family members, and friends, and in their overall sense of what it was to be a man. These shifts could occur in a matter of months, sometimes even weeks. To be sure, the change was only partial, and much in the men remained as before. But they could feel themselves significantly altered, and in many that change could be sustained and built upon over a considerable period of time. I recalled that Erik Erikson had come to some of his views on identity change in connection with work with World War II veterans. And for me the rap group experience became part of a long-standing interest in the potential for significant change in adults, as opposed to dogmatic assumptions sometimes made by classical psychoanalysis to the effect that the first six years are so crucial to the formation of self that everything that follows is more or less superstructure.

Of course it was not only the veterans who changed. Something important was happening to me in my sense of myself as a psychiatric professional. I was surrendering the last vestiges of my professional armor. To be sure I had been somewhat innovative in my work in Hong Kong and Hiroshima, but I had still functioned in those studies as a more or less proper psychiatrist. Now I was going further in overcoming professional distancing—still focused on psychological motivation but bringing that focus closer to the vantage point of the veterans themselves. I could closely share their death encounter and their survivor mission of exposing and ending the war. I was becoming a very different kind of professional, one who could permit himself to combine specialized knowledge with passionate plunges into moral and political realms. I don't think I've ever changed back.

While we never had more than a few groups going in our project, it had reverberations that went far beyond those grungy rooms in the VVAW office and the Catholic seminary. Vets and shrinks from many different cities got in touch with us about forming groups of their own, and when the Veterans Administration belatedly evolved to the point of recognizing the special alienation of Vietnam veterans, it began an "outreach program," in which thousands of veterans participated, largely modeled, we were told, on our New York project. (It was run for many years by Arthur Blank, a psychiatrist and Vietnam veteran who had himself opposed the war, and who had been a younger faculty colleague at Yale with whom I had given a couple of seminars on the war for psychiatric residents.) The rap groups also produced a few psychologists, notably Arthur Egendorf, who was to write illuminatingly about the psychological experience of his fellow Vietnam veterans. The rap groups became part of a larger healing process among Vietnam veterans as well as a piece of the history of the veterans' antiwar movement.

12

_____

"The Sixties"

THE AMERICAN STRUGGLE with Vietnam was inseparable from something called "the Sixties," whose historical currents extended well into the seventies. Whatever you said or felt about the war took you quickly to raging debates concerning larger moral and political questions. Expressions of the sixties, moreover, were worldwide, perhaps the first historical example of global rebellion. Given my interests, it was not surprising that my own experience of the era was international—involving Japan and England as well as my own country. It has become convenient for many to view the sixties as simply a period of excess. But that ignores the serious social movements that emerged: movements opposing war, nuclear weapons, and colonialism, and advocating feminism, social justice, and, of special psychological importance, the bold questioning of authority. One thinks of the sixties as a time of the young, and it was certainly they who released most of its energies. But not enough attention has been paid to the experience of those of us who were adults. I turned thirty-four in May 1960, and the decade's rebellious currents have strongly affected all of my subsequent life. But the sixties, more than any other era, confronted me with a tandem of rebelliousness and totalism. I was hardly free of confusion, but tried to keep my bearings by embracing much of the rebellion while taking a critical stance toward the totalism.

A Japanese Sixties

Apart from my Riesman prologue to the sixties, my first exposure to the rebelliousness of the decade took place in Japan. I arrived in Tokyo in mid-January of 1960 to begin my study of Japanese university students and their interaction with history, and there they were, four months later, demonstrating in front of the Diet (the parliamentary building) in the thousands, swelling to the hundreds of thousands as they were joined by working people, professionals, businessmen, and just about everyone except the high government officials and powerful industrialists who, in corrupt collusion, ran the society. Demonstrators saw themselves as defending democracy against what could be called the "totalism of the old," in this case the immediate act of the prime minister (Nobusuke Kishi), who had been a war criminal associated with emperor worship, and then a postwar conservative politician. Kishi had just performed an outrageous postmidnight parliamentary maneuver in ramming through a ten-year extension to the much-contested United States–Japan Security Treaty. The depth of feeling was expressed in the full month these mass demonstrations were sustained with a remarkable absence of violence.

BJ and I, like many others, were struck by the beauty of the daily evening scene of (as I wrote then) "students marching exuberantly past, shifting into their celebrated zigzag dance, their flags held aloft, the whole thing looking like the work of an artist whose genre of socialist realism could not contain his highly romantic impulse." At one point a very slight and young-looking university student emerged to talk to BJ and me and boldly cleared a path for us among the demonstrators to meet the leader of his group; we never made it to the leader but I took our guide's name and address and he soon became a regular participant in my research.

But there developed frustrations (the demonstrations had little immediate political effect) and that early nonviolence did not always hold. Some years later my friend Takeo Doi wrote me about encountering violence on the part of one of the extremist factions of Zengakuren (All-Japan Federation of Students' Self-Governing Societies), which included being forcibly held in his office for a period of time. I had interviewed students in that faction and written about their "totalism of the new" in the form of a vision of pure communism, and had witnessed their "mock-military" battles with police in which the students armed themselves with long poles, helmets, and shields. I spoke of such protestors as establishing "Japan's claim to the most militant of all youth rebellions and the most polarized and troubled of all national university scenes."

A Japanese sixties conflict came close to home in the form of two friends of mine, both literary figures still in their twenties, who had once been almost brothers but by the time of my Tokyo stay in 1967 had become bitter public antagonists. I had met both Jun Etō, the prominent literary critic, and Kenzaburo Oe, the remarkable novelist who would later win a Nobel Prize, in 1961 in connection with my work on youth and history. I was first friendly with Etō, who taught me much about rebellious literary currents among the young, for which he was in fact something of a spokesman. But Etō, from the mid-sixties, began to express, both in person and in correspondence, more conservative views, especially in relation to the emperor. He even told me how at a literary ceremony, when shaking the emperor's hand, he felt a "shiver" run through his entire being. In contrast, Oe had never ceased to be a fierce critic of the emperor system with what he called its "omnipresent shadows" within all Japanese. I became friendly with Oe a little later, partly because of our strong mutual interest in Hiroshima, and was deeply sympathetic to his outspoken political stands, in which he insisted on the accountability of Japanese for their war crimes. When BJ and I invited them to our Tokyo home for a dinner of reconciliation, they both responded warmly, and the dinner itself was full of good feeling as they nostalgically recalled, in many toasts, their earlier friendship. But in keeping with the Japanese tendency to avoid direct confrontation, there was no discussion of the impasse between them or the issues that divided them.

Sadly but not surprisingly, the dinner did little to actually reconcile them; their friendship was not resumed, though perhaps there was a touch of greater civility in their disagreements. The emperor as a symbol continued to radically divide them. Oe felt sufficiently strongly about its harmfulness to take the unprecedented step of declining the Imperial Order of Culture (awarded after he had received the Nobel Prize in literature in 1994) because it was given in the name of the emperor. For that he received constant death threats from right-wing groups, to the point where he had to take extensive personal precautions. He and I became closer over the years, read most of each other's work, and when he came to the City University of New York to speak at the Center on Violence and Human Survival, he declared himself, with his puckish smile, my "disciple." But it was he who taught me about the kind of courage required, in the face of personal danger, to confront not only one's country's leaders but a centuries-long imperial tradition. Etō, in contrast, reembraced that tradition with its totalistic temptations. Their friendship was a casualty of the sixties, a Japanese version of what I and many other Americans were to experience.

A British Sixties

R. D. Laing, the quintessential sixties psychoanalyst, helped give a somewhat wild but professional cast to my British sixties. I was myself struggling with how to incorporate what I had experienced in Hiroshima into my way of being a psychiatrist, and was working on heretical theory involving death and death symbolism. I had admired Laing's book *The Divided Self* as a remarkably sensitive and sympathetic exploration of the schizophrenic mind. I was to learn a great deal from him about professional rebellion and the perils of absolutizing that rebellion.

Our family was in London for six months in late 1966 for me to participate in John Bowlby's Tavistock Clinic seminar on issues of attachment and loss. After I was introduced to Laing by friends, we had lunch together, during which we talked about our respective deviations from professional orthodoxy. Laing then invited me to have dinner with his group at a place called Kingsley Hall in East London, where he had put together an experimental community that included people who had been diagnosed as schizophrenics, others who treated them, and "anyone else who wants to live there." He was demonstrating his conviction that, as he put it, "there is no such thing as schizophrenia," and that the word itself (literally, "split-mind") is nothing more than "a misplaced metaphor." But upon arriving there, we found the place in disarray and Laing explained that we would go elsewhere for dinner because one of the people living there had smashed up all the china. So about fifteen of us assembled at a nearby Chinese restaurant, where we had lots of good food and drink. Toward the end of the dinner, Laing, now rather drunk, began to ruminate about the lecture trip to the United States on which he was about to embark: "What shall I shay to the Americans? What should I explain to them about schizophrenia?" And then, in what was surely a Zen moment, a plate thrown in his direction crashed into the wall behind him, and the woman who had thrown it cried out: "Just take me along! I'll show them what it is!" She was of course the same woman who had broken the dishes in Kingsley Hall. She was telling Ronnie that schizophrenia did indeed exist and could be a form of madness. Shards of the shattered plate caused small cuts on Ronnie's face. He smiled silently, and BJ thought he looked quite beautiful, something like a bleeding Jesus. Very quickly, conversation was resumed as though nothing had happened, and we all finished our dinner.

To me the dish thrower was loud and clear in her warning not to romanticize schizophrenia, but determined revolutionaries do not heed warnings. In his subsequent book, *The Politics of Experience*, which was to become his most famous work, Ronnie elevated those we call schizophrenic to the status of sage. The book contained valuable insights about the experience of transcendence—these were never absent from Laing's writings—but its careless, self-indulgent style contrasted sharply with the rigor of *The Divided Self.* The disciplined clinician struggling with the authority of an existential tradition had given way to the omniscient guru who recognized no authority but his own.

During subsequent meetings in the United States I found him to alternate between strict spiritual discipline (he had undergone mystical Buddhist training in Sri Lanka) and alcoholic sloppiness. I gained the impression that the alienated seeker in him had a strong impulse to escape from patients, disciples, and everyone else. He was fragile and, sadly, deteriorated during his last years to a point where his medical license was revoked for alcoholic displays with patients. Yet I was enriched by my friendship with Ronnie, who, at his best, brought intellectual power to a constant questioning of received psychiatric assumptions. But I came to see his professional and personal rebellion as having spilled over into still another version of totalism. Schizophrenia was, after all, more than a "misplaced metaphor."

Revolution at Yale

During most of the sixties I was based in New Haven, and the May Day (May 1, 1970) uprising at Yale brought student protest to my own back-yard. The Yale rebellion was in a sense late—Columbia had exploded in 1968 and Harvard in 1969—at a university without much history of political radicalism. But the May Day event posed the most danger of all because it combined antiwar sentiment with support for the Black Pan-ther leader Bobby Seale in connection with his controversial New Haven murder trial. A few prominent Panthers made ominous threats of "burn-ing buildings" and even "taking lives." Yet while Columbia and Harvard officials seemed confused by events and ended up calling in police, which created legacies in their universities of painful schism, Yale was able to ride out its crisis through a form of leadership that was both progressive and pragmatic.

From the early sixties Yale had undergone a kind of reformation—in admission policies that reached out to a broader representation of Ameri-can society, including women (beginning in 1969), and a spate of faculty appointments of people with relatively more critical and progressive lean-ings. I had never been much involved in administrative matters, having always seen myself as having one foot in my university and the other in the wider world. In my antiwar focus, I was intense but hardly a wild man. I was sympathetic to antiwar passions of students and to the aspirations of black leaders (though concerned about violence and extreme rhetoric on the part of some of the Panthers), but I was concerned that Yale and other American universities weather the storm and keep going.

At the same time I was involved in quieter reflection with faculty and students. BJ and I had formed a faculty group called Serendip, in which we explored, during monthly meetings at each other's homes, speculative ideas in each other's disciplines. And I belonged to another discussion group at the Yale Divinity School (hosted by its dean, Colin Williams) where we considered relationships between life and work in our psycho-logical and spiritual efforts. I also created "reading courses" with under-graduates in which we could examine critically the ideas of writers who were then influential, including Norman O. Brown and Abraham Maslow in psychological areas, Joseph Campbell on mythology, and Mircea

Eliade on religion; and sometimes, equally critically, current writings on practices of meditation. But as tensions built at the university, issues surrounding them increasingly entered into all these reflections.

As the Yale campus prepared for the May 1 demonstration, I became a member of a loosely knit group we called the "Concerned Yale Faculty," made up of people sympathetic to much of sixties protest. We did not play a large part in things but might have had an influence slightly beyond our limited numbers because, unlike many on the faculty, we could and did talk to students. We saw ourselves as taking a stand against what my friend Ken Keniston called "the rage of the old toward the young."

The two heroes of that Yale moment were Bill Coffin, the university chaplain, and Kingman Brewster, its president. They were well aware of the danger that the Yale event would encapsulate a national confrontation between, on the one hand, the Nixon administration, which had denounced the Panthers and, many believed, sought a violent confrontation, together with the FBI under J. Edgar Hoover, which was employing every form of manipulation and infiltration to discredit and disrupt the Black Panthers; and on the other, the more belligerent among the Panthers and the students (including the Weathermen, a split-off from SDS) who were prone to violence. Coffin and Brewster responded with a systematic outreach that was respectful toward all parties.

William Sloane Coffin was from a wealthy old-Yalie family and had been associated in his youth with the Office of Strategic Services and its successor, the CIA. But he was to become one of the steadiest and most courageous voices of the civil rights and antiwar movements. He and I became friendly at Yale and shared a number of antiwar platforms. We talked a lot about social change that could avoid violence, and Bill discussed principles of Gandhian nonviolence at the monthly group ("Serendip") BJ and I had formed. I don't think I ever saw Bill without a twinkle or a smile, always conveying a sense of sufficient spiritual confidence to avoid contempt or rage toward adversaries.

Bill could turn a phrase as well as anyone, and his Sunday sermons— scriptural, antiwar, and tender—were celebrated events on the campus. BJ and I had a special experience in 1966 at one of those sermons that had little to do with its content, but much to do with Bill's openhearted style as a preacher and human being. Having no babysitter for our infant daughter Karen, we took her along, but she apparently did not appreciate the sermon as much as we did, as in the middle of it she burst into a wail whose decibel was of such magnitude that it even drowned out the formidable baritone of the preacher. Bill paused, looked up to locate the source of the interruption, saw us moving rapidly toward the exit, smiled benignly, and declared: "Don't go. It's okay. Babies are what it's all about!" We did leave, but only to calm our daughter, and returned in time to hear the conclusion of a biblically infused antiwar message.

Bill found it more difficult to manage his personal life. During a period when his marital difficulties were spilling all over the Yale community, I went to see him, together with our close mutual friend Arnie Wolf, to express our love and support for him in the face of his wife Eva's increasingly indiscriminate denunciations of him throughout the community. (Of course, much could have been said from her vantage point, since Bill was far from an ideal husband and they were soon to be divorced, but he was the one who was our friend.) That visit was unusual for me, since I have made it a point, particularly as a psychiatrist, to avoid intervening in people's personal struggles. But Arnie and I sensed Bill's vulnerability, and he was clearly grateful for the talk. It brought about an added dimension to our friendship.

Bill brought his commitment to nonviolence to the buildup of Yale's May Day event. As a university official who had participated in the burning of draft cards, had marched with Martin Luther King, Jr., and had also served with the CIA—and as a human being who inspired trust in just about anyone—Bill was uniquely qualified to mediate among student radicals, Black Panthers, Yale administrators, and the New Haven police. Only later did I learn how systematically he went about creating a "monitoring committee" that worked out concrete arrangements of protest and response, especially between the Panthers and the police. Bill was everybody's chaplain at Yale, mine too. When a few conservative alumni objected to his activities and pointed out that Yale was his employer, another responded by reminding them that Coffin was in the employ not of Yale but of God. I knew what he meant. Bill taught me a great deal about what we call "spiritual authority." Like the Berrigans, but in a very different way, he lived the life of a spiritual hero, and what he did contributed greatly to the outcome of Yale's crisis.

Kingman Brewster, as president, was the fulcrum. Our concerned faculty group, somewhat self-importantly, formed a three-man delegation to visit Brewster and convey to him our advice. In addition to myself, the delegation included Peter Brooks, the humanities professor and my good friend; and Kenneth Mills, the West Indian–born philosopher and authority on third-world revolution, who was already holding constructive meetings with black students and faculty, Black Panther representatives, and university officials. We had decided to make two simple recommendations to Brewster: first, that the Yale campus be opened up completely to demonstrators to encourage dialogue among all groups; and second, that he make a principled statement about the Black Panther trial. Brewster listened to us in a friendly fashion but seemed a bit restless, even a little bored, as though he expected something more. He told us that he had already made up his mind to do both things we suggested, and we left the meeting with the strong impression that he was well ahead of us in his thinking and planning.

We were not entirely surprised. When he assumed the presidency of Yale in 1963, shortly after my own arrival, I shared the view of many that he was a patrician lightweight who had not particularly distinguished himself intellectually. But over time we became aware of the large role he played in the real revolution at Yale—that of opening up the university to minorities and bright students from anywhere in society—and of his admirable support for Bill Coffin when the Yale chaplain was put on trial for civil disobedience and angry Yale alumni demanded his resignation. By 1970 it had become clear to most people at Yale that Brewster—or "the King," as he was called—was a thoughtful, progressive, and fair-minded university president.

Not long after our delegation's visit, Brewster released the important statement he had already planned to make about the trial: "I personally want to say that I am appalled and ashamed that things should have come to such a pass in this country that I am skeptical of the ability of black revolutionaries to achieve a fair trial anywhere in the United States." The Yale campus would indeed be opened to everyone that day with a great show of institutional hospitality. Once more, Yale faculty members had underestimated Brewster. Nor did we know he had consulted extensively with his friend Archibald Cox of the Harvard Law School (another humane and progressive WASP Republican) about how to avoid the mistakes Harvard had made in responding to student protests, particularly that of closing down its campus and eventually calling the police. Brewster himself had arranged meetings with all parties, including a special post-midnight gathering, just hours before the scheduled demonstration, that involved such movement leaders as David Dellinger, Tom Hayden, William Kunstler, and Jerry Rubin, at which much agreement was achieved on how to keep things peaceful. That postmidnight meeting was all the more important in the wake of the announcement just the day before of America's "incursion" into Cambodia.

An overall atmosphere of nonviolence was furthered by Brewster's actions and meetings, Coffin's monitoring committee (working closely until the last moment with both Panthers and police), the Yale faculty's decision to "suspend normal academic expectations" for the day of protest (a cautious but important compromise), and the Panther leadership's decision in turn to seek to avoid violence. I came to realize how much Brewster had contributed to all this, and what a remarkable blend of ethical sensitivity, political savvy, and overall steadiness and courage he had managed to call forth.

What I remember was mostly a granola event—a spread of health foods and soft drinks, rock music, the Yale campus overflowing with students, demonstrators, and good feelings. The speakers demanded a fair trial for the Panthers but were on the whole more welcoming than inflammatory. That idyllic atmosphere was temporarily interrupted in a manner that could have been dangerous. A couple of young whites, who turned out to be provocateurs (probably employed either by the FBI or a branch of local law enforcement), screamed falsehoods into microphones about black people being arrested and beaten up, and did succeed in arousing demonstrators to challenge the police, who, in turn, used a certain amount of tear gas. When that occurred it was none other than Doug Miranda, a young Panther captain, who (in Panther street talk replete with expletives) pleaded for peace and told his people to respect the university and seek learning of their own if they wanted to make true revolution.

The image that stays with me was the beneficent figure of Allen Ginsberg, propped in zazen position before a second-story microphone, chanting melodious oms, defying the tear gas with the help of a couple of students who dutifully applied wet towels to his eyes and face. Ginsberg also recited a poem he'd written honoring May Day and Yale as well as demonstrators and the Panthers ("Spring green buildings . . . May Day picnic . . . O holy Yale Panther Pacifist Conscious populace"), while gently castigating war-making authorities ("O President guard thy sanity . . . and end your violent War Assemblage").

The murder charge against Bobby Seale was eventually thrown out by the judge. There had been a murder in the Panther movement, apparently ordered by the then-"field marshal" George Sams, Jr. Sams had spent time in a mental hospital and was widely believed to have been an FBI informant and agent provocateur (it was he who had tried to implicate Seale). On May 4, just two days after the end of the Yale demonstrations, four students were shot and killed at Kent State University by members of the Ohio National Guard during an antiwar protest. Yes, the good feelings were indeed "evanescent" (as Peter Brooks was later to write) but for me that moment at Yale mattered and gave at least a glimmer of the possibilities for change.

It turned out that Brewster had more surprises for me. We had two additional encounters, the first of which was no more than glancing but still important to me. In the spring of 1972, I decided to telephone him to inform him that a group I headed, called "Citizens' Committee for Redress of Grievances," which included a number of people on the Yale faculty, was going to engage in antiwar civil disobedience in the antechamber of the U.S. House of Representatives the next day. I explained that most members of the group would be arrested after refusing the police order to leave, but those who wished to avoid arrest could obey that order. Then without having planned to do so, I heard myself ask, "Would you like to join us?" I felt free to be a bit provocative because I knew Brewster to be strongly against the war and he and I had become friendly acquaintances from the time of the May 1 event. After my question there was a brief silence at the other end of the line before Brewster made his reply: "No, thanks, Bob. You do it your way, and I'll do it mine." That was the better side of Yale-style sensibility—gentlemanly encouragement of independent action, each in his own fashion, with perhaps a faint suggestion of class distinction. I imagined Brewster conferring about the war over brandies with the likes of George Ball and McGeorge Bundy while I and my fellow protestors were being herded into police vans outside the Capitol building. But I also experienced it as a member of the Yale faculty receiving a blessing from his university president in relation to the American practice of civil disobedience. I loved him for that answer, and it became another part of our family mythology. Whenever BJ or I wished to do something a little differently from the other, one of us would say, with a deflating smile: "You do it your way, and I'll do it mine."

The other encounter should have been a happy one but turned out to be strangely sad. It took place in late 1978 in the American Embassy in Paris. BJ and I had been invited to stay in the living quarters of the embassy while recovering from fractures we had received in an automobile accident (all of which I'll explain in the next section). While there, we were included in a large dinner party held as part of a conference for American ambassadors to Western European countries. Brewster was then ambassador to England, and after dinner he and his wife, Mary, and BJ and I were able to have a friendly reunion and retire to a small sitting room to discuss old times at Yale. We talked at length about the May 1 event and I expressed to Kingman my admiration for his skillful and humane handling of such an overwhelmingly difficult occasion. But he seemed to take no joy in my praise. If anything, he looked increasingly distraught. He said that he remembered those days as extremely painful—death threats to him and his wife, angry disagreements with students, faculty, black leaders, and the New Haven police, and then vicious denunciation by influential alumni. Rather than associations of triumphant resolution, or even satisfaction over having avoided violence, he and Mary looked back on the whole experience with considerable pain and melancholy.

BJ and I were surprised and troubled by what we heard. We had underestimated the many dimensions of stress Brewster had been under at the time. But I came to view his reaction as that of a survivor who had been publicly acclaimed a hero while inwardly self-critical in relation to what he had done or not done. The closest analogy I came to was a strange one: that of the soldier who restrained from firing at My Lai, had also been embraced as a hero, but could not cease condemning himself for not having done more to stop the killing. There had been no killing at Yale, but

Kingman might well have been haunted by what he considered personal failings that could have contributed to large-scale violence and even to the destruction of a great university.

Kingman Brewster and Bill Coffin exemplified what could be called heroism through decency. Bill had long honed the ethical and pragmatic discipline required for that kind of heroism and could take Yale events in stride. Kingman had to do much "learning on the job" in mobilizing some of the best of American resources to cope with the country's antiwar rage and racial pathology. What was remarkable was that he succeeded. I should not have been surprised by the personal price he paid.

Vietnam on the Dunes

Wellfleet had to figure in my Vietnam-centered American sixties. On August 6, 1971, at the request of friends, BJ and I hosted a fund-raiser on the dunes just beyond our Wellfleet house for the "Harrisburg Eight," a group of Catholic antiwar activists who had been put on trial for their civil disobedience, pouring blood on government draft files, and alleged conspiracies to "sabotage" government property and even to "kidnap" government officials. We thought it appropriate to schedule the fund-raiser on the Hiroshima commemorative day. The event brought the Vietnam War to our Wellfleet sands, had unexpected repercussions of illegitimate FBI behavior, and provided a lesson for me in the function of the Jesuit order.

The occasion was spectacular—a cloudless late afternoon on which more than two hundred guests sat in folding chairs facing the ocean just beyond the large dune standing some three hundred yards from our house. A number of the defendants were present, including Elizabeth McAlister, the nun who was to leave her order to marry Phil Berrigan. The main speaker was Dan Ellsberg, who had just achieved heroic notoriety by making public the top-secret Pentagon Papers on the war. There were also powerful antiwar readings by two gifted actors: our close friend Harris Yulin, and Faye Dunaway, who was then staying on the Cape with Harris.

At the center of the event was a young disciple of the Berrigans, a charismatic priest named Joe O'Rourke, who coordinated everything with a compelling combination of kinetic energy, spiritual passion, and low-key humor. And on the next morning we went back to the dune with O'Rourke, where he conducted a much smaller peace mass, whose participants, in addition to our family, included McAlister, Yulin, Dunaway, and various peace movement leaders, among whom were Dave Dellinger and Howard Zinn. Each of us read a piece or made a statement having to do with war or resistance, interwoven with O'Rourke's elegant rendering of Catholic ritual. The same day we arranged a meeting in my study for the considerable number of activists who had come for the event, and talked about ways of strengthening our opposition to the war. The fund-raiser itself brought in a respectable amount of money for the Harrisburg defense committee, and BJ and I were pleased and nourished by the events of the whole weekend. Then came the reverberations.

People who had been guests at the event began to write or call to tell me of being visited by FBI agents asking about the content of Ellsberg's speech but also about "Lifton's politics." I had the impression that the FBI had been caught off guard in learning about the fund-raiser only after it was over, and was trying to catch up with things. Then I received a rather folksy phone call, one that went something like this: "Hi, Dr. Lifton. How's it going? I'm John Jones, your Cape Cod FBI agent. When it's convenient for you, I'd like to drop in and chat about the meeting you had on August 6. I just want to see whether what I read in the paper [there had been a brief article in a Provincetown weekly] was accurate." To which, with equal friendliness, I gave the kind of reply I'd learned in the antiwar movement: "I'm terribly sorry but I won't be able to see you. I just do not feel it would be proper to discuss with you anything about people who had been guests in my home." After a brief back-and-forth in which I repeated my refusal, he responded cheerily: "Okay, Doc, I understand. Maybe some other time."

One side of me was amused by the phone call, and I took some delight in telling people about the local FBI man's folksiness, wondering whether the FBI sent its less aggressive agents out to pasture on Cape Cod. But I also experienced a sense of uneasiness and anger concerning the bureau's overall interest in our event and in me. Nor was I pleased by the caller's anticipation of a visit "some other time." I discussed the whole situation with people in the antiwar movement, including two lawyers, Ramsey

Clark and Leonard Boudin. They urged me to collect more evidence on FBI behavior, so I asked the Harrisburg Defense Committee assistant who had handled invitations to write to everyone on the guest list asking them in detail about any approach by the FBI. Six of the guests reported that agents had questioned them both about Ellsberg and myself. Several mentioned implied threats by the FBI that failure to cooperate might require one to appear before a grand jury. (About a year later we began to hear odd sounds on our telephone and discovered that the FBI had tapped our line, and were told by an employee of the building that they used a "black box" technique of bringing in people from the outside falsely identified as telephone company employees to do the dirty work.)

My way of responding was hardly bold or militant. I decided to express my complaint within the American political system by writing to various members of the U.S. Senate, and then to make some kind of public statement of protest. The senators I wrote to included Alan Cranston and George McGovern, because I knew them to be strongly antiwar, and Edward Kennedy and Abraham Ribicoff, because they were from the two states in which I lived. In my letters I described the event on the dunes as "peaceful and thoughtful," mentioned its distinguished sponsors (scientists George Wald and Salvador Luria, the poet Stanley Kunitz, and the artist Robert Motherwell), and complained about the FBI behavior as harassment of Ellsberg, a violation of constitutional rights of peaceful assembly, and infringement on my own individual rights. I asked that they "look into the matter and take action against this kind of abuse of government function." I had not realized that, according to protocol, each of the senators would initiate something on the order of an investigation by writing to J. Edgar Hoover, then in the relatively final days of his infamous reign over the FBI (and over just about everyone else), summarizing or forwarding my own letter.

A few of the senators sent me copies of the correspondence, which included Hoover's patently false response claiming that "the sole purpose" of the FBI interviews had been to determine whether Ellsberg had made reference to the top-secret Pentagon Papers and insisting that no reference had been made to "Lifton's politics" and that there had been no element of threat. I made similar points in an op-ed column I wrote for *The New York Times*, stressing the FBI's "harassment of supporters and sympathizers of the Harrisburg and Pentagon Papers defendants," its contacting of guests as well as myself, all in the service of what I called "the psychology of intimidation." The *Times* accommodatingly titled the article, "To Frighten and Stifle," words I quoted from one of the offended guests.

Thinking back on the fund-raiser and its consequences, I was again impressed by the lengths to which the government would go to undermine opposition to the war coming from the Catholic left. But at the same time I was struck by how, in protesting this behavior, I could have access to mainstream officials and institutions, to senators and the op-ed page of *The New York Times*, taking advantage of my respectability as a professor of psychiatry at Yale. I was fighting back, but from a position of high privilege, and certainly taking no risks. I confess to having experienced another moment of David-versus-Goliath pleasure—along with my characteristic dose of absurdity—in combating the legendary FBI despot, J. Edgar Hoover. I knew at the time that I was hardly dealing with an earthshaking event, but I was calling upon American constitutional rights and political traditions that have always meant a great deal to me. No wonder that, as part of a later *Nation* magazine symposium on patriotism, I wrote, "Scratch a radical critic and you find an America lover."

There was still another sequel, this one having to do with the admirable dune priest. I had lost contact with Joe O'Rourke for about two years, until receiving letters from him and others in the Berrigan community with troubling news. O'Rourke was being put on trial by the Jesuits and was in danger of being expelled from the order. The story was this. A Catholic church in Boston had refused to baptize the baby of a woman who, although herself Catholic, was a leading pro-choice advocate. O'Rourke thought the refusal to be wrong and proceeded to baptize the child on the steps of the same church. He was being put on trial not because of the act of baptism but because he performed it after a superior had ordered him not to. At issue was the fundamental Jesuit vow of obedience.

O'Rourke and his friends were trying to mobilize support for him in connection with the official trial, and I was asked to write on his behalf to the current "Father General" of the order, Pedro Arrupe. O'Rourke wanted very much to remain in the Jesuits, as has his mentor, Daniel Berrigan. At the time I knew just one thing about Arrupe: he had survived the atomic bomb in Hiroshima, having been there as a missionary at the time. I later learned that he had trained as a physician and had quickly formed a medical team to help save lives, had become head of the Jesuits in 1965, and was known as a progressive leader who insisted on combining justice with faith. I went to some pains to write a strong letter to Arrupe trying to convince him of the importance of keeping Joe O'Rourke in the Jesuits. I undoubtedly was a bit hyperbolic in speaking of Arrupe's "spiritual kinship" with me in connection with the atomic bomb, of my professional encounters with Jesuit priests, of O'Rourke's modeling his behavior on that of St. Ignatius of Loyola, founder of the Jesuits, and of the importance to me as a secular Jew of O'Rourke's "sensitive Catholic conscience." But I meant all of it, along with my conclusion that, by expelling O'Rourke, "your Society will be made infinitely poorer."

In stark contrast, Arrupe's reply was a lesson in brevity. It was, in fact, something on the order of a cruel work of art. He thanked me for my interest in the Jesuits, pointed out that obedience was the basic vow of the order, and concluded with one of the pithiest sentences to appear in all of my thousands of pages and millions of words in notes and correspondence: "Father O'Rourke is undoubtedly a good man, but need not be a Jesuit." O'Rourke was being kicked out. Perhaps he had been less skillful than Dan Berrigan in dealing with the Jesuit hierarchy while carrying out radical actions. I was left with a combination of resentment of the injustice done to O'Rourke and awe in connection with this terrible display of authoritarian clarity on the part of the Jesuits and their otherwise progressive leader. I had a new sense of why the Jesuits had been around for so long.

As for O'Rourke, I'm happy to say that he never succumbed. He remained an activist, married, and became an advocate of married priests and the first president of Catholics for a Free Choice. He died in 2008 at the age of seventy, but my lasting image of Joe is of that young, smiling, spiritually passionate priest of the dunes.

My Journey with Motherfuckers

In my writings during the late sixties and early seventies, I tried to suggest some of the upheaval of that time, as in a small book I called *Boundaries*, with a subtitle, "Psychological Man in Revolution." I included in it short essays on the breakdown of boundaries in various areas in which I had worked: boundaries of destruction (as in Hiroshima), of life and death in general (in connection with nuclear threat), of the self (in the protean style), of revolution itself (the excesses of the Chinese Cultural Revolution), and of the contours of American society (what I called the "New History"). I did retain my allergy to totalism by warning of the dangers of *eliminating all* boundaries (sought by some young rebels and advocated in one strand of the writings of the classicist-turned-sixties psychoanalytic visionary Norman O. Brown) as opposed to questioning and recasting them.

That last chapter was derived from a longer essay, "The Young and the Old—Notes on a New History," which best conveyed my sixties sensibility. Part of my focus in the essay was on the mocking and self-mocking humor of the young as a restraint on totalism, best exemplified by the phrase "Up against the wall, motherfucker!" which took on classic proportions in student rebellion. That focus was to lead to an unexpected series of events involving not universities but a New England high school and one of its teachers. I traced some of the psychological and cultural journey of the slogan from use of the word *motherfucker* (increasingly unhyphenated) in black youth subculture to suggest either extreme transgression or admiration; to a contemptuous creation of the whole phrase, "Up against the wall, motherfucker" by white policemen when ordering (mostly black) suspects to take their places in the police lineup; to the reclaiming of the full phrase by the black poet LeRoi Jones (later Amiri Baraka) by adding to it in a poem the words "This is a stickup!"; to a radical group of Yippies naming themselves "Up-Against-the-Wall, Motherfuckers"; to the embrace of the phrase as a central slogan of rebellion by the Columbia University SDS student leaders in their 1968 uprising; and finally Lionel Trilling's pun in characterizing the striking students at his own university as "Alma Mater-fuckers." I was clearly having fun, but I did include a serious analysis of the phrase, which took it beyond the Oedipus complex and viewed it as "a way of playing with an image of ultimate violation and of retribution for that violation."

The essay's appearance in so respectable a journal as the *Atlantic Monthly* (September and October 1969) was what probably emboldened Robert Keefe, a high school English teacher in Ipswich, Massachusetts, to assign it to his class as a source of information on things happening in American society. But the parents of one of the students became incensed at their child's exposure to such obscene language and complained formally to the principal and school board. Keefe was suspended from his teaching job. He sued for reinstatement and was represented by a lawyer named Philip A. Mason, who belonged to a Boston firm with the imposing letterhead of Brown, Rudnick, Freed & Gesmer. Mason wrote to me asking that I help Keefe's case by providing a brief justification of my use of the word and phrase in the article, and I responded with a very sober statement on the significance of language and its relationship to humor and mockery in cultural and generational conflict. I then received regular progress reports, always in staid lawyerese ("As you may or may not have heard, Mr. Keefe has been granted a trial, which will be held on November 12 . . ."). In his last report Mason wrote triumphantly of the outcome: "As you may or may not have heard, Mr. Keefe has been fully reinstated and the school board's position has been completely rejected." But now there was an added flourish: "This is a victory for Mr. Keefe, for Brown, Rudnick, Freed & Gesmer, and for Dr. Lifton, and a defeat for the motherfuckers." Clearly the word was contagious.

I learned new things about the episode in 2008 by turning to the Internet via Google and typing in "Keefe," "Up against the wall, motherfuckers," or, most enjoyably, "Lifton, motherfucker." It turned out that the phrase entered the music world, providing lines and titles and, in one case, lyrics to a song that consisted solely of the repetition of "Up against the wall, motherfuckers!"

But more important was the legal sequence. The appeals court decision in the Keefe case invoked the principle of academic freedom and termed my essay "a valuable discussion of 'dissent, protest, radicalism, and revolt,'" which was "in no way pornographic." That Massachusetts decision, in turn, was applied to another case involving a student at the University of Missouri who distributed an underground newspaper with the headline version of the phrase, and the Missouri decision condemned the banning of such words as a form of government control over educational institutions. Beyond my pleasure at the way in which the two briefs viewed my article, I believe it fair to say that the decisions represented democracy at work. Legal authorities were able to step back from the intense, sometimes violent passions of the sixties and affirm not only academic freedom in teaching and learning but also the legitimacy of expressions of humor and mockery, even when offensive to some, as forms of protest.

The Dark Side of the Sixties

One of the more bizarre sixties events (though it occurred in the mid-seventies) in which I became involved was the Patricia Hearst trial. The trial and the events leading up to it reflected the caricatured extremes rebellion could assume, as well as the confused and fearful reactions of American society and the self-aggrandizing manipulations of those confusions in the courtroom. Hearst was kidnapped in February 1974 by a tiny cult (with a charismatic black leader and a handful of white followers) who proclaimed themselves revolutionary members of the Symbionese Liberation Army. About two months later she was photographed by a hidden camera holding an automatic weapon at a bank robbery staged by the group in San Francisco, became a fugitive for a year after most of the group had been killed in a shootout with authorities, and was arrested in September 1975 and tried in San Francisco early the following year.

Because the chief defense lawyer, F. Lee Bailey, argued that Hearst had been subjected to a form of "brainwashing" or thought reform, I was asked (together with two other psychiatrists and a psychologist who had also studied the process) to be an expert witness on her behalf. Hearst to me had always been a dirty word—it meant William Randolph Hearst, her grandfather, whom I understood to be a strident, amoral reactionary and corporate manipulator of yellow journalism to the extent of bringing on the imperialistic Spanish-American War of 1898. But a psychiatrist already working with the defense, whom I knew and respected, told me by telephone that Patricia Hearst had not only been kidnapped and abused but subjected to systematic mind manipulation; I thought that, whatever her family heritage, she was entitled to a defense that considered a form of psychological victimization that I knew something about. I was apprehensive about the sensationalism surrounding the case, but perhaps also attracted to the national prominence it was receiving.

Inside the courtroom a vicious adversarial contest was staged. The prosecutor, Robert R. Browning, was young, nasty, legally effective, and politically ambitious. Bailey, perhaps the country's most famous criminal lawyer, was extremely intelligent but had something of the style of a con man, drank too many martinis at lunch, and turned out to be commuting back and forth from legal seminars he was giving in Las Vegas.

I spent a number of hours interviewing Patricia Hearst and found much to support the idea that she had been subjected to a crude version of a thought reform–like procedure. Kept in a closet for almost two months, she was constantly threatened with death or permanent captivity, continuously accused of selfishly exploiting her privileged status at the expense of poor people (a convincing accusation in relation to a member of the Hearst family), pressed to make damning self-criticisms, and subjected to a sexual relationship, which might subsequently have become consensual. In my testimony I stressed parallels between her experience and what I had observed in my military work with American POWs and with Chinese and Westerners in Hong Kong.

I could also have mentioned the phenomenon of the "Stockholm syndrome" (the tendency of people held hostage, initially at gunpoint, to become sympathetic to their captors and their cause, partly because of being deeply impressed by their dedication and partly because of having shared an ordeal with them in being pursued and sometimes under attack by authorities). Also relevant was a concept I came to later, that of "doubling," the capacity of people in response to extreme situations to form a functional second self that can be ethically at odds with the prior self (Patricia Hearst turning into "Tanya" the revolutionary, and then back to Patricia Hearst when arrested).

My later conclusion was that Patricia Hearst should never have been tried. Ideally there should have been an agreement, possibly one containing a guilty plea and a recognition of extreme mitigation in connection with her physical abuse and severe and systematic psychological manipulation. But both prosecutors and defense lawyers undoubtedly opposed any such arrangement, given their ambitious personal agendas in creating "the trial of the century."

In the courtroom there was a zero-sum atmosphere that was unrelentingly adversarial; expressing the slightest nuance became an occasion for attack and ridicule by the opposing lawyer. Matters were further confused by testimony arranged by the prosecution, including that of two "forensic psychiatrists" who could say with straight faces that Hearst had voluntarily joined the SLA out of deep rebellion against her parents, that she was "a rebel in search of a cause." There was also in the courtroom a populist resentment of the defendant as a Hearst, as coming from the rich and privileged, and as the writer Diane Johnson put it, a disapproval of "radicals in general" and "in particular, undutiful children and rebellious women."

It also turned out that Bailey and his defense team made an egregious legal error by trying to argue simultaneously two separate and ultimately contradictory defenses: that of the "gun at the head," the sense of being directly coerced into the bank robbery by SLA members whose guns were pointed at her; and that of "brainwashing" or being subjected to a manipulative psychological process which caused her to internalize the group's views and join in their actions, and to fail to take advantage of opportunities to escape. Still I was shocked by the verdict: guilty of armed robbery and the use of a firearm to commit a felony. She served twenty-two months in prison until her seven-year sentence was commuted by Jimmy Carter, and later (in January 2001) she was given a full pardon by Bill Clinton at the end of his presidency. I would like to believe that our psychological testimony contributed to the commutation and eventual pardon.

I wrote an op-ed column soon after the trial explaining the thought reform–like pressures to which Hearst had been subjected, and I wrote to Dave Riesman that my participation in the trial was "a way of reasserting [my] stance" against totalism and coercion that had been so important to me since my beginning work on thought reform.

Although my testimony and the *New York Times* piece were well enough received, I did not escape unscathed. Together with the other psychiatrists who testified, I was fiercely attacked in the *New Republic* by Thomas Szasz, a libertarian psychoanalyst not given to evenhandedness, as part of his long-standing crusade against psychiatric testimony of any kind in the courtroom. But my most embarrassing moment came on the *Saturday Night Live* television show when I felt myself an object of ridicule as an actor represented my testimony in such a broadly pedantic manner that I could almost join in the laughter. My fifteen-year-old son, however, congratulated me effusively, thrilled that a character representing his father appeared in any capacity at all on his favorite show.

Falling Out with Friends

Many friendships ended during the sixties. Not surprisingly, I had a number of bitter conflicts with colleagues at Yale. But the most painful effects of the buildup to the May Day protest involved friendships with people who had nothing to do with Yale.

I wrote to Dave Riesman about events at Yale, and when he responded I was taken aback by his antagonism toward the students. Our friendship had always thrived on full expression of any kind of thought, always with the expectation that it would stimulate interesting ideas in response, and that there would be quick mutual sympathy and a feeling of common ground. Now we both seemed to have to tread carefully on each other's sensibilities on questions having to do with student radicalism. In the past Dave had been a strong and often lonely advocate of student expression and student rights. But he was in many ways a traditionalist and was deeply offended by students' violation of order and civility, and ultimately of adult authority. I recently saw a letter he wrote to his friend Erich Fromm in which he said, "In the late 1960s Lifton went over to the far left, and resents any criticism of communism whatsoever; at any rate, Chinese communism." The conflict in so close a friendship was painful at the time and it was now sad to discover so great a misrepresentation of my views in one with whom I had had such remarkable mutual understanding.

In retrospect, I do have a little more sympathy for one aspect of Dave's position, his warnings about the vulnerability of American society to political backlash against radical movements, warnings that proved all too cogent during the decades following the sixties. What I had not understood was that he himself was psychologically vulnerable to joining that backlash—hence his recoil from prior receptivity to radical attitudes of the young, and his experience of a personal resurgence of conservative views. But even when ill at ease about these conflicts, we kept on writing and talking to each other. Eventually we were able to return to much of the overall sensibility we shared, whether about nuclear threat, war and peace, or, most important, our aversion to totalism. We could also recover a great deal of our personal warmth and spontaneity. Our political disagreements did not disappear, but our affectionate, lifelong friendship could survive this uneasy interlude.

The most shocking example of the Yale uprising's impact on a personal friendship had to do with Diana and Lionel Trilling. BJ and I met the Trillings at Norman Mailer's Brooklyn home in the mid-sixties. The four of us quickly became good friends, had a number of dinners in New York, and spent time together in Wellfleet and later in London. While we were all aware of political disparities among us, my work on thought reform and Lionel's on liberalism gave us much common ground. We were also drawn together by our shared affection for Mailer, our fascination with his imagination, and also by our concern about the bizarre, almost mad directions his mind could seem to take in both his writing and his life (what Diana called his "crazy side"). Lionel himself could be a bit zany, on one occasion recounting to us, with a mixture of irony and pleasure, his childhood fantasy of being descended from British royalty. When we were together, BJ would frequently be paired off with Lionel and I with Diana. By that time Diana had moved into a hardened anticommunist and anti-youth-rebellion position. But she and I liked each other and enjoyed each other's minds, and could manage our differences by means of a certain mutual tactfulness. Diana had a marvelous capacity for playful (not a word one tends to associate with her) forays into all levels of discourse—from soap opera plots to presidential politics to a friend's hangover, to the decline of Marxism and rise of psychoanalysis, and the increasing importance of celebrity in American society. Our sensibilities were in many ways similar, and we were a kind of test case for openness and friendship between people of highly antithetical political views. The experiment seemed to succeed, at least for a while.

We did feel a strain on our four-way friendship in connection with the student rebellions of the late sixties, especially the Columbia University uprising of 1968. Columbia was, after all, Lionel's longtime institutional home. I could understand his softly expressed resentment toward students who seemed to want to bring down the university. And he could understand my feeling that the students were reacting to a dreadful war in which they could be asked to fight and die, doing so as a generation threatened with nuclear annihilation, and combining serious political purpose and theater in their occupation of the president's office. I myself was not without some doubt about the choice of the university as a field of battle. I learned later that Lionel had allied himself with faculty members seeking mediation and the avoidance of police involvement, although he said little about this at the time. And his witticism about "alma mater-fuckers" expressed a certain balance on his part.

That was hardly the case with Diana. For her the rebellious students were little more than thugs who imperiled the university. In terms of our friendship, it was the Yale uprising, or at least the buildup to it, that became sadly decisive. *The New York Times* had run an article about that buildup, in which I had been quoted as being among those faculty members advocating that Yale open up its campus and engage in dialogue with the protestors. A few days later, at a large reception given by Dave and Evey Riesman in their Cambridge home, Diana came up to me with fire in her eyes and declared, in a tone of self-righteous contempt: "You have betrayed the academic profession!" She then histrionically turned around and marched away. What I felt was a mixture of confusion, hurt, and anger. I too felt betrayed—in my case by a friend from whom I had in the past experienced only affection and respect. And I was appalled that a commonsense suggestion of open dialogue on a university campus could so trigger her rage.

Over time I was to wonder whether the earlier affection and respect had been real, concluding that it had, but that our friendship had required disciplined restraint on each of our parts, which finally was undermined by the fiercely polarizing currents then sweeping through American society. There were probably thousands of friendships that suffered similar fates. A year later, at the home of a mutual friend, I was able to speak to Diana and tell her how unreasonable I thought she had been, and of my own anger and resentment. She spoke quietly but unapologetically, saying at the time she saw me as "a symbol of that kind of betrayal [of the academic profession]." I responded, also civilly but a little less softly, saying that I objected to being made by her into a symbol of anything, and that she ought to have looked at me instead as a person and a friend with his own considered point of view. She did not disagree, but said, in effect, that she felt so strongly about the matter that she could not help seeing me as a symbol. (It struck me later that her position was something on the order of the legal defense known in forensic psychiatry as the "irresistible impulse"—however wrong the action, the perpetrator was innocent because of lacking the psychological capacity for restraint.) The conversation resolved nothing. Our friendship with the Trillings was over.

Deeper Intellectual Divides

I had conflicts with other intellectuals who were antagonistic to many of the currents of the sixties. In that regard I had a revealing encounter with Irving Howe. We were together at a small meeting in 1971 at the Greenwich Village apartment of William Phillips, editor of the *Partisan Review*. William was a stubborn survivor of the New York intellectual wars and called the meeting for the ostensible purpose of recreating an influential group of "New York intellectuals" (I learned later he had called a number of such futile meetings, mostly involving people who were connected with or had written for the *Partisan Review*). I had long admired Howe as an unusually articulate social democrat who stood mostly for the things I did. But during earlier conversations I had with him on Cape Cod, he always seemed irritable, especially so about young rebels. From Todd Gitlin and Tom Hayden, former sixties student leaders who became friends of mine, I learned of Howe's continuous conflicts with younger-generation radicals. While some of his criticisms of their excesses were undoubtedly justified, he emerged as something of an Old Left curmudgeon, denouncing some of the qualities I found appealing in young rebels, including their mixture of protean experimentation with political commitment.

At that New York meeting a personal conversation with Howe did much to clarify our differences. I mentioned my admiration for his writing and agreement with most of his political stands but wondered why he was so consistently critical of student rebels and so uncritical of much of American Cold War behavior. He told me that for him communism, and its betrayal of the ideals that led so many people to support it, was the great issue of our time. The students had to be confronted on their failure to take a stand on communism. And Cold War policies that resisted communist goals should be supported. I told him that I understood what he was saying but for me the great issue of our time was Hiroshima and the general threat of nuclear annihilation. So I believed strongly that we should join the students in their opposition to belligerent Cold War policies. Our exchange was quietly civil and did little to alter the thinking of either of us.

There was something generational here, though Howe was only four years older than I was. But he, like many other New York Jewish intellectuals, had been drawn very early into passionate communist or Trotskyite affiliations, and experienced the brutal betrayal of that idealism in a direct and highly personal fashion. I had never invested idealistic energies in communist visions. Those energies were to be claimed by Hiroshima and nuclear threat. It was a matter of the particular traumatic historical involvement one has survived, and the meaning and mission one derives from that survival. Howe's views on nuclear weapons undoubtedly had many parallels to my own, and my sense of communist brutality (strengthened by my study of Chinese thought reform) undoubtedly resembled Howe's. But inevitably our strongest political and ethical passions went in different directions. To Howe, the rebellious students often seemed naïve about communism and unwilling to denounce it, and at times themselves to resemble totalitarian movements. While I agreed with that last concern, to me the students were crying out against a mentality that had created a world in which nuclear extinction seemed likely, and against a war created by a similar mentality. My exchange with Howe was particularly excruciating because we otherwise shared so much.

A number of the New York intellectuals were deeply threatened by the rebellious currents of the sixties and embraced the anticommunist purpose of the Vietnam War. I knew a few of them before they got there and was appalled by the stands they came to assume: cruel views toward social justice in American society, and the most dangerous kind of military belligerence internationally. Irving Kristol was a troubling case in point. I remember him from the early sixties when he was an editor at Basic Books, and BJ and I became friendly with him and his wife, the historian Gertrude Himmelfarb. In our conversations Irving was soft-spoken and thoughtful, and could be quite humorous in making fun of others and himself. He had emerged from a Trotskyite past into years of anticommunist struggle, and in the fifties had been a founder and editor of *Encounter* magazine in London. But soon he went further, and I was aghast at the turn his politics took as he became one of the main theorists of the neoconservative movement and seemed to divest himself of the compassion I thought of him as possessing. But then he broke the stereotype in a way that is bound to dissolve any writer's critical faculties. He wrote a sympathetic review in 1970 in *The New York Times* of my essay collection, *History and Human Survival.* He praised my way of addressing human beings in connection with larger historical issues, expressing only mild reservations about some of my ideas. Given how much our political views had diverged by then, I thought the review quite remarkable in its generosity. I never discussed it with him and hadn't seen him in decades when he died in 2009.

Kristol said something important about himself as late as 2008: "Ever since I can remember, I've been a neo-something: a neo-Marxist, a neo-Trotskyite, a neo-liberal, a neo-conservative; in religion a neo-orthodox. . . . I'm going to end up a neo-that's all, neo-nothing." *Neo,* of course, means new, or a new version of. Kristol has constantly sought out a new version of an old ideology, in each case finding it ultimately unsatisfactory, and himself suggests a deep intellectual emptiness that culminates in "neo-nothing." He did become sufficiently entranced with neoconservatism to articulate its crass doctrine all too effectively, while living out an alliance with power so characteristic of former communist neoconservatives and being awarded the Presidential Medal of Freedom by George W. Bush. In reading him one sometimes gets the sense that, though his neoconservative passions were strong, he was at the same time aware of playing an intellectual game in which he could be variable and volatile.

There has been much speculation over what caused a significant group of Jewish intellectuals, many of whom had been Marxists, to embrace neoconservative ideology and policies. I don't think that there is a single cause—there never is in connection with human behavior—but I agree with those who point to concerns about Israel as a significant factor. I would go further and suggest that, more than just Israel, there could be involved a primal fear of another Holocaust, of personal and collective annihilation, in which case domestic callousness and military belligerence could be seen as humane and life-enhancing. Of course this is only speculation, but it is likely that extreme emotions of this sort are behind the conversion to the totalistic extremes of the neoconservative position.

Kristol collaborated in some of his enterprises with Daniel Bell, the historically minded sociologist, but Bell, though often a critic of the left, has avoided the neoconservative path. He had been at Columbia in 1968 and was with Lionel Trilling, part of the faculty group advocating mediation with the students. He and I have been friendly acquaintances since the late fifties, and I have a nice memory (perhaps from the mid-sixties) of Dan and his wife, Pearl, and BJ and myself walking down Riverside Drive on a late Sunday morning following an Upper West Side brunch, with Dan skillfully spinning out a series of very funny Jewish jokes. But we were always in disagreement about youth rebellion and its significance for American culture. Dan tended to see harm or pathology in the young, and in one written exchange expressed the fear that they would go so far as to violate the incest taboo and thereby create extreme social chaos. I raised the opposite possibility, namely that the hedonism was part of what I called proteanism, forms of experimentation that contributed to preserving the self during a period of great historical confusion. I was moved to discover in the library papers a warm personal letter from him in response to my father's obituary in *The New York Times* in 1966. I think that Dan, as a City College graduate, was affected by the obituary's emphasis of my father's lifelong involvement with that institution.

A couple of decades later, during the early eighties, Dan and I were to share a Japanese boondoggle, which included the French anthropologist Claude Levi-Strauss, through the largesse of the Suntory Foundation, endowed by Japan's biggest producer of whiskey. We were lavishly entertained and had exchanges with a considerable number of leading Japanese intellectuals. The high moment came when, before a large audience and television cameras, we were each asked to make a statement advising the Japanese about the future—which we did with utmost predictability: I urged the Japanese to confront the Hiroshima and Nagasaki atomic bombings as a basis for taking the lead in efforts at international nuclear disarmament and peacemaking. Dan urged them to concentrate on developing a viable middle class and building up their military strength. Levi-Strauss urged them to pay attention to their own cultural tradition, to "be yourselves." The activist psychiatrist called for atomic bomb witness, the centrist sociologist for Cold War stability, and the wide-ranging anthropologist for preserving cultural identity. I do not think the Japanese learned very much from us, but we surely learned a lot about a developing cultural resurgence in Japan that was taking on conservative, countersixties coloring.

I was struggling at the time with my relationship to anticommunist intellectuals. My work on thought reform brought me into that realm, but I wanted to avoid it as a self-definition by combining critical exposure of communist totalism with strong opposition to the Vietnam War and support for student protest. My involvement with anticommunist intellectuals culminated in my participation, in 1969, in a vastly self-important conference, whose theme was something on the order of "the intellectual in society," held in a plush hotel in New York City and sponsored by various groups, including a number of major American foundations and the Congress for Cultural Freedom. The latter was undoubtedly the most ambitious of the intellectual groups organized to combat duplicitous but at times effective communist propaganda. The Congress for Cultural Freedom was international and not only organized conferences in Europe and the United States but created influential journals, such as *Encounter* in England and *Der Monat* in Germany, which attracted prominent European and American writers of fairly diverse views. Those initially included such highly respected people as Kenneth Galbraith, Czeslaw Milosz, Hannah Arendt, Dwight Macdonald, and H. Stuart Hughes. But during the late sixties there were several exposés of a CIA link. It turned out that the Congress had been created by the CIA to provide intellectuals with an alternative to the influence of communist or communist front groups. That CIA tie tended to invalidate the enterprise, except for the more narrowly anticommunist figures (including Arthur Koestler and Irving Kristol) who knew about and accepted the idea of CIA support. I did not, but justified my attendance at the conference by its much broader backing and the opportunity provided to assert my views on Hiroshima and nuclear weapons.

Neither my memory nor my notes record anything of great moment that transpired during those two or three days, but I do recall a personal encounter that came to matter to me. My sense of absurdity in connection with the conference discussions gave rise to one of my bird cartoons. I had been drawing these little figures—what I called bird images rather than actual birds—from at least the late fifties. Often one bird (usually the bigger and presumably older one) would say something pretentious and self-serving and would be deflated by the other bird; or else one would ask a seemingly naïve question and the other would provide an unexpectedly revealing answer. To me the birds express the fallibility of just about everyone and everything, and the absurdity we are likely to encounter around us and within ourselves.

I can't remember the exact cartoon I drew at the conference but it could have been something like one bird asking the other, "Why are your ideas so fuzzy, circular, and contradictory?" And the other replying, "Because I'm an intellectual." Whatever the particular cartoon, during a lunch break I passed it to a friend at an adjoining table who I thought would enjoy it. I was observed doing so by Israel Shenker, a *New York Times* writer assigned to cover the conference, who happened to be sitting at that table. Shenker was amused by the cartoon and even more by the phenomenon of my drawing and giving words to these creatures. He took me aside and proposed that he do a feature story on me in connection with this "avocation." I resisted the idea, having always considered the birds to express private sentiments that I shared with people around me, and also because I foolishly feared that I would be seen as trivial or lightweight. But something in me was also intrigued. So we compromised and agreed that Shenker could interview me about the birds and write an article, which he would show me with the understanding that if I did not like it, nothing would be published. In fact, I loved the piece he wrote, which was run as a *Times* feature story with a heading "Erudite Professor Draws Absurd Little Birds" and illustrated by a couple of examples.

The article presented me to the world in a new way. For the first time, it was publicly suggested that I was a man who evoked laughs. But the laughter could be an uneasy response to gallows humor. The two books of cartoons I published (*Birds* and *Psychobirds*) were dominated by responses to Vietnam and the sixties but could also reach out to a more "existential" sense of absurdity. Consider two of the cartoons.

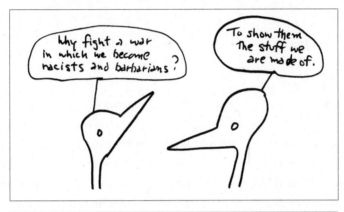

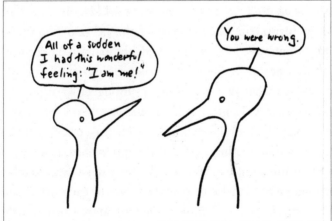

BJ, always a great enthusiast of the little creatures, gave me the kind of mixed compliment about them that only a spouse could offer: "The birds are what you'll be remembered for." I would just say that they are my intellectual underbelly, much related to but extending beyond Vietnam and the sixties.

13

<hr style="width:10%"/>

Home from the War

Redress of Grievances

The Vietnam War dragged on. My involvement with antiwar veterans taught me more and more about what it was doing to our soldiers and to the country at large. I was increasingly affected by the "existential evil" I had earlier identified. The war was at the heart of the divisions and antagonisms dominating the society. And all too often, blame was focused either on the peace movement for stirring things up, or simply on Vietnam veterans for what they had done, as though the larger society and the people who made decisions to fight and extend the war had no moral and legal culpability. I felt increasingly that it was time to get beyond my study, and even the meeting places of the rap groups, and become more seriously involved in protest. So when two younger activist acquaintances, Fred Branfman and Carl Rogers, came to me in early 1972 with a suggestion that we create a group of prominent American intellectuals and professionals to engage in civil disobedience, I could not have embraced the idea more enthusiastically. Fred and Carl were in their twenties and their vision was one of their well-connected elders joining the young in (as the language of the time had it) "putting their bodies on the line." We were to do something like that, though in the most gentle fashion, in what I myself came to characterize as "fat cat civil disobedience." It was my enthusiasm more than anything else that caused me to become the group's closest approximation to a leader.

We began to call around to friends, and with the help of antiwar lawyers, we built our group around two very American concepts: the First Amendment constitutional right of the people to petition their government for "redness of grievances" (our official title was "Citizens' Committee for Redress of Grievances," though we mostly called ourselves "Redress"); and the Nuremberg principle of opposing an "aggressive war" and the "war crimes" of one's own government.

Our theories took us to the House of Representatives, specified by the Constitution as the place for citizens to seek their redress. We did that on a sunny April day in 1972, and have a wonderful photograph in our Redress archives of the folksinger Judy Collins and myself, walking toward the Capitol steps, while displaying together a giant scroll on which was printed our petition demanding that Congress end the war. Judy is elegant in her floor-length dress and shoulder-length hair, and has an expression on her face that is ardent, almost beatific. I am wearing a light summer jacket and bow tie, my hair also on the long side, and look both determined and distracted. We are followed by a long line of perhaps a hundred and fifty people, looking pleasant and well dressed. They were professors (Martin Duberman, Peter Brooks, Howard Zinn, Richard Falk), writers (Francine Gray, Dwight Macdonald, Kenneth Koch, Garry Wills), leaders in the peace and women's movements (Benjamin Spock, Gloria Steinem, Bill Coffin), university presidents (John William Ward of Amherst and Harold Taylor, formerly of Sarah Lawrence), and actors and producers (Joe Papp, Barbara Harris, Candice Bergen, Isaiah Sheffer).

There was much of the mock-heroic about us, and most of my memories of Redress are odd and humorous. For one thing, we were careful to steer clear of the actual House chamber, the entering of which would be considered a felony that could lead to years of imprisonment, rather than the lesser misdemeanor with which we were prepared to be charged for refusing to leave the antechamber. The night before we held a meeting of the group in the Dupont Plaza Hotel, where many of us were staying, to make our final preparations and go over details. I was chairing things and found myself something of a group therapist in seeking to alleviate people's fears about breaking the law and being arrested. (Our eleven-year-old son, Ken, had expressed such fear for BJ and me when we were explaining to him why we would be away for a couple of days. First, referring to scenes he had viewed on television, he implored us: "Don't go! The police will hit you over the head and beat you up." When we explained that everything was carefully planned and would be orderly, he touchingly declared: "Then let me go with you!") In truth, my only fear was that the whole thing would fail, people would drop out, the event would not occur, or that whatever we did would go completely unnoticed.

Fortunately, someone had had the inspired idea of inviting Dick Gregory, the black comedian, to address us. Gregory is not only one of the world's funniest men but has himself been an indefatigable practitioner of every kind of civil disobedience in opposition to war and poverty. Gregory had witnessed our discussion and our demeanor, and now addressed us as a friendly uncle: "Looking around at you middle-class white folks, I can see that some of you are a bit *scaared*. Look, that's okay. The first time I went out to break the law I was pretty scared myself. So you know what I did? I found myself a couple of nuns and walked behind them." Then he added a piece of advice: "Look, don't take what I'm saying the wrong way, but I gotta tell ya, this is one time you can't call the *police*." Gregory's riff gave us the perspective we needed.

We were welcomed on the Capitol steps by friendly congresspeople such as Bella Abzug, Herman Badillo, and Ron Dellums. We then entered the antechamber and, as previously arranged, Speaker Carl Albert came out to receive our petition. I presented it to him, declaring in the most authoritative tone I could muster: "We demand that you call the House of Representatives into emergency session in order to pass a bill ending all funding of the war in Indochina!" Albert, a short man who seemed to take up little space in the room we had come to dominate, looked up at me with glazed eyes and said, "I will refer the matter to the appropriate committee." That seemed such a caricature of bureaucratese that I was literally dumbfounded and unable to think of anything to say. Fortunately, standing right behind me was Paul O'Dwyer, a progressive lawyer from a prominent New York political family, who had defended the Harrisburg Eight, and who now whispered loudly into my ear, "Tell him that we find his reply unsatisfactory." So I raised my head and my decibels and boomed out: "We find your reply *unsatisfactory!*" I've never forgotten that lesson in political robotism. Shortly after that the police made their announcement ordering us to leave; a small number in our group (who for one reason or another did not wish to be arrested) complied; the rest of us stood our ground.

We were arrested very peaceably—no handcuffs, just an individual policeman assigned to each of us and guiding us firmly but not unkindly by the arm to a paddy wagon. Later I wondered how there could be a hundred-plus officers available for this task, and I learned that the Washington, D.C., police department thought it a good opportunity to use us for training new recruits on how to arrest people. They needed quite a few paddy wagons as well, and when those vehicles arrived at their destination, Ben Spock and I found ourselves walking at the head of the group from the parking area to the Washington lockup. When we got there, the chief warden came out and greeted Ben warmly: "Hiya, Doc. How's it going?" Spock replied in kind, as to an old friend, and the warden added: "Now you tell the folks that we run a good shop and everybody will be treated okay," to which Spock smiled his assent. Spock was then close to seventy, still a vigorous protestor, and I had the feeling of his passing the mantle not to the very young (they were protesting on their own) but to middle-aged adults like myself and my friends. (In the lockup, things were a bit crowded because of all the people we caused them to arrest. So there were inconveniences—eight of us in a cell so small that we couldn't all lie down at the same time, and a single toilet that allowed for no excretory privacy. But nobody was cruel or even unpleasant toward us, though BJ later told me that male guards on the female side had a slightly more abusive attitude. I do remember having a glimmer of what it was like to be totally controlled by a particular institution, much attenuated by my awareness that it would be just for one night.

Mostly the experience was very upbeat. Everyone seemed to settle in easily enough, and there were playful emanations from neighboring cells. The poet Kenneth Koch called out to me, "Hey, Lifton, you got us *in* here. Now how about getting us *out*?" In his case there was pain underneath the humor, as I later learned that he was claustrophobic and that it had taken some courage for him to seek arrest. Isaiah Sheffer mimicked Hollywood gangster films by grabbing his cell bars and shouting,

"Where's me mout'piece?" In my cell we had a spontaneous all-night seminar in which we explored, convivially and enthusiastically, such matters as historical and political sources of disastrous American policies, parallels in ancient mythology, and the merits of various efforts to bring about change. I remember Garry Wills being especially lively on classical models; also holding forth in the cell were articulate lawyers, professors, and foundation heads. We each took breaks for a half hour or so of attempted sleep, but the jailhouse seminar kept going and its ocean of words did not cease until we left the cell the next morning. There was lots of talk on the women's side as well, but apparently more personal. BJ later told me about her conversation with the actress Candice Bergen, who talked of life with her father, the ventriloquist Edgar Bergen, and the jealousy she experienced toward her father's dummy, Charlie McCarthy. As prisoners we not only enjoyed ourselves but were quite well behaved, except for one little transgression. Someone decorated a cell wall with a large graffiti message that read, "Don't fuck with redress!"—another bit of self-mockery, considering our highly intellectualized and ultranonviolent character.

The charge against us, as it is in such matters, was "unlawful entry." We each appeared before the judge to make our plea of nolo contendere, meaning that we did not contest the verdict. Richard Falk, whom we had designated to make a statement on behalf of all of us, spoke of our being motivated by the "situation of intolerable cost for the peoples of Indochina and of unpredictable peril for American society," associating our "small action of defiance" with principles of individual responsibility in connection with the Nuremberg obligation.

We carried out a second act of civil disobedience a month later, this time in the room adjoining the U.S. Senate chamber. At our pre-arrest evening meeting, we decided that we would not simply refuse to leave but would lie down in order to symbolize Vietnamese and American dead. In addition to going over our plans, I again had the quasi-therapeutic task of responding to fears and doubts. There was one particularly memorable exchange in which someone else replied for me. An elderly woman questioned the plan because, as she put it, "Lying down isn't really dignified," and before I could say anything in response, I heard Garry Wills's resonant words from the rear of the room: "Neither is dying!"

We were addressed briefly by a few antiwar senators, including Ted Kennedy, Mike Gravel, and Jacob Javits, before their regular session in the Senate chamber. But when they and others emerged to find our supine bodies pretty well covering the floor of that outer room, they did not seem delighted to see us. We seemed to be more acceptable standing up than lying down. I expected no more from prowar senators, our antagonists, but was taken aback by the antiwar senators who also were intent on avoiding us. They in particular didn't think it politically wise to be seen with or photographed among lawbreakers like ourselves. The only senator who strode unhesitatingly among us was Barry Goldwater, the archconservative, militarily belligerent bête noire of all antiwar activists. He explained that he was looking for a friend of his, his former speechwriter Karl Hess, who had gone over to our side and joined the protest. I remember trying to help him as he came near me, raising my head from my prone position and pointing in the direction where I thought Hess could be found. Goldwater then stepped over and around our bodies, an unself-conscious visitor from another world. When he finally found Hess, they shook hands warmly, exchanged a few pleasantries, and Goldwater once more made his way among our inert forms to leave the room. The war's most extreme advocate, and no one else, had "socialized" with us.

We were hardly a national sensation, but we did receive a certain amount of attention from newspapers, radio, and television. I felt that we had made a small contribution to the amorphous potpourri of American antiwar sentiment by conveying the message that people of standing in the society could feel sufficiently outraged by the criminality of the war to cross a threshold into civil disobedience.

My leadership was in many ways propelled from below (younger people involved in organizing included not only Branfman and Rogers but also Tom Davidson and Anita Dworkin) and guided by our lawyers (Arthur Kinoy, Richard Falk, Peter Weiss, and Saul Mendlovitz). Much of my Redress effort had to do with listening and persuading on the telephone and bringing together radical activists (who provided much inspiration), left liberals (who made up most of our group), and centrist liberals (whose conscience I could often tap). The effort could be tedious but also joyous in finding another métier for antiwar expression.

Our activities after our two forays in the Capitol—antiwar conferences and other public stands—were somewhat anticlimactic and the group's energies waned after about two years. I sensed that, and wrote a note to myself in late 1963 titled "Redress without Tears" in which I expressed a yearning to go back to theoretical work on the psychohistorical model (or paradigm) of death and the continuity of life that I was trying to develop. Redress had always been fluid, improvisational, and uncertain, and many of us could now sense its imminent demise—though from time to time there have been rumblings among people associated with it about reconvening the group and reasserting its practice of civil disobedience to oppose the war in Iraq or the war in Afghanistan.

I had two "Redress dreams" in which these matters were expressed in amusing but significant ways. In one of them I was the leader of a small Redress-like group, which included Margaret Mead. She was in favor of our mounting an action in Spain to contest the violation of human rights there. I listened to her suggestions and encouraged the others to express their views, but then strongly objected to her proposal. I pointed out that the Spanish police, as part of a totalitarian state (Spain was still under Franco's rule), would suppress our action before it could have any effect. But I wondered whether I was being overfearful in my objection.

In another dream the Redress-like group I was leading sought to make a "dramatic public demonstration," this time in America, and we were searching for a theme around which to do so. Someone suggested that the theme be "Home from the War," which seemed a good idea to most of those present. But I objected, pointing out that, since it was my book title, people would think that the event was a promotion for the book itself. I proposed instead that the theme be "Back from the War," and the group agreed to this change.

The two dreams reflected my conflicts not only about activism versus book writing but also about dedication versus self-aggrandizement, and about personal issues of risk, courage, and fear. I can't say that I've ever resolved these conflicts, but I've never stopped being aware of them, or of their humorous underbelly, and that has helped.

Neither Victims nor Executioners

Home from the War is not only the angriest of my books but also the one that is most, in itself, an act of protest. More than that, it records a shift in my own identity toward combining my professional efforts with a more radical social perspective. So the last sentence of the original preface reads: "I cannot say that I underwent the same transformation as the Vietnam veterans I describe, but I did not emerge from this study unchanged." I originally called the book "Neither Victims Nor Executioners," the two roles Camus urged human beings to avoid, roles into which Vietnam veterans had been thrust and from which they sought to extricate themselves. It could well have been a confusing title and *Home from the War* is probably a better one, but "Neither Victims Nor Executioners" came closer to the gut feelings I wrote about.

The heart of the book lies in the rap group experience, and I dedicated the volume to the nineteen veterans and five shrinks who had been most active with me in our particular group, listing all of them by their first names, and adding one more name as well: that of a Vietnamese child who survived My Lai. But here too I followed my mosaic principle of including larger background matters that illuminate immediate findings, in this case having to do with war-making, change, and healing. The book is both dark and hopeful: dark in depicting not only the nature of the war itself but also the elements of American society that brought about the war and its atrocities. What is hopeful is the theme of transformation that is so prominent throughout, in which the changes undergone by individual veterans represent larger possibilities for American society. Most of the book tells the story of the rap groups and the veterans' struggles with guilt, rage, and violence, the counterfeit world of the Vietnam War, and the experience of renewal many described in connection with being a man, "learning to feel," and finding meaning in their lives. I viewed the antiwar veterans as embodying a potentially prophetic function for the society as a whole: questioning the warrior ethos, suggesting modes of change, and recasting moral questions for professionals like myself.

With the war still on when the book was published, it was reviewed everywhere, more widely than any book of mine before or since. Responses were sharply divided in tone, largely depending upon the reviewer's convictions about the war. A little more than half of the reviews were strongly favorable, saying I'd captured terrible truths about Vietnam. But there were plenty of attacks, accusations of bias in my attitudes and in my limiting the study to antiwar veterans (though I had made clear I was doing just that, and not claiming to represent veterans in general). So *Newsweek* lauded the book for probing "deeper and more widely into the perversion of the warrior ethos," while *Time* denounced it for being "a polemic in which moralizing smothers analysis." Centrist liberal critics could be offended by the book: for instance, Christopher Lehmann-Haupt of *The New York Times* said that returns on the Vietnam War are not yet in (it might prove "necessary to the survival of American civilization") and added that he would want his psychiatrist to be more neutral on the subject. I had failed to convince such reviewers that a psychiatrist could combine moral passion with accurate psychological investigation. But I was buoyed by the almost uniformly enthusiastic reviews by psychiatric colleagues who seemed to recognize the depth of the war's psychological cost and accept the value of working specifically with antiwar veterans and chronicling their change.

Beyond reviews, I had more hostile reactions to me than in connection with any other book. One anonymous group sent me a certificate containing a drawing of an upside-down peace symbol whose edges resembled the claws of a chicken, with my name on top; I was the winner of "The American Chicken Award" for advocating that we quit this war. And a menacing telephone caller asked me: "How do you feel, Dr. Lifton, now that you lost Cambodia?" What I felt, leaving aside the wild exaggeration of my influence, was that it was time to unlist my telephone number.

My struggle with responses to the book was expressed in an August 1973 exchange of letters with Susan Sontag, a friend who was not yet a cultural icon. After receiving an advance copy she wrote to me from France, saying that the book was "good . . . the experience of reading it a harrowing one, as well it should be." I wrote back about having to get used to the fiercely polarized emotions the book seemed to arouse. I then mused further on whether people like ourselves could "have it both ways" in being "radically critical (even subversive) of certain currents in our society," and expect to be "enormously rewarded by that society for our efforts." I said that in recognizing the contradiction I felt "a glimmer of liberation." But I would now emphasize the existence of at least a corner of American society deeply responsive to calls for reassertion of dormant ideals of that society, and *Home from the War* was in fact a finalist for the National Book Award.

Despite its wide response, the book sold quite modestly. But it does seem to have had a long-range impact as writers, activists, and professionals of various kinds have conveyed to me, over the years, a sense of the book's importance in their lives. It also shaped my subsequent reactions to American war-making, and in a 2005 reissue of the volume I wrote a new introduction in which I made systematic psychological connections between Iraq and Vietnam. When I was told by a leading Israeli resister (part of a group that refused to fight in occupied areas) that *Home from the War* had influenced his decision, I could feel that the book had become part of an international body of literature contesting atrocity-producing situations anywhere. So yes, perhaps the book, and the work with veterans that created it, provided me with a "glimmer of liberation" after all.

Part Four

Nazi Doctors—Did It Really Happen?

14

Strong Enough Stomach?

GOING BACK TO research on Nazi doctors is different from doing that with my other studies. In reimmersing myself in work on thought reform, on atomic bomb survivors, and on Vietnam veterans, I rediscovered the suffering and staying power I had witnessed and some of my own mixture of pain and intensity. But with Nazi doctors the universe that had to be reentered was so extreme and grotesque that I still find it hard to believe I spent so much time in it.

The difficulty any mind has in taking in the Nazi project was made clear to me by Dr. Viktor T., a distinguished Jewish psychiatrist and admirable human being who had been an Auschwitz inmate for a year and had then embarked upon decades of professional work on the effects of incarceration in Nazi camps and on treatment of survivors. As we sat down together in his modest office to begin one of our interviews, he looked at me with a quizzical expression and said, in characteristically quiet tones: "You know, Robert, I've been involved in this problem for more than forty years, and I still can't believe that it really happened—that anyone would try to round up all the Jews in Europe and then send them to a place to kill them."

Of course he knew very well that it had indeed happened, but in a portion of his mind, he periodically experienced disbelief in its actual occurrence. Those who seriously investigate Nazi killing can have moments of just that kind of incredulity. And in my case, if part of my mind said the Nazis couldn't really have done what they did, then I couldn't have studied them and written a book about them. This difficulty everyone has in taking in the actuality of Nazi behavior can render people susceptible to the falsehoods of Holocaust deniers. The deniers, often Nazi sympathizers, exploit this tendency to incredulity in their preposterous claims that the Nazis engaged in no systematic killing of Jews, or perhaps only killed a small number of them. But my psychiatrist-survivor friend taught me that recognizing in oneself such periodic disbelief can energize one's efforts at full confrontation of truth.

When turning to this portion of the memoir, I experienced a sense of dread and a tightening in my chest. And I began to have unpleasant dreams, resembling those I had when I first embarked on the work, dreams involving bleak, threatening landscapes. At the same time there was another part of me that was quite willing, even eager, to reexamine this period of my life. I recall it as a time of great significance for me, and have memories of working in high gear to complete the most difficult of my projects.

When first talking to people in the late seventies about my interest in the work, they frequently responded with a metaphor of the stomach. They would ask, "Do you have the stomach to do it?" or "Do you have a strong enough stomach?" I noted that within just a few days' time "at least three psychoanalysts put the [stomach] question rather menacingly," which "alarmed me a bit." I thought later about how the Japanese used "stomach" as we use "heart," meaning the center of spiritual or psychic energy. But from the way Americans were using the stomach metaphor, it was clear that such meanings could transcend cultural differences. In any case I was by no means sure that I had either sufficient stomach or heart for what I was getting involved in. I know now that I greatly underestimated just how demanding the enterprise would be in order to protect my decision to go ahead with it.

There was another issue raised to me, having specifically to do with engaging evil. A friend, arguing against my going ahead with the study, referred to a principle of Jewish moral tradition that required one to avoid any contact with evil; one should keep one's distance from it, just let it lie. I rejected her argument and held to an alternative principle of probing the sources of highly destructive behavior in order to combat that behavior, and of seeking knowledge more generally about any kind of human motivation. I understood that to be a principle of both the Enlightenment and the psychoanalytic movement, and I still firmly adhere to it. But I sensed even then that her warning was not entirely without merit, and it was to take on troubling relevance in connection with my interactions with Nazi doctors.

There was a related warning that was intellectually more complex and more difficult to deal with. It had to do with the concern that, in probing the minds of Nazi doctors, my psychological "understanding" of them would become a form of justification and would replace moral judgment. Or else I would make a clinical diagnosis of Nazi doctors, and the language of psychopathology would replace that of moral transgression. I had observed this problem in connection with a study done by a friend in which he probed the motivations of Soviet psychiatrists who incarcerated political heretics in psychiatric institutions by labeling them as mentally ill. When a respected advisor on his manuscript told him that his psychological explanation would be viewed by readers as vindication of these psychiatrists, my friend decided against its publication.

Here I was helped by an aversion to reducing behavior in general to psychopathology, and particularly behavior involving large historical forces. In previous work I had not been reluctant to make moral judgments, but I knew that with Nazi doctors I had to be especially clear about my ethical approach. I assumed that Nazi evil was a given, and came to understand my research as an exploration of psychological and historical currents conducive to evil. With that model, uncovering influences and motivations in no way replaced or interfered with an ethical focus. I became convinced that *evil* was a term I needed in connection with the work, contrary to the inclination of many in the social sciences to avoid the word because it defies precise definition and tends to be subjective. But I would insist that language requires reverberations beyond pure logic, and there is no better word to evoke extreme transgression producing extensive death and suffering. At the same time I viewed evil as specifically human, rejecting the frequent religious view that it derives from a supernatural source such as the Devil. A conversation I had with Elie Wiesel touched on those issues. We were discussing Nazi doctors—I had begun to interview them and he had observed a few from a distance in Auschwitz—when he posed this question to me: "Tell me, Bob, when they did what they did, were they *men* or were they *demons*?" I answered that, as he well knew, they were human beings, and that was our problem. To which Elie replied, "Yes, but it is *demonic* that they were *not* demonic." He was saying that everything would have been much simpler if the evil were in some way supernatural or at least nonhuman.

Looked at externally, my involvement in the work seemed to come about by accident. It began with a phone call from John J. Simon, who had been my editor at Random House for *Death in Life* and was now with a different publisher, Quadrangle Books, which was owned by *The New York Times*. John told me with some excitement that Quadrangle had gained access through the *Times* to extensive documents on Josef Mengele and other Nazi doctors at Auschwitz, assembled by a judge who had done elaborate investigations for criminal trials in Frankfurt. The judge was to arrive in a couple of days, and John and his colleagues wanted to talk to me about doing a study of Mengele. Was I interested? I was, and met the next day with John and another editor, and again the following day with them and Judge Horst von Glasenapp. Glasenapp, a lively, intense man who spoke excellent English, had been in the German army, then a POW in the Soviet Union, and in the process of becoming a judge developed a strong interest in Nazi crimes. His focus was influenced by having married a doctor and also by having undergone psychoanalytic therapy in Frankfurt with a member of the institute headed by Alexander Mitscherlich. Glasenapp knew a great deal about all aspects of Nazi doctors and was to become an essential source of information for me. He was not without his quirks, partly related to German culture (once when I telephoned him in the evening, he righteously declared that I should never telephone a German home after 9 P.M.). But he was wonderfully generous not only in providing documents and conveying all he knew, but in tracking down additional material. He contributed much to my getting the research going.

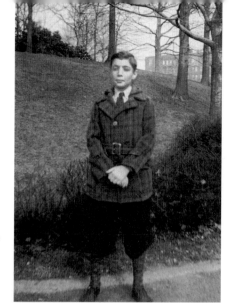

In Prospect Park in
Brooklyn, circa 1935,
wearing the "knickers"
of that time.

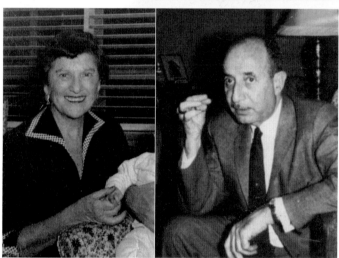

Ciel Roth Lifton and Harold A. Lifton, circa late 1950s.

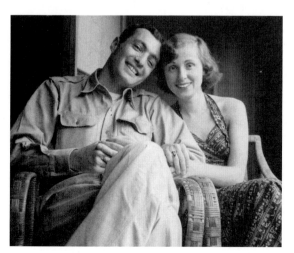

In uniform
(though hardly in
combat) with BJ,
in Saginomiya,
Tokyo, Japan,
1952.

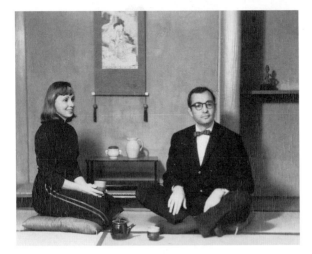

With BJ, Japanese-style, Tokyo, circa 1960.

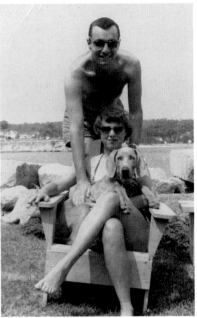

With BJ and Runcible,
in Provincetown, 1959.

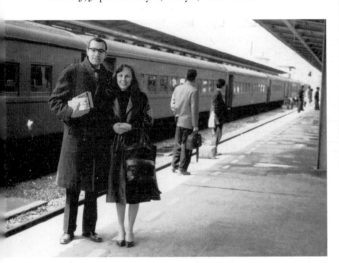

BJ and I arriving at Hiroshima station, 1962.

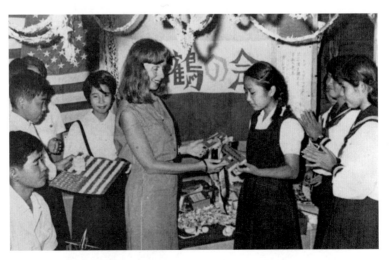

BJ with members of the Folded Crane Club, Hiroshima, 1962.

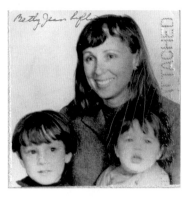

BJ's 1967 passport photo with Ken and Natasha.

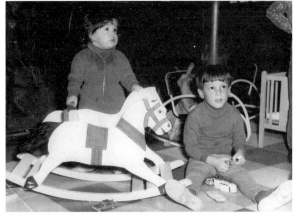

Natasha and Ken aboard the Queen Elizabeth, 1967.

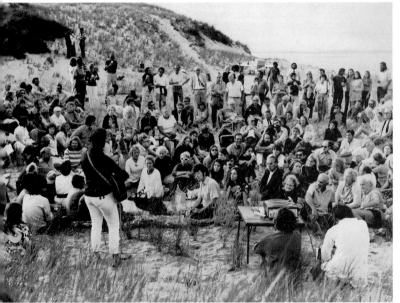

Antiwar fundraiser on the dunes. Robin Howard is singing. I am sitting with my back to the camera next to Harris Yulin (in white shirt), Wellfleet, 1971.

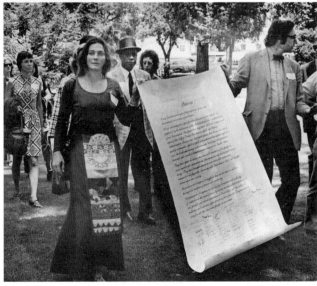

Holding Redress banner with Judy Collins, followed by fellow protestors, on the way to the House of Representatives for our act of civil disobedience, Washington, D.C., 1972. *Photograph by Lorraine W. Gray.*

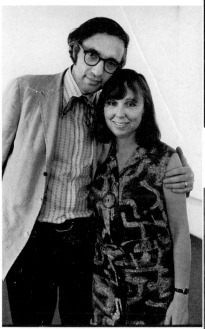

With BJ at a gallery, New York City, 1972. *Photograph by Eikoh Hosoe.*

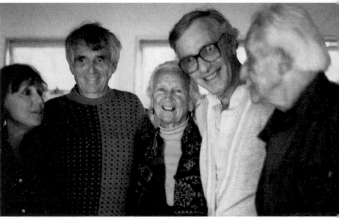

With BJ, Dan Berrigan, Joan Erikson, and Erik Erikson, at Wellfleet meetings, 1977.

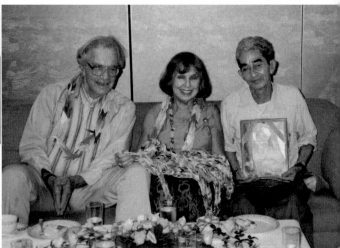

With BJ and Ichiro Kawamoto, Hiroshima, 1980.

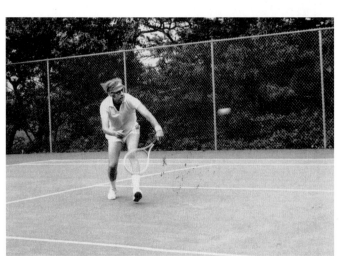

Setting myself for a backhand, Wellfleet, circa 1980s.

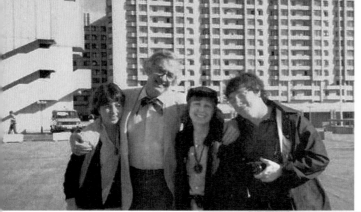

With Natasha, BJ, and Ken in Moscow, on a trip sponsored by the International Physicians for the Prevention of Nuclear War, 1983.

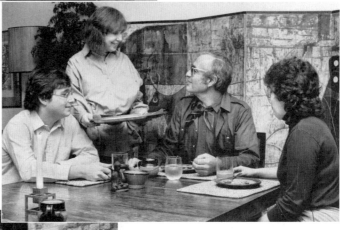

With Ken, BJ, and Michelle, New York, circa mid-1980s.
Photograph by Mike Fuller.

With John Mack at a conference in Prague, 1990.

Dan and Natasha, New York City, circa mid-1990s.

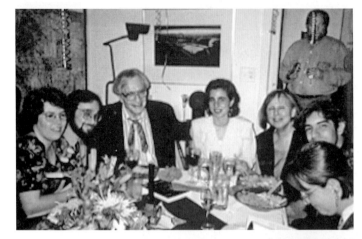

With Michelle, Ken, Natasha, BJ and others at my 70th birthday party, New York City, 1996.

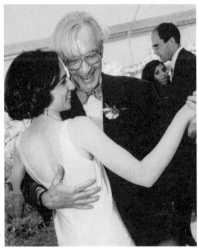

Dancing with Natasha at her wedding held at our Wellfleet home, 1997.

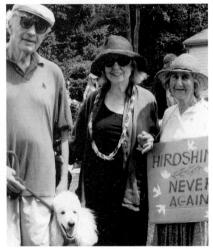

With BJ and Jingly at annual Hiroshima vigil, Wellfleet Center, August 6, 2005.

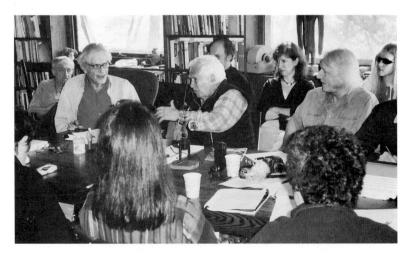

Around the table at a Wellfleet psychohistory meeting, with (facing camera) Norman Mailer and Chuck Strozier and (backs to camera) Cathy Caruth and Hillel Levine, circa 2004.

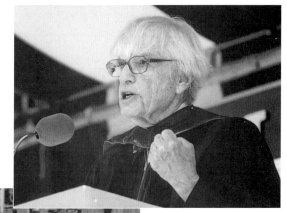

Receiving honorary degree and giving graduation address at Stonehill College, Easton, MA, 2008.

BJ and I celebrating our reunion with Iring and Elisabeth Fetscher, Frankfurt, 2009.

With filmmakers Hannes Karnick and Wolfgang Richter, and BJ at preview showing of documentary on my work on Nazi doctors, Frankfurt, 2009.

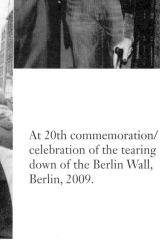

At 20th commemoration/ celebration of the tearing down of the Berlin Wall, Berlin, 2009.

With grandson Dmitri, following his cello concert, Cambridge, 2009.

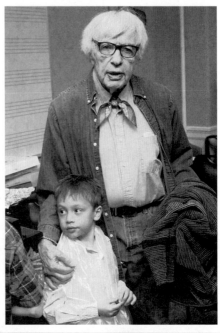

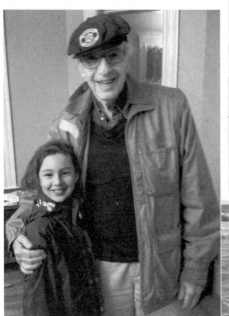

With granddaughter Lila after returning from a Red Sox–Yankees game, Cambridge, 2008.

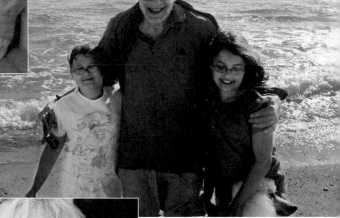

With granddaughters Jessica and Kimberly, and Jingly, on Wellfleet beach, 2008.

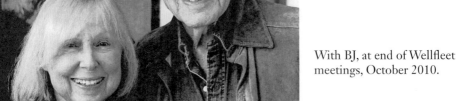

With BJ, at end of Wellfleet meetings, October 2010.

Yet well before John Simon's phone call, I had been heading toward a Holocaust study. My decision during the mid-sixties to compare psychologically Hiroshima survivors to survivors of Nazi camps was an early step in that direction. At that time I met frequently with psychiatrists working with Holocaust survivors (notably William Niederland, Henry Krystal, Emanuel Tanay, Martin Wangh, and Ulrich Venzlaff) and first presented an overall statement on the psychology of the survivor in 1965 to a workshop on massive psychic trauma, sponsored by Krystal and held at Wayne State University in Detroit. I also immersed myself in the literature of Nazi camps, especially in memoirs of survivors. Holocaust survivors were, from the beginning, integral to the conceptual grid I was developing.

In one sense my rabbi friend Arnie Wolf was right: Hiroshima was my path as a Jew to the Holocaust. But it was equally true that I associated these two events with new, mid-twentieth-century destructive forces that threatened all existence. For me the Holocaust and Hiroshima became a constellation of world destruction, and in taking on the new study I became aware of my unusual opportunity to bear psychological witness to both. I have since struggled in my mind with the relationship of the two, always aware of the naked, hands-on evil of Nazi mass murder, as opposed to the technologically distanced—but also evil—atomic bombings. I was much later to explore with Eric Markusen the differences and similarities between these two forms of "genocidal mentality" in our book by that name. I was shifting from a focus on survivors to one on perpetrators, and told friends at the time that I sensed I would soon become involved in a Holocaust study and this time wished to focus on the killers.

I had a series of dreams during the summer and early fall of 1976 (before John Simon's telephone call) in which there were prominent appearances of friends I associated with the Holocaust and with Jewishness. In one of them Elie Wiesel and I meet by chance, have dinner in a city in New Jersey that, according to Elie, "is a wonderful place to leave from for Europe," and then participate together in a Jewish ceremony that "is a bit strange to me and I do not really understand it." In another dream, I travel to a distant commune with a man who resembles Hillel Levine, another friend, a sociologist and rabbi, with whom I had been actively discussing my interest in Holocaust study. I noted that "there is a certain restlessness in our trip" and when we get there "a number of people I meet ask me—and I ask them—'What are you doing here?'" Like all dreams, these had many layers concerning different aspects of my life and work. But what they seemed to have in common was a quest or a journey that was compelling to me but at the same time confusing, and was bound up with my Jewishness. The convenient port in New Jersey for getting to Europe in the first dream reflects my sense of the appropriateness for me of this inner psychological movement toward the Holocaust, whatever its uncertainties.

One way or another, I now believe, I would have undertaken a Holocaust study. The Simon/Glasenapp encounter was serendipitous in the way that deep inclinations bring about what seem to be chance occurrences. Rather than a "strong stomach" (or any other kind of stomach), what was involved was an inner feeling on my part that it was right—even necessary—for me, both as a scholar and a Jew, to undertake this kind of study.

"Retooling"—New Kinds of Interviews and New Guides

In response to some of my early impressions of the work, my friend Arnie Wolf made another wise pronouncement, this one during a meeting of our small group at Yale Divinity School: "You have in the past studied mostly victims. Now you are studying a different group, the victimizers, and perhaps you have to retool for that purpose." Arnie pointed out that Hannah Arendt had to do the same in connection with writing about Adolph Eichmann, had to prepare herself for confronting a victimizer.

Clearly my "retooling" would involve my mind-set as an investigator, and especially in connection with my actual interviews with Nazi doctors. In the past I had been sympathetic to those I talked to, whether survivors of Chinese thought reform or the atomic bomb or the Vietnam War. I was not sure exactly how I would feel toward the former Nazi doctors I sat down with, but I knew that it would be far from sympathetic. I would in fact be seeking information about their behavior in a murderous project. I would not be directly confrontational but would be persistently probing. Wary of potential deception, I would seek to learn all I could from every possible source about a particular doctor and the groups and activities in which he was involved. Rather than the kind of alliance with survivors in my earlier studies, I anticipated a contest between the Nazi doctor and myself, between two people with antithetical backgrounds and purposes, in which there would be considerable antagonism.

Yet I also knew that in any such psychological interview, even with a Nazi doctor, there would have to be elements of civility and cooperation, and of nuanced feelings. That is why Erik Erikson could say to me, concerning the work, "You might even make contact with their humanity." Elie Wiesel, for similar reasons—and because Nazi doctors might shock and surprise me in ways that I could not anticipate—referred to my work as "a dangerous project." Those comments made me uneasy—and with good reason, as it turned out, as I was to experience no little conflict over precisely what they suggested.

Seeking Counsel—Alexander Mitscherlich

An important part of my "retooling" was connecting with a whole new group of knowledgeable people for guidance and intellectual exchange. I first turned to Alexander Mitscherlich, as he, with his colleague Fred Mielke, had been responsible for the original exposé of Nazi doctors on the basis of evidence at the Nuremberg medical trial in 1947. Mitscherlich, a longtime anti-Nazi and towering intellectual figure during the post–World War II era, had reintroduced Freudian psychoanalysis in Germany and written, sometimes with his psychoanalyst wife, Margarete, highly influential books on Nazism and German society. Indeed, it was my impression that, while classical psychoanalysis in many other places was declining in energy and influence, it could thrive in Germany precisely because, under Mitscherlich, it had a powerful subject to explore. I first met the Mitscherlichs during the mid-sixties when Alexander was invited to Yale to lecture on his work. When Fritz Redlich introduced him, he declared that welcoming Mitscherlich to Yale was one of the high moments of his entire career.

Alexander was outspoken, could be crusty, and was extraordinarily knowledgeable and historically minded. Margarete was in every way his intellectual equal, always elegant and articulate. Both were passionately committed to the humane political and social principles that dominated their lives. BJ and I became friendly with the Mitscherlichs and invited them both to speak at a Wellfleet meeting in the early seventies, he on the psychology of Nazism and she on her work on psychoanalysis and feminism. I also wrote an introduction to the American edition of their important book on post-Nazi Germany, *The Inability to Mourn*, lauding their shared background of courageous anti-Nazi activities no less than their powerful psychohistorical work. But all that took place well before I had shown any intent to do research on the Nazi era in general or on Nazi doctors in particular.

When I wrote to Alexander about the study I was embarking on, he responded with a characteristic blend of caution and encouragement. He pointed out that after so many years it might be difficult for me to reach "the right persons" (meaning the relevant Nazi doctors) but that he knew I would make careful preparations and that he and his wife would do everything possible "to support your plans." As for his own records, he said that "Unfortunately, the mother of my co-author Fred Mielke . . . burned up all my files of the Nuremberg trial . . . because she was living in very cramped quarters." During my talks with Alexander on my first research trip to Germany (in December 1977), he emphasized that what he and Mielke uncovered about medical crimes and the collaboration of doctors with the Nazis was only "the tip of the iceberg" and that there was much more to be learned about the whole problem. With each subsequent conversation, he and Margarete recalled more of their own experience and expressed increasing enthusiasm about my project.

In those early conversations, Alexander told me something of considerable significance for the work I was starting. He said that most Germans of his generation—the Nazi generation—could not psychologically confront the evil they had been part of, that the human psyche is incapable of inwardly experiencing its own involvement in evil of that magnitude. Hence, he added, former Nazis tended to resort to various defense mechanisms and evasions, often that of seeing themselves as victims. Alexander accurately anticipated my experience with Nazi doctors. It turned out that not one of them was able to say to me that he had been part of something evil that he deeply regretted. Virtually all of them attempted to represent themselves as beleaguered men more or less victimized by circumstances.

Alexander also told me something important about his encounters with German medicine in the postwar era. He had attended the 1947 medical trial in Nuremberg at the request of leaders of the national medical society; aware of his anti-Nazi credentials, they "wanted to polish their image," meaning that they expected him to say that there were a few bad apples but the profession itself was clean. In fact he said the opposite, emphasizing not only individual crimes but the overall collusion of the profession: "When I found out the terrible things doctors had done, I knew I had to write about it. I also knew that it would ruin my medical career."

And indeed, even in postwar democratic Germany, the profession never quite forgave Alexander for his truth telling. As he further explained to me: "When the German edition [of his and Mielke's book, *Doctors of Infamy*] came out with a printing of 10,000 copies, they were suddenly all gone. The medical society had bought them up and destroyed most of them." Although Mitscherlich distinguished himself first as a neurologist and even more as Germany's leading psychoanalyst, he was never offered a medical professorship. He did hold a chair in Frankfurt, but it was in social science rather than medicine.

I also admired Alexander for making use of his subsequent psychoanalytic knowledge to confront the Nazi era in general. I know of no other psychoanalyst or psychological professional who, through influential writings and public statements, has played such a large part in his country's democratic struggles. The philosopher Jürgen Habermas, Alexander's friend and public political ally, called him "the people's pedagogue." When Alexander died in 1982, I had completed most of my research in Germany and was in the middle of writing it up. I dedicated the German translation of my book to the Mitscherlichs and a few years later was enormously pleased to be invited by the institute he founded to give the first Mitscherlich Memorial Lecture. That deepened my sense of continuity with this remarkable man. Whatever difficulties I encountered in my work, they were nothing compared to what Alexander faced—and overcame—in his own society.

Elie Wiesel

I also turned quickly to Elie Wiesel. He was strongly associated in my mind with any Holocaust study, as my dreams made clear. I had met Elie during the late sixties when he was living in a lonely room on the Upper West Side. At the time I was drawing upon his Auschwitz masterpiece, *Night*, for my section at the end of *Death in Life* on the psychology of survivors. Elie recorded in *Night* (written in the late fifties) his experience, as a fifteen-year-old prisoner, of desperately trying to keep his father alive. He was unsparing in his self-condemnation at the relief he felt when his father died, for having experienced "in the recesses of my weakened conscience" something close to "Free at last!" He told how after being liberated he looked into a mirror, and "a corpse looked back at me. The look in his eyes as they stared into mine has never left me." Elie and I talked about this form of "death guilt" and about its paradoxical nature in being suffered by survivors. Then, in 1969, he was part of a poignant group of Auschwitz survivors meeting to discuss making a statement on the My Lai Massacre, which had just been publicly revealed. I was invited to join the discussion and was struck by how painful for them that was: survivors wanted to condemn the slaughter at My Lai as coming too close to their own experience with the Nazis, but were at the same time reluctant to criticize too severely the country that had provided new life for them.

Elie and I became good friends, and could tease each other about our differences. He spoke of initiating a project "to make Bob more Jewish." And I raised the question of whether he would have been capable of embarking on the kind of ten-day trip BJ and I had taken with Florence and Richard Falk to southern Mexico, during which we spent a great deal of time drinking rum. He smiled but seriously pondered the question and said, almost regretfully, that it would not be possible for him because he would feel too guilty. (But a few years later, when BJ and I were enjoying the facilities of a rather vulgar hotel in St. John in the American West Indies, we were amazed to spot at some distance across the dining room a figure BJ thought looked very much like Elie. I said it couldn't be Elie because "what would a man like that be doing in a place like this?" It turned out that he and his wife, Marion, were on an Israeli ship, which awarded prominent Jewish literary figures free cruises.)

By December 1976, when I discussed my Auschwitz project with him, he had become a well-known figure in connection with the Holocaust but not yet its preeminent spokesman. He was fascinated by my study, and we began a dialogue about it that lasted through the writing of my book. He said: "What you are doing is even harder than what I have been doing— you have to enter the mind of the oppressors." He was enthusiastic about introducing me to other survivors, about books he thought I should read, and about foundations I might apply to for support. He declared that there was "no project more important," and added something that completely surprised me: "It will be a great adventure." By which I think he meant that I would have to cope with terrain that was strange, demanding, and illuminating. He even at one point suggested that we might travel together to Auschwitz, as though joining me in that adventure and in some sense reclaiming his own experience (he had not yet revisited the death camp). But, he warned: "You must not make one false step."

That worried me, as it seemed to be a requirement for perfection that no one could meet. It also perhaps foreshadowed a certain amount of tension that was later to occur between us. The tension had to do with his unease concerning some of what I wrote about the complex psychology of Auschwitz survivors; with our differing political views and especially my more critical stance toward Israel; and with Elie's becoming a considerable celebrity, a status that renders interactions with others more difficult. Yet Elie never ceased to be a haunted survivor, and when I plunge back into this work I recall how much I gained from our conversations about very difficult matters and from his unstinting and imaginative support.

Raul Hilberg

I learned much from Raul Hilberg by reading sections of his intellectual masterwork, *The Destruction of the European Jews*, one of the few truly great studies of the Holocaust. I soon got in touch with him, and at our first meeting he surprised me, not with his detailed knowledge about the Nazis and their behavior—that I fully expected—but with his lively intellectual curiosity about new approaches to the Holocaust, and about much else. He also had a droll sense of humor. For instance, noting that the Nazis had sustained remarkable zeal in carrying out the Final Solution until the moment of their defeat, he imagined their leaders asking themselves the question: "What's the use of our whole movement if in losing the war we didn't at least kill the Jews?" That kind of gallows humor both conveyed insights and was a way of coping with the obscene Nazi universe he had long inhabited and I was now entering.

Hilberg had not been subjected to the kind of excruciating suffering experienced by Wiesel, but he and his family had been harassed by the Nazis in Vienna, where his father was temporarily imprisoned, prior to their escape (when Raul was thirteen) first to France and Cuba, and then to the United States. He told me that, as a child of twelve, he was not only fearful of the Nazis but also fascinated by them and thought to himself that "I would some day write about them." He was the consummate recorder of Nazi bureaucratic killing machinery, emphasizing how it encompassed Nazi officials at all levels as well as ordinary people. That approach had enormous relevance for my work on Nazi doctors and my focus on their socialization to killing. In a sense, I could fill in psychologically much that Raul had laid out functionally. Hilberg was a passionately committed, single-minded man who essentially wrote, and constantly revised over decades, one extraordinary book. At the same time he was a wide-ranging intellectual and scholar, highly responsive to insights coming from any direction. (He recommended a book, *Into That Darkness*, by the journalist Gitta Sereny, which some others had considered insufficiently scholarly, because it shed important light on the role of German psychiatry in the Final Solution.) He urged me to keep "an open mind" about everything I encountered, and to record my findings however they might offend certain people.

I came to consult with Raul frequently, and he was generous enough to take on the role of advisor, to me and my publisher, in the completion of my book. When he died in 2007 in Vermont, where he had taught for many years, I felt the loss of another giant who had provided such firm shoulders for me and others to stand on.

Among the many additional Holocaust scholars I met, I was struck by the identical comment about my work made by two of them. One was Lucy Dawidowicz, author of *The War Against the Jews*, who was American born but had lived in Poland and done considerable work on Jewish cultural history. The other was Fritz Stern, the Columbia historian and author of *The Politics of Cultural Despair*, who came from a distinguished German family that had converted to Protestantism and who left with his parents at the age of twelve. Each of these scholars strongly endorsed my study, emphasized its importance, and then added with considerable feeling, "I myself couldn't do it." They were saying that they had been too close to the Holocaust to be able to sit down and talk with Nazi doctors as I proposed to do. I realized that my undertaking that kind of study had to do with being a Jew but one who had been at some protective distance from the mass killing of fellow Jews. That combination could hardly enable me to avoid personal conflicts in carrying out the work. But it did allow me to combine intense motivation with at least a modicum of detachment of a kind less likely to be available to people with more direct experience of grotesque Nazi cruelty.

A Different Erik Erikson

Although close to him at the time, I did not immediately turn to Erikson for advice on the work. Of course I knew of his Bavarian Jewish upbringing, and of his early essay, "The Legend of Hitler's Childhood," in which he described how the Führer, in *Mein Kampf*, mythologized his childhood, blending history and fiction, in ways that connected with passionately shared German feelings and enabled him to create the figure of a national savior. But in our many conversations, he had not said much about the Holocaust. I became aware that it was somewhat awkward for Erik to discuss Jews and their victimization, which I understood to be related to his deep ambivalence about his own Jewishness. Although raised as a Jew by Jewish parents (his mother and stepfather), he long nurtured a fantasy (which could well have been consistent with historical truth) that his missing biological father was a Danish Christian. And I knew of Erik's deep attraction to early Christianity and his adolescent conversion-like experience. While I respected his right to complexity in all this—he was a man who transmuted his own identity confusions into profound insights about identity in general—neither of us was ever fully comfortable in talking about Erik's being, or having been, a Jew. That discomfort undoubtedly prevented our discussions of

Nazis and Jews from having the openness and spontaneity we brought to other subjects.

Until, that is, a visit BJ and I made to his Cape Cod home in Cotuit in 1978, shortly after my return from the research trip during which I began my interviews with Nazi doctors. I told him about my early encounters with Nazi doctors, how, despite their evasiveness, they revealed a great deal. And I described how inmate doctors were allowed to do limited medical work but had to placate Nazi doctors in trying to protect patients from being sent to the gas chambers. I was astonished by his excitement about my descriptions of those meetings. He wanted to know everything—how I went about the work, how the doctors behaved, their defenses and contradictions. He would call out to his wife, "Joan, listen to *this*. What Bob is doing is *amazing*!" More than that, he began to recall his early life in Bavaria. Partly associating to my descriptions of inmate doctors, he referred to his stepfather as "a kindly Jewish doctor." He seemed to combine critical observations on German psychology with aspects of personal nostalgia.

I had never heard Erik talk so fervently about his German childhood. It occurred to me that, beyond his conflicts over Jewishness, he had invested enormous psychological energy in his forward-looking American experience. He had thrived here and found an "American voice" to a degree that very few émigré psychoanalysts or intellectuals were able to do. He had in the past described his experiences of returning to Germany for talks or conferences as always fraught with ambivalence. Paradoxically, my study of a terrible subject evoked surprisingly tender associations of his German and broadly European past. My work reawakened much in him that had long been suppressed.

He was fascinated by my focus on healing and killing and on interviewing physicians, emphasizing that I could talk to them "doctor to doctor." His suggestion that this gave us a certain affiliation made me a little uneasy but I understood what he meant. That and my other work, he added, made me "the best person" to do the study. He mused on the issue of German obedience, likening it to a form of religious worship. We talked more generally about how any nation could be capable of its own form of genocide. But then Erik leaned forward and said, with a kind of impish gallows humor that he knew to be politically incorrect: "Don't tell anyone I said so, but this just *had* to be *German*." He and Joan reflected on how these physicians' young adult identity must have become bound up with the Nazi movement, and it was in this context that Erik mentioned the possibility of my making contact with their "humanity."

Soon afterward, the four of us had a more wide-ranging conversation, shifting about from Nazi doctors to Freud to Jesus (whom Erik was beginning to write about) as a Jew. Erik said that Freud wrote about Moses (in *Moses and Monotheism*) "because it was his way of insisting upon looking into precisely what people of his time did not want to expose," meaning controversial aspects of the creation of the Jews. He then turned to my own work and said that I too—in the case of nuclear weapons, Vietnam veterans, and now Nazi doctors—"probed the things people do not want to probe." I then asked Erik what he thought Freud would be investigating if he were alive now. But before he could answer, BJ took Erik's hand in one of hers and my hand in the other and said: "Freud would be investigating Jesus and investigating Nazi doctors—he would be doing both." BJ was of course partly teasing Erik and me, but also suggesting a sweet moment of communion in our work, our sensibilities, and our lives. My study of Nazi doctors created a new bond between Erik and myself.

Healing and Killing

From the beginning I was struck by the bizarre Nazi interweaving of healing and killing, and over the course of the work that convergence took on increasingly profound significance for me. Doctors are supposed to heal; Nazi doctors killed; but they killed in the name of healing. They did this at two levels. There was the involvement of ostensible healers in the nitty-gritty killing of Jews, most notably in Auschwitz. And there was the vast ideological metaphor of "healing the Nordic race"—and ultimately the world—by means of a "Final Solution to the Jewish problem." I noted the "creepy feeling" I experienced in being a member of the same profession. Yet that very discomfort undoubtedly sensitized me to the bizarre Nazi behavior at both levels.

A key moment in my interviewing occurred when a leading Nazi administrative physician told me that he joined the Nazi Party after hearing Rudolf Hess, a prominent party leader, declare in a public speech: "National socialism is nothing but applied biology!" He was saying that scientific biological truths lay behind all Nazi policies. Over time I came to see the essential motivation of the entire Nazi enterprise to be not so much the attainment of political and military domination as the realization of a biological mission of getting rid of all "bad genes"—whether by murdering mental patients in the "euthanasia" project, or Jews in Auschwitz. Since those bad genes had weakened the Nordic race, it could be cured only by their removal; and since the Nordic race was the only creative race, its cure would ensure a brilliant human future. In that sense the entire Nazi undertaking was a biological and ultimately a medical project, the expression of what I called a "biomedical vision." No wonder, then, that the death camps themselves were mostly set up by transferring personnel and equipment from "euthanasia" killing centers. One could, in fact, view all of Nazi mass murder as "medicalized killing," with Hitler as (in the words of one commentator) "the highest ranking physician."

I remembered Margaret Mead's observation that "doctors are frequently on the edge" in the sense of making "triage" decisions concerning who will live and who will die. I became interested in doctors' transgressions in other places: Soviet psychiatrists diagnosing dissidents as mentally ill and incarcerating them in hospitals; Japanese doctors performing vivisection and their own medical experiments on prisoners during World War II; white South African doctors falsifying medical reports on blacks tortured or killed in prison; the Tuskegee syphilis experiment, in which doctors of the U.S. Public Health Service, over forty years (1932–72), studied the progression of tertiary syphilis in nearly four hundred black men without offering any treatment; and American doctors performing unethical, and sometimes lethal, experiments with drugs and mind manipulation on behalf of the CIA. I thought of doctors as retaining a shamanistic legacy, as arbiters of life and death; the witch doctors, from whom we are descended, could make use of their magic either to heal or to harm. That legacy can still include an aura of omnipotence, which despotic groups have been all too ready to exploit with the collusion of doctors themselves.

I came to learn that doctors have been involved from the beginning in this healing-killing duality, as expressed in Greek medical mythology. Asclepius, the first skilled healer and son of Apollo, made use of a magic potion, which when drawn from the right side of the Gorgon (a monstrous female form) would kill; from the left side, cure. Asclepius, in turn, was killed by Zeus, who saw him as becoming too powerful in his capacity to revive the dead, but then agreed to make him god of medicine. Asclepius's duality is still represented by the snake coiled about his staff, a symbol not only of divine fertility but also of the threatening underworld. (As a frontispiece for *Psychobirds*, my second volume of bird cartoons, I made this drawing of a two-headed snake, representing this unhealthy duality.

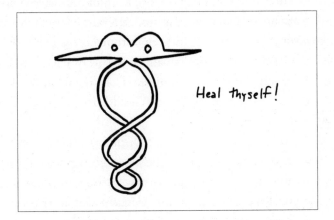

I had Nazi doctors on my mind but I was also playing with a sense of a broader potential for duality—or what I was later to call "doubling"—in doctors in general.)

I was later to discover that the Faust legend derived from a learned German physician and necromancer of the fifteenth and sixteenth centuries: that is, the man who offered his soul to Mephistopheles in return for superhuman powers was, at least in his original appearance, a physician. It would seem that the physician is seen as one who either seeks or possesses dangerous power, especially power over death. And others, including genocidal political leaders, can claim this "medical" power in carrying out vast killing projects to "heal" their own people.

Bad Dreams

In December 1977, with the help of research grants, I made a sixteen-day trip to Germany, my first intense immersion in the research. I wrote ahead to Glasenapp and to Johannes Borger (a young German teacher introduced to me by my friends Karl and Ruth Deutsch, who worked closely with me early in the research), asking them to help arrange meetings with various people, some of whom I had written to. These included German physicians who had worked with the Nazis, Auschwitz survivors who had been on medical blocks, and writers and archivists knowledgeable about Nazi medicine. In sixteen days I could see only a limited number of people from any of these groups, but I managed to spend time in a number of German cities and had intense encounters everywhere.

It was on that trip that I had my first interview with a Nazi doctor, Ernst B. (whom I'll mention again as important to the work), which was both invaluable and shocking in its painful details of what Auschwitz was really like. In the midst of my sensations from that and other extraordinary experiences, I thought of Elie Wiesel's prediction that my work would be "an adventure."

But the adventure would take its toll. During the trip and immediately after it, I had a series of dreams. Details varied, but I would inevitably find myself in a wretched landscape with everything destroyed. Even the extensive barbed wire had rusted and blackened. The landscape might include vaguely outlined figures of barely discernible people. In some dreams I was alone; in others BJ would be there, either next to me or at some remove; and at times our children as well were behind the same barbed wire. The dreams were particularly real to me, and upon awakening it took a few minutes for me to extricate myself from them and realize, with great relief, that it was "only a dream."

During the trip itself, however dreadful the material I was exposed to, I was focused on carrying out the work and even buoyed by a sense of accomplishment. But when I returned to New York I found myself in a very different psychological state. I was agitated, struggling with images of my German encounters, and felt isolated from people around me. The Auschwitz dreams continued, and awakening from them brought me less relief. There seemed to be no one I could talk to about my experiences and my feelings. BJ did not want to hear about details of the trip. She told me that she had shared everything with me in the past, but not this time—this subject was too much for her (though before long she was to undertake a Holocaust study of her own, which I will come to later). It was hard for me to be with people in general because I found it impossible to convey to them what I had been through—it was much too complicated, they would surely not understand, and probably didn't want to hear about such things anyhow. Yet there was nothing else I wished to talk about. I was in a version of a post-traumatic state: I could neither talk nor not talk about the trauma. And to complicate matters, the trauma was bound up with a deeply valued experience. Then two meetings with friends helped me to emerge from that state and indeed, gain useful perspective from it.

When I telephoned John Simon, my editor, he immediately suggested that we have a drink together, which we did at a hotel bar. I ordered only Perrier, as I seemed to have a need to be completely clear. For about two hours I simply poured out every detail of the trip that I could remember—my impressions of specific Nazi doctors and their convoluted behavior, the grotesqueness of everyday life in Auschwitz, bizarre interactions between Nazi and inmate doctors, contradictory impressions of Mengele on the part of both Nazi colleagues and Jewish survivors, my strange feelings about moving back and forth between the Nazi era and contemporary Germany, and even stranger feelings about bringing back this Nazi world to New York City. John asked a few questions here and there but I must have done 90 percent of the talking. In the process I found myself not only enormously relieved but also aware, as I noted, of "structuring the experience a bit, rendering it real, carrying it forward, including even a preliminary outline for the book." And that night, for the first time since my return, I had no Auschwitz dreams.

I also went to see Elie Wiesel. He wanted to hear everything, especially what I had learned about Auschwitz and the Nazi doctors there. I somehow wanted him to know about my dreams. My tone in mentioning them was slightly dismissive (I was very much aware of talking to a person who had *really* suffered in Auschwitz) though I was not without a touch of self-pity. I said: "Elie, I greatly appreciate your enthusiasm about my work, but I do have to tell you that I've been having terrible dreams about finding myself in a place very like Auschwitz. Worse, my wife and my children too are sometimes there as well." He was silent for a moment, then looked at me steadily, with neither unkindness nor special sympathy, and said quietly: "Good, now you can do the study." I understood what he meant—that Auschwitz had to inhabit me psychologically, as was beginning to happen, if I were to do serious work on it. I was paying my dues.

I had one more dream a bit later that, mercifully, did not include Auschwitz. It was a dream I was even fond of, which I recorded in this way:

I am driving in my car and a policeman stops me for speeding. As we talk I explain to him my various theories about the human mind. It is my way of coping with him and of trying to avoid a speeding ticket. He becomes interested in what I am saying and I apparently do not get the ticket.

To me this dream, in a slightly humorous way, had an element of confidence. I understood it to be saying that I was "speeding" a bit emotionally in my plunge into Nazi behavior, had to find inner restraint and balance with the help of outside authority, but could cope with the problem by calling forth a combination of ingenuity and psychological knowledge.

Our Munich "Home"

I decided to spend the 1977–78 academic year in Germany, together with BJ and Karen (Ken was to stay at his prep school in Vermont) to carry out my interview work. But I wasn't sure which city to choose. In correspondence and discussions with German and American friends, and visits of my own during earlier trips, I considered the pros and cons of such places as Munich, Frankfurt, Heidelberg, and Berlin. It was clear that Berlin would be the most cosmopolitan and pleasant city, but it posed formidable logistical problems at a time when the city was divided between the two Germanies, while Munich's strong Nazi past (along with its easy access) made it convenient for the work but potentially uncomfortable for us to live in. An important factor in deciding on Munich was the appointment offered me there by my friend Paul Matussek at the Max Planck Institute of Psychiatry, which he headed. Paul had studied Auschwitz survivors and was eager to exchange ideas on the subject with American colleagues. I had been on several panels with him in the United States, and had invited him to Yale for a lecture. The fellowship at his institute included a modest honorarium, had few requirements, and, most important, provided a professional connection within German society in carrying out the work.

The connection enabled us to work out an arrangement in which Paul sent out the first letter to any Nazi doctor my assistants and I located, using language he and I jointly composed. In the letter he introduced me as a "prominent American psychiatric researcher" who was now studying the "stresses and conflicts" of German physicians under National Socialism. The doctors in question knew what was behind the euphemistic language but it gave them a certain breathing space. The letter also mentioned my earlier work on Hiroshima and Vietnam, enabling me to be seen as someone concerned with his own country's destructive behavior as well. When a doctor wrote back agreeing to meet me, or to consider doing so, I sent him a letter promising anonymity and affirming his right to discontinue our interviews at any time, which would both be included in the informed-consent document we would later sign. This was in keeping with what became known as the Nuremberg Code of researchers' responsibility to those they study, as required in my case by the Yale Committee on Research with Human Subjects. Of course I was aware of the irony of being held to that code while studying the very people whose transgressions had brought it into being, but I also thought it entirely appropriate.

As it turned out, about 70 percent of those approached agreed to see me. In a society still preoccupied with hierarchy and authority, they were probably influenced by the medical standing of the physician introducing me. In addition, many were intent on creating a personal narrative of self-justification, and some saw an opportunity to talk about experiences that had long been unmentionable. In making these arrangements and offering advice when complications arose, Paul was always shrewdly sensitive to the mentality of fellow German physicians of that era (he had himself served as a medical officer in the German army). We remained steady professional associates but never became warm friends.

A closer friendship that also contributed to my decision for Munich was with Fritz Friedmann, a German Jew who fled during the Nazi era and then returned to his country after the war to establish an institute for American studies. Passionate in his intellectual goals and intent on showing us "the other Germany," Fritz introduced us to the community of bright and progressive people he assembled, a number of whom, most notably Brigitte Fleischmann and Christiane Clemm, were to assist and advise me in my research. At the same time he and his wife, Elizabeth, did everything to make us comfortable in Munich and treated us as members of an extended German Jewish family.

Yet BJ, Karen, and I were to have serious difficulties in Munich. We were there only because of my research on Nazi doctors, which meant that the three of us were constantly immersed in Nazi imagery. And all of us frequently associated what we experienced in the Munich of the late seventies with terrible events of the Nazi era. For instance, there was a dry cleaning plant across the street from our apartment with smoke spewing from its chimney. As BJ and I looked out the window one day, we both admitted having the painful daily experience of seeing in that smoke the crematoria of Auschwitz. On another occasion when I was by myself and boarding a bus, I saw that the driver's hands were occupied, so, instead of handing her my ticket as one was supposed to do, I thought I would make things easier by reaching a little farther to place it in a small ticket pile. As I did so, she screamed at me and slapped me sharply on my wrist. My very limited German did not permit me to explain myself, so I simply retreated to a rear seat. But she kept on shouting in a mocking tone while pointing her finger at me, as if to make sure that other passengers were aware of the idiot who had behaved so badly on her bus. She was a heavy-set middle-aged woman, and in my mind was quickly transformed into a sadistic female head of a block or *lager* in a concentration camp. I was shaken by the incident for days and had fantasies of arriving at her camp as an American military liberator, ordering her seized and imprisoned, and even executed. I discussed the experience with a few friends in terms of its representing an authoritarian or even violent aspect of German culture, not to mention my own violent images in response.

BJ had an incident of her own, in which a friend took her to an antique shop where they were shown a large collection of menorahs and other ritual objects. BJ was upset at seeing them, pointedly asked how they were obtained, and became more angry when the salesman pleaded ignorance. She came home livid at this casual display of what was all too clearly murderers' booty. Our thirteen-year-old daughter, Karen, had nightmares about the Nazis and told us about her fears of being captured by them. When we tried to reassure her that the Nazis had been defeated and were not around anymore, her heart-wrenching response was "They must still be around because Daddy is talking to them." She also found it difficult to be the "new girl" at the international school she attended. Worse, on one occasion she was told by a couple of girls there that they would no longer have anything to do with her because she was Jewish.

BJ had a much more difficult time in Munich than I did, partly because at the time she had no project of her own. I became quickly immersed in my research, and traveled a great deal. Even horrendous information became grist for the mill, and I knew that I would eventually have my say about it in the book I would write. (I have sometimes referred to writing a book as "the intellectual's revenge," but have been advised not to put that image in this memoir because it can be so readily misunderstood.) From the beginning I was helped, intellectually and spiritually, by an ever-widening group of young and not so young Germans who, in supporting my work, were making their own confrontation with their country's recent history. BJ too became fond of many of them but could not rid herself of her sense that "the German soil has been polluted for a thousand years." Her attitude did not change until she began systematic work on her biography of Janusz Korczak, the Polish Jewish pediatrician, writer, educator, and Holocaust martyr, who refused to leave the children in his care and was killed with them in Treblinka. In pursuing that remarkable project, BJ was actively constructing a Holocaust narrative and became less vulnerable to German remnants. But by then she was no longer living in Germany with me.

After four months in Munich, we decided to make a two-week trip to Israel, where I would interview Auschwitz survivors and work at the Yad Vashem archives, and we would also take a short vacation with a little swimming and beachcombing. We did all that and thrived, and BJ was especially happy to be out of Germany. Two nights before we were scheduled to leave, she and I watched an important television documentary on Mengele. When it was over BJ looked at me and said quietly, "I can't go back there." I understood what she was saying and felt badly that I had subjected her to so much pain by bringing her to Germany. But I also experienced a slight sense of abandonment. So we made a fundamental change in our family arrangements and found a comfortable place in Jerusalem for BJ and Karen to stay. I went back to Munich, packed and sent most of their things, and carried more of them with me when I returned to Jerusalem three months later. (The only problem was our two cats. I obtained the required medical certificates for them, which I presented to veterinary authorities in Jerusalem, but the cats then disappeared into the bowels of the airport. Nobody seemed to know where they were—until I happened to notice their two cases going round and round on one of the baggage carousels.)

Overall, the arrangement worked out reasonably well. BJ immersed herself in research on Korczak, and was able to interview a number of Israelis who had been either children or younger teachers in his Jewish orphanage. (She was later to travel extensively in Poland, where she could interview non-Jewish Poles who had been teachers or children in his separate Polish orphanage, and uncover previously unknown details of Korczak's life.) Karen had some difficulties in connection with switching schools but made new friends as she and BJ settled into their life there. I made frequent trips from Munich to join BJ and Karen in Jerusalem and could have compelling intellectual exchanges with Israeli scholars and Holocaust historians such as Yehuda Bauer and Saul Friedländer, as well as two extraordinary psychiatrists who became our close friends, Hillel Klein and Shumai Davidson. All of them belonged to an unofficial category of Israelis who were immersed in Holocaust issues, peace-minded and critical, increasingly uneasy with their country's political and religious intransigence, and inclined to spend a good deal of time outside Israel.

In Germany, without my family, I was needy but responsive to and increasingly sustained by friends like the Friedmanns in Munich and the Mitscherlichs in Frankfurt, along with a widening circle of thoughtful Germans I came to know throughout the country. I continued to travel from Munich to all major German cities, made two intense trips to Poland, and did additional interviews throughout Western Europe and Scandinavia. It was perhaps logical that Germany and Israel became pivotal countries for my research, but our arrangement caused them to be further juxtaposed in my mind as places of nurturing intellectual and personal ties. From these travels I would return to my always temporary, never quite relaxed, but increasingly comfortable and manageable Munich "home."

15

Sitting Down with Nazi Doctors

The Repentant Anti-Nazi

After moving to Munich, the first German physician I interviewed was an *anti*-Nazi doctor, introduced to me by a close colleague at Yale, Steve Fleck, who was himself a German Jewish émigré. I told myself that I did so in order to get another point of view, which was true enough, but it was also to bolster my spirit, my courage. The interview turned out to have its own important revelations.

I encountered an animated man in his mid-sixties who greeted me as a friend—and then quickly lapsed into a surprising rhetoric of self-condemnation. He told me that he came from a family of Social Democrats and could quickly recognize the Nazis as thuggish and dangerous. During his medical training he refused to join the Nazi student groups and therefore was excluded from a university connection. He was able to find a small research institute where a physician unenthusiastic about the regime could work quietly and avoid trouble. But a problem arose for him in being required periodically to serve in hospitals where patients included both civilians and military personnel. There he heard rumors about terrible Nazi atrocities, rumors he sensed to be true, but which he felt he could do nothing about. He said that an appropriate response would have been absolute resistance, but that would have meant punishment, possibly death—and, he added softly, "I am not a hero." As he saw it, "In not resisting [and in] participating in their profession . . . I helped them"—which was a way of saying that the medical profession as a whole came to belong to the Nazis and simply working within it was a form of collaboration.

During the Nazi era he felt himself alienated from classmates and former friends, almost all of whom seemed to go along with what the Nazis asked of them. Then, after the war, he experienced a different kind of alienation within his own family when his younger daughter accused him of having been a Nazi follower, "because nothing happened to you." As he explained his daughter's view, "I survived so I couldn't be against them." He mentioned that there had been much talk in the postwar years about the older generation's difficulty in communicating with their children, and commented, "If we can't communicate, it is because *both* generations are unable to do so."

At that point his son-in-law, present because they thought we might need an interpreter, intervened and said that he was being too hard on himself, that no one could have expected him to actively resist. But he refused to be solaced and said that, in reaching his sixties, he had come to the terrible self-judgment, "You have badly used your profession and your life," and added, "The worst feeling is when you can't do anything, and the second worst that maybe you *could* have done something."

The son-in-law continued the conversation when he drove my interpreter and me to the nearby station. He again insisted that his father-in-law had been much too self-critical, and that "it is human nature for everyone to make concessions at such times." But then he seemingly contradicted himself with an additional comment that was more sweeping and more ambiguous: "Yet I must say that it is difficult to really understand anyone from that period—it is difficult to speak about their problems. The whole period is strange to us." He was saying in effect that any German who lived during the Nazi period had to be tainted by it in a way that was remote from, and not quite fathomable by, subsequent generations.

I was later to discover, to my chagrin, that none of the actively Nazi doctors I interviewed expressed the kind of guilt and negative self-judgment I heard from this anti-Nazi doctor. There was a certain psychological parallel here with the man who had not fired at My Lai, and with Kingman Brewster, who had so admirably guided Yale during its time of crisis. People who behave well in highly threatening situations can be more prone to berate themselves—to experience feelings of guilt— than those who behave badly. This is partly because the former (heroes and victims) allow themselves to take in psychologically, and apply their demanding conscience to, the painful realities involved, while the latter (perpetrators and their collaborators) call forth every form of defense mechanism to avoid inwardly experiencing precisely those realities.

"Hey, This Bastard Is One of Them!"

My "retooling" for Nazi doctors was helpful only to a point. Situations arose that I could not prepare for, and I experienced feelings and conflicts I had not expected. The first Nazi doctor I sat down with for a detailed interview was unusual in having been introduced to me by a Frankfurt trial prosecutor with whom he was on good terms. He had been favorably described by prisoner-doctors who said he had saved their lives in Auschwitz, and had declared himself eager to meet and talk with me. He greeted me like a friendly host in his attractive sitting room, which looked out on a lovely Bavarian landscape. I remember having the thought that this man was likable and that it was congenial to be with him. But I was immediately horrified by that thought and reminded myself, still silently but anxiously and even angrily, "Hey, this bastard is one of them!"

Paradoxically, it was when he was being very forthcoming that my feelings toward him shifted toward anger. He told me how Nazi doctors were horrified upon arriving in Auschwitz, in some cases experienced considerable anxiety and nightmares, and then were helped to adapt to the place by old hands who, almost like therapists, guided them through their first "selections" assignment, in which the doctor divided those Jews who were to be sent to the gas chamber (the great majority) from those relatively intact young adults who were to be admitted to the camp to perform slave labor. When he described how the newcomers joined the old hands in heavy drinking, I asked him to convey to me the kind of words that were exchanged among them. He said that an old hand would justify the place with the following question: "Which is better, to die in shit, or to be sent to heaven by the gas?" I remember the rage I felt toward him as he told me this, even though in doing so he was acceding to my request for concrete description.

A year later, after listening to that passage on the interview tape, I noted feeling "repelled, speechless, immobilized" and again "enraged." Then, as well as at the time of the interview, I also felt demeaned: because, as a Jew, I was part of the victimized group he was talking about; and because I spoke so politely with the man who was saying these things. I noted hearing on the tape something "like a cross between a sigh and a groan, coming from me, even as I tried to keep the interview going, and said such things as 'Yes,' and 'Right.'" My sense of the required discipline at the time of the interview meant suppressing expressions of moral judgment. That undoubtedly made sense from the standpoint of the research but nonetheless seemed a hideous compromise.

I was helped through the process by my sensitive interpreter/assistant, Matthias Scheer, a young Harvard-trained German lawyer who worked very closely with me and became a good friend. When the Bavarian doctor uttered those despicable words, Matthias nodded sympathetically toward me, saying in effect, "I understand how painful this must be for you and I'm completely with you in what you are doing."

Atmospheric Variations

In most of my interviews there was a very different kind of atmosphere. The Nazi doctor and I would engage in an exchange that was at first somewhat formal, then would slowly build into back-and-forth comments and associations as he would seek to explain his version of events and defend his actions. There was an adversarial element, all the more so when he recognized from my probing questions that his efforts to gain an alliance with me as a fellow physician were not succeeding. My interpreter in those cases became both a connecting link and a buffer between us. He had to convey the words of each of us from the perspective of the speaker, but both questions and responses had to be filtered through his sensibility. Where there was antagonism or overt skepticism, he took some of the blows in ways that helped keep the conversation going.

A more relaxed atmosphere could offer its own pitfalls. For instance, a distinguished German anti-Nazi psychiatrist whom I respected urged me to meet with Dr. Hans T., whom he described as "a very nice man even though he has a Nazi past." Dr. T. turned out to be very nice indeed, gracious in his hospitality (served me apple strudel, which he called a "Viennese ritual") and very forthcoming in providing me with a view of Nazi "racial science" from the inside. With equal pleasantness he glossed over his step-by-step intellectual and moral corruption in his description of his rise in Nazi medicine to become director of an Austrian research institute on "racial biology." After our second interview, I noted that "I had a very strong reaction to the interview [because] he was someone who really wanted to recreate the whole Nazi period for me . . . to work closely with me in that way . . . but was totally without moral insight about what he had done." I added that the interview "hit me hard" because he was "now supposed to be in our camp," and seemed in many ways to have a similar sensibility to my own. That in turn made me wonder whether "what he did, others, maybe I myself, might have done."

I had the opposite kind of problem—a particularly tense moment—with a doctor undergoing a prolonged court trial because of what he had done at a "euthanasia" killing center. (Doctors were still being tried in German courts, but increasingly infrequently, as the legal system, like the country in general, was tiring of the issue.) I questioned him about the gassing of mental patients, and then asked specifically whether he himself had turned on the gas cock. He became agitated and shouted at me: "I thought you were a *psychologist*. That question sounds like a *prosecutor*!" I explained that it mattered psychologically whether he, or any other doctor, actually opened the gas cock. He would say no more about the subject, though his outburst seemed to answer my question. Yet, almost to my surprise, he was willing to continue with the interview, perhaps associating it in his mind with his legal defense.

Another doctor who had been at a "euthanasia" killing center began his interview with me on a particularly absurd note. As a bit of a chocoholic, I appreciated the quality of German dark chocolate, and frequently carried bars with me for physical and psychological nourishment. This doctor noted considerable chocolate on the back of my pants—it was a warm day and the bar had melted—and rushed me into his inner office, where he made something of a surgical event out of washing and scraping off the chocolate. I felt humiliated both because the whole thing was too personal and friendly, and because he seemed to be more or less taking over our meeting. Matthias was convinced, probably correctly, that the doctor was mainly concerned about his furniture. In any case, I quickly recovered from the indignity and questioned him aggressively about his behavior at the killing center. It turned out that he had managed to arrange a quick transfer from the center, felt morally less culpable than the doctor who had shouted at me, and was therefore able to behave with me in the relaxed way that he had.

Friends I talked to about the work were curious about the atmosphere of my different interviews. I remember a conversation with Michael Reich, a thoughtful political scientist who had been a student of mine at Yale, in which I found myself distinguishing the very different atmospheres that prevailed.

With Jewish survivors things tended to be very congenial—one could say gemütlich—a quick sense of mutual sympathy and common purpose. The experience could be therapeutic for them, both in finding expression for painful matters and in giving further meaning to their suffering through exposing and combating the overall Nazi project. And for me the clarity of that research alliance was psychologically nurturing in its contrast with the draining, evasive maneuvers of Nazi doctors. When I discussed with my friend Michael my sense that, except for a few accidents of history, I could readily have been one of those Jewish physician-survivors, he wondered whether each of them could be called my "double." That is, the physician-survivor and I became interchangeable parts of a common "self."

With non-Jewish survivors, mostly Polish but also German, there could also be a strong and rewarding alliance, though with less personal identification. The atmosphere would depend upon whether I perceived the Polish survivor (partly on the basis of what other survivors told me) as having had a close, cooperative relationship with Jewish inmates, as opposed to retaining significant elements of Polish anti-Semitism (in some cases becoming almost inseparable from Nazi doctors). In the latter situation the atmosphere of our interviews was much more formal and mutually guarded.

In the case of Nazi doctors, the atmosphere was one of tension, with wariness on both sides, whatever the apparent civility. But here too there were distinctions. There was a definite relationship between our discomfort and the degree of the doctor's moral culpability. But there could be considerable uncertainty about that, in both his mind and mine, which led to equal uncertainty about how to behave toward one another. Or he could speak rather freely about himself, but in a dissociated way, as though he and I were making observations together on a third person. Where a doctor (or a high Nazi official like Albert Speer) had been close to Hitler, the interview could be dominated by the virtual presence of the Führer.

These atmospherics could contain various mixtures and many contradictions. I tried to be flexible while always keeping in mind my rigorous research function. I came to have confidence in my approach as it enabled me to weather just about any development. At the same time I had awkward and painful moments, as I will further describe, and experienced some conflicts that could never be completely resolved.

Dream Signals

My dreams at that time reflected this sense of carrying on despite my conflicts. One dream took me back to Auschwitz, where I was again a prisoner, but my overall situation was "not quite as bad as I would have expected Auschwitz to be." Another prisoner there turned out to be a friend of mine with whom I could converse freely. In my associations at the time I thought, somewhat uneasily, of some "relatively friendly" interviews with Nazi doctors. But I also referred to a sense of energy derived from my "subjective sense of being a Jew in doing this research" and my "fundamental identification with victims." Overall, the dream expressed a sense of acclimation to the work.

The second dream involved walking through a house, apparently looking for a Nazi doctor, when someone said to me, "Well, he is here with his mother." I proceeded with my efforts to arrange the interview. I noted that the dream somewhat humanized Nazi doctors—they too had mothers—without curtailing my research intensity. The dream also took me to associations about "the woman" in Nazi behavior, and in the life of the investigator as well.

And in that regard, I had a series of erotic dreams involving beautiful young women, though noting later that "the scene remains controlled," suggesting restraint even in the dream. Then and later, when relaxing with friends or even giving a public talk, I would sometimes bemoan the grim subjects of my research and would say such things as "My next study will be about love, sexual pleasure, and human goodness," or about "the varieties of human orgasm." Underneath that little "joke" about changing my subject to something more pleasant was a hunger for erotic, life-affirming images to counterbalance my immersion in cruelty, dying, and killing.

Agonizing Contradictions

The Nazi doctor who taught me most about Auschwitz was also, morally, the most excruciatingly enigmatic. During the thirty hours I spent with a man I called Ernst B.—five day-long interviews over the course of two years—I was never without a moment of intense ambivalence toward him. Entering into this ambivalence was my sense of his extraordinary value to the research and my determination to keep the interviews going.

He was the previously mentioned Bavarian doctor who had been so hostlike in receiving me and so revered by inmates for having saved lives. Yet although unique among Nazi doctors in being a hero to many former prisoners, he was at the same time a close comrade and outspoken admirer of Josef Mengele, one of the most murderous of Auschwitz figures. How could that be? I'm not sure I ever completely answered that question, but in pursuing it I learned a great deal not only about him and the Nazi project but also about the extreme contradictions that can prevail in the human psyche—in his, and in mine.

Dr. B. saved lives in a number of ways: by giving inmate doctors jobs doing laboratory work in the "Hygienic Institute," where they had manageable working conditions and an adequate diet; by rescuing a number of them from the gas chambers when they had been "selected"; and by arranging for good medical care when they became ill. Simply being courteous to them—introducing himself and shaking hands, as though among equals—had a stunning impact in the brutal Auschwitz environment. One former prisoner called him "a human being in an SS uniform," and another spoke of prisoners' reverence for him to the extent of form-ing "a cult of Ernst B." When B. was tried in Poland after the war, he was acquitted on the basis of testimony by inmate doctors, particularly by a respected Czech professor, that he had saved their lives.

Dr. B. described to me a remarkable incident, which I found hard to believe—until it was confirmed to me by a prisoner doctor I also inter-viewed. Soon after arriving in Auschwitz, while still agitated by what he found there, B. thought he spotted, among the miserable-looking prison-ers, a close friend of his named Simon Cohen, his companion on long bicycle trips during his youth. He asked everyone around him, including both Nazi doctors and prisoners, how he could find Cohen but received no help from them. The prisoner doctor I talked to told me how shocked he was when B. burst into his laboratory in the Hygienic Institute, inquir-ing loudly about Cohen, and how he had urged him to quiet down, fearful that such behavior would be dangerous both to Dr. B. and himself. He told him that thousands of Jews came through Auschwitz, many of whom were named Cohen, and it would be impossible to find this man, but was at the same time very moved by him "because I never before heard an SS man pronounce the name of a Jewish friend." B. never found Simon Cohen—he later came to think that seeing him was an illusion—but he did have disturbing dreams in which his deteriorated Jewish friend looked at him accusingly, asking him how he could "belong to those people" and declaring, "That can't be you!"

Yet this same man not only acknowledged his friendship with Mengele but never ceased to express his admiration for him as "the most decent colleague I met there." He stressed their shared intellectual background, their "objective" discussions about such things as "racial biology" and "the Jewish problem." He explained that to understand Mengele one had to realize that he embraced early SS ideology concerning the necessity of exterminating the Jews "for the recovery of the world." He viewed his colleague as "a man of perfect integrity, one who lived out his convic-tions." When I mentioned Mengele's cruelty, B. at first dismissed this as rumor and said it "would be contrary to the personal impression I have of him." I then asked B. whether he would change his opinion if I pre-sented him with clear evidence of Mengele's practice of sending one or both twins he was studying to the gas chamber in order to obtain autopsy reports. B. immediately replied that he would not because such behavior took place in the context of Auschwitz: "One must be aware that in the Auschwitz milieu, where thousands were being killed continuously, such a thing was nothing at all, in no way extraordinary . . . but as an outsider one cannot understand this."

B. stressed the importance of Mengele's scientific work, along with his "sense of responsibility" in correcting "technical mistakes" in the gassing in order to enable the process to be carried out in a more "humanitarian" fashion. When I asked B., given their differing postwar paths (he was cooperating with German legal authorities, while Mengele was in hiding in South America), how he would feel if they were to meet in the future, he replied that he would be delighted to see his old friend and they would enthusiastically resume their "rational" discussions.

In talking about Mengele and other SS doctors, he made it clear that they were his comrades, that whatever their differences he was fundamentally one of them. He explained the higher regard that prisoner doctors had for him as resulting from no more than a superior "bedside manner" on his part. He was intent on avoiding performing selections, and could do that (with the help of a superior in Berlin) by insisting on his bureaucratic separation, as a member of the Hygienic Institute, from the camp doctors responsible for the selections. His adaptation to Auschwitz also required him to drink even more heavily than was the norm for Nazi doctors. B. had dreams of fleeing from the camp with an attractive Jewish laboratory assistant and together joining Polish anti-Nazi partisans. Yet he managed to function well in Auschwitz, becoming, as he put it, "integrated into the whole thing," did not take advantage of opportunities to leave, and came to feel that "I had a task there to fulfill."

Over the course of our interviews my feelings toward him ran a full gamut from admiration to rage and everything in between, and his feelings toward me were apparently just as complex. Looking back I would divide our strange interaction into three phases. The first, taking place during our long initial interview, was one of surprising rapport. Here were two people from extremely antithetical backgrounds quickly entering into an elaborate exchange concerning the most grotesque matters. I was surprised at the intensity with which he poured out his Auschwitz experiences, including relations with inmate doctors and friendship with

Mengele, and pleased by the pains he took to make me aware of complicated details. I had the sense that he found in me a suitable recipient for a long-suppressed need to vent these experiences in depth. I was greatly impressed by his life-sustaining help to inmate doctors (supported by accounts of many of them); appalled by his friendship with and sympathy for Mengele; and utterly fascinated by his every word, as I saw immediately in this man a treasure trove of material for my research. After we left Dr. B.'s home, my interpreter expressed his amazement at the extent to which the two of us could communicate with one another at that first meeting.

The second phase was one of steady cooperative effort, extending through two subsequent marathon interviews. Now he poured out intricate observations concerning not only his own experience but every kind of interaction in the camp. We settled into our interviews, my enthusiasm for their value in my work mounting even as I found myself troubled by increasing evidence of his Nazi sympathies. Then came the third phase—roughly the last two of our all-day interviews—characterized by an atmosphere of antagonistic ending. He began to complain that the interviews were becoming a burden, attributing the problem to his wife's fear that they would somehow result in harm to him, but giving me the impression that he himself was becoming uncomfortable about them.

Now B. began to mention the Nazi era with a certain amount of nostalgia. He would say that, yes, the Nazis had their excesses, but at least people knew where they stood and what they believed, as opposed to the absence of belief and discipline in today's youth. He added that his position toward Auschwitz had "hardened," by which he seemed to mean that he had come to accept a kind of logic to the place. As he put it, "If you look at Auschwitz objectively, you cannot oppose the selections"—that is, if you accept Auschwitz as a murder factory and a slave labor camp, selections make complete sense. When I replied with a question as to why, then, he himself had gone to such effort to avoid selections, he said that it was a matter of his "emotions"—which came close to the Heinrich Himmler position that any inability to join in the Nazi mission of killing Jews was a matter of "personal weakness."

Clearly he had hardened in his attitude toward me as well, and seemed intent on destroying any common ground that might have existed between us. (He probably knew, or at least suspected, that I was Jewish, and certainly saw me as a strongly anti-Nazi American.) He went out of his way to shock me, by claiming that many SS doctors at Auschwitz sympathized with Hitler's idea that the Jews had to be exterminated because all other methods (ghettos, restrictions, forced emigration, etc.) had failed; and added that, like Mengele, he would have been quite ready to offer his services to improving the efficiency of the burning of bodies. And when he spoke of visionary SS views held by Mengele—National Socialism as a "world blessing" in absolute contrast to the Jews as "ultimate evil"—he himself did not seem very removed from those views. From that perspective, he explained, Auschwitz was not a moral issue but a technical one concerning the efficiency of burning of bodies. Whatever sympathy I had previously experienced toward this man was now replaced by something close to seething anger. Earlier, B. had warned me to be on guard against people like himself reconstructing their experience in self-serving ways, and from that standpoint his damning personal admissions were a kind of gift to me. But I hated myself for participating in, and even valuing, this dialogue. By the end of the interview he was clearly eager to leave, and I was not sorry to see him go.

Just about that time I had another encounter that threw more light on B.'s relation to inmates. After a talk I gave in London on the psychology of the survivor, a pleasant middle-aged woman came up to me to express special interest in my work on Nazi doctors. She identified herself as the daughter of the Czech Jewish medical professor whose testimony on behalf of B. at his trial in Poland had been crucial to his acquittal. When we met the next day to discuss the matter, she told me how her father talked constantly about B. as the kindest of men and told her in detail how he had saved his life by means of specific actions not once but three times. She described how Dr. B. became a mythic figure in her life, a man with almost godlike purity and goodness. So much so that when her father died a few years earlier, she began to think about B. as taking his place, had dreams about B., and even considered looking him up to tell him of this special love she felt for him.

Yet one thing about the relationship between her father and B. puzzled her. After the trial in Poland, B. wrote her father to thank him warmly for his testimony. Her father wrote back saying, in effect, you saved my life in Auschwitz and I was happy to save yours at the trial. But that was the end of the correspondence. Her father surprised her by neither maintaining the correspondence nor making any arrangements to meet again with B. She asked me if I had any understanding of why he behaved that way. I decided that I could be psychologically helpful to her by telling her more of what I knew about the overall situation. I said that B., whatever he did for her father, still represented for him a Nazi doctor in Auschwitz. I explained that B. had remained close to a number of his Nazi colleagues, including Josef Mengele (I was not violating B.'s confidentiality, as he was on public record in his trial documents as having said this); that her father, however grateful to B., must have sensed this; and that he had a strong personal need to separate himself from Auschwitz and from the accommodations inmate doctors had to make in order to survive. By helping to save B.'s life in Poland he had not only balanced the moral scales between them but had affirmed his own autonomy and life-power by reversing the Auschwitz situation in which he had depended upon B.'s beneficence for survival. She told me that our talk would relieve her of some of her uncomfortable fantasy about B., and I knew also that it would contribute to her understanding of what her father had been through. Our conversation gave me further perspective on the complications that surround even the most merciful outreach of perpetrators toward victims in an institution whose function is atrocity.

I came to recognize in B. an important psychological combination for much Nazi behavior: embrace of at least fragments of Nazi ideology (having to do with national greatness and personal life-power) along with intense group influence, or what I came to call socialization to evil. Because of early family conflicts, B. had a particularly strong need to ingratiate himself with any group he encountered: with fellow students as an adolescent when drinking with them; with Nazi university authorities by joining their student organization and demonstrating how an indigenous product could serve a biological function as a culture medium; with the rural community in which he first practiced medicine; and when in

Auschwitz, with fellow Nazi doctors *as well as* inmate doctors. He continued that pattern with American military captors and Soviet legal authorities after the surrender; with the community in which he practiced after the war; with the prosecutors in the Frankfurt trial to extricate Mengele even as he continued to defend his friend and Auschwitz colleague; and in his interviews with me, at least until close to their conclusion. Though he was more a pragmatist than an ideologue, the pervasive Nazi message stayed with him, as made clear during his last two interviews with me and in subsequent public statements (possibly associated with senility but significant in any case) in which he expressed reluctance to condemn Auschwitz. His susceptibility to group influence was extreme, but some such susceptibility is universal and tells us much about the Nazi capacity for achieving widespread socialization to evil and enlisting the services of very divergent kinds of people.

The behavior of Nazi doctors like B. led me to my concept of "doubling." The term connotes a form of dissociation in which the self divides into two separately functioning wholes: an "Auschwitz self" enabling one to live and work there and engage in mass killing; and a relatively more humane prior self enabling one to return to Germany during leaves and behave as an ordinary husband and father. What was remarkable about B. was that he included in his Auschwitz self and its Nazi components (in a way that no other Nazi doctor I knew of did) a considerable measure of lifesaving humanity.

I also came to see B. as emblematic of the "decent Nazi"—quotation marks are crucial—one who is relatively well educated, presentable, friendly, and even kind in immediate human relationships, often seeing himself as combating the more thuggish Nazis around him. Such people were nonetheless convinced Nazis and, because more capable than others, did much of the work of the regime. They could sometimes create, as B. did, a humanitarian pocket within the evil project they ultimately served. B. was also a kind of Nazi doctor "everyman"—neither brilliant nor stupid, never particularly a leader but always bent on fitting in. One of my assistants angrily spoke of him as the most dangerous of Auschwitz types because, as he put it, there are always a few fanatics like Mengele, but the larger problem came from followers who should have "known better." B. leaves me with a dual sense of ugly Nazi adaptation on the one hand, and on the other a laudable capacity to hold out a lifeline in a death camp. B. demonstrated the capacity of the self to roam far and wide in its contradictory behavior. That capacity was exploited by the Nazis in their time, and created much ambivalence in me. But that same capacity enabled B. to grasp every nuance of contradiction within Auschwitz itself and thereby contribute as he alone could to my knowledge of that death camp.

Breaking Bread—"How Far Do You Go?"

Dr. Karl S. was the most overtly Nazi of all the doctors I interviewed. He provided me with a remarkable account of the Nazification and biologization of the German medical profession, and also caused me to experience some of the most awkward moments of my research.

S. had been a high-ranking medical administrator and welcomed his chance to tell me his version of things. He also regaled me with interesting details about his family tree and its rural past going back for centuries, of his father's encounter with Bismarck, and his own dueling-fraternity dominated student life. I noted that he tried to be congenial but was also on the edge of senility. During three grueling interviews totaling about twenty hours he would swing back and forth between coherent descriptions that were of considerable interest to my work, and what I called "mad Nazi soliloquies," usually coming at the end of a long session.

For instance, in a sustained rant late in our first interview, he denounced "false stories" and "propaganda" about concentration camps, insisting that only hundreds of thousands and not millions had been killed, and that technical analysis refuted claims of extensive gassing. He chuckled derisively at the ineptitude of these propagandists. Later Matthias told me that over the course of this diatribe I looked as though I were "about to explode." S.'s home where all this took place was in a very isolated rural area and was situated at some distance from the road. By the time the interview ended, the land surrounding the house was in total darkness, and S. produced a powerful flashlight to illuminate our way to our car. As we walked, we heard only the deep barking of what sounded like very large dogs.

Matthias and I were at first shaken by the experience, but over a drink we soon could see the gallows humor in this weird caricature of a sinister Nazi scene. Matthias called it a "Simon Wiesenthal situation" (referring to the famed Nazi hunter) and observed that Dr. S. was living up to the most extreme version of "the horrible German." I likened it to a grade-B Hollywood movie about Nazis. With some amusement we imagined the incredulity of friends of ours—Jewish intellectuals on the Upper West Side in my case, German colleagues in the Social Democratic Party in Matthias's—about our presence in such a scene.

But there was something else about the experience with Dr. S. that made me considerably more uncomfortable. It had to do with the luncheon break after a long morning of productive exchange. Usually in such situations, my interpreter and I would have lunch at a nearby restaurant and return in an hour or so, providing everybody with something of a respite. But Dr. S.'s home was so isolated that there was no restaurant at all nearby. Going off to find one would have consumed most of the afternoon and left little or no time for continuing the interview. S. was aware of this and urged us to stay and have lunch with him, making clear that his wife had prepared food for us. What went through my mind was this: I really wanted to get away for lunch, needed an hour's relief from this hateful Nazi, and above all did not want to "break bread"—share the ritual of a meal—with such a person. I was also concerned about Matthias requiring such a break in his difficult role of psychologically minded simultaneous interpreting. But on the other hand I was fascinated by the interview, had the impression that this man was telling me things I could hear from no one else, and that by refusing his luncheon invitation I might be depriving myself of that rich vein of research material. I consulted with Matthias, who, understanding the situation fully, strongly favored our joining S. for the meal.

The next hour was one of the most difficult of my entire research experience. Divested of our rather clearly defined interview roles, we were suddenly thrust into a social situation and reduced to making small talk. S. partly filled the gap by telling stories of his family, one of which concerned his father's visit to Bismarck to present the compliments of his university fraternal organization (to which Bismarck himself had also belonged). The group was joined by Gerson von Bleichröder, Bismarck's Jewish banker or "German Rothschild," who, in his old age, had diminished vision. Bleichröder wished to kiss Bismarck's ring but mistook S.'s father (much younger but also bald) for the great man and began to kiss his ring instead. S.'s punch line: "When my brothers and I tell this story, we always say to my father, 'Couldn't you have asked him for a little money?'" I stifled my anger at the anti-Semitism of the tale and said nothing.

Later Matthias and I talked about having been compromised by our pleasant demeanor before this Nazi. As Matthias put it, "Our being so polite to him, telling him to thank his wife for giving us lunch—sitting down and eating with him—how far do you go?" I had the same question, the same self-condemnation (as I noted) for being on "such seemingly affable terms with this man and his monstrous ideas." Again I told myself that my planned book—having the ultimate say—justified our behavior, but that did not prevent me from feeling unclean in connection with this "socializing."

I was not wrong about the value of these interviews. S. gave me a unique sense of what it was like to be an active participant in the very formation of Nazi medicine. He did so as a combination of a medical street fighter and what could be called a biological intellectual. Everything dated back to World War I, from which his father had returned wounded. Too young to participate in that war, S. joined the Freikorps (Free Corps), the voluntary right-wing paramilitary units made up mostly of demobilized soldiers who saw themselves as an alternative to communist revolution and a source of social order at a time of national chaos. S. described his ideas at the time as *"völkisch,"* focused on creating a powerful, even mystical German community. He believed that "the war experience had made a people of us" and retained what he called this "people's nationalism" over the course of his medical studies. It was as a physician that he joined the Nazi SA (Sturmabteilung, or Storm Troopers), which he considered a continuation of the Freikorps. Besides marching proudly and belligerently through the streets while singing the Horst Wessel song, he and other doctors in the SA were to form the nucleus of the National Socialist Physicians' League, which did much to shape Nazi medical behavior.

From childhood S. had been deeply immersed in biology, influenced by German writers who combined a biological and *völkisch* worldview. He could therefore have something of an epiphany when hearing the prominent Nazi leader Rudolf Hess declare that National Socialism was "nothing but applied biology." S. and others then held forth, in speeches and writings, a concept of "biological socialism" that claimed for the Nazi movement both scientific truth and populist realization. He promulgated among other doctors the equally mystical concept of being physicians to the "people's body" (*volkskörp*) and told me proudly that "never over the centuries have doctors enjoyed such a high position as in the Third Reich." He believed that doctors like himself were to be the vanguard of a new, all-encompassing German (and ultimately world) gemeinschaft, or community. As I listened, I had the sense that, precisely because he was a half-mad ideologue, S. could convey to me, even if in slight caricature, something close to the essence of Nazi medicine and its potential for killing.

Interestingly, S. viewed these visionary ideas as beyond politics, as part of a movement rather than a state or party. He claimed that things began to go wrong for the Nazis when issues of race and biology were taken away from the doctors with their noble vision of serving a mystical German *volk*, and instead dealt with legalistically (as in the race laws). He even claimed that the Nazi Party originally promised that it would dissolve itself once National Socialism came to power. In this and all else, he saw his views as consistent with Hitler's, describing the Führer as "a genius" who was ultimately betrayed and manipulated by people around him, and possibly even poisoned by a notorious quack doctor upon whom he became very dependent. S. tried to identify his visionary self as closely as possible with Hitler, declaring only half humorously, "Hitler and I were the only real National Socialists."

In contrast, S. saw Heinrich Himmler as misguided and ignorant, substituting a kind of "veterinary breeding" for a true biological worldview. It was Himmler, not Hitler, who was responsible for the concentration camps, and for ruining what S. considered a beautiful medical movement. The Nazi project failed, he insisted, because he and other doctors were given insufficient opportunity to disseminate their biological truths— their revolutionary medical projects aimed at eliminating bad genes—so that "the tragedy of National Socialism was that it was never realized."

This dedicated Nazi purist became so discouraged with what was being done to his movement that he decided to leave everything—his high administrative position and his wife and seven children—to go to war on the eastern front. He was partly making up for his not having been able to serve in World War I. As he told me, "I wanted to experience war. I knew that you proved yourself in war." And he wrote (in a later book) of his experience as a physician to an SS tank unit as providing him with "sacred happiness." In this embrace of war as a form of purification and an experience in the "metaphysical realm," he was living out a more general fascist vision.

S. and I were to have one more grotesque personal exchange. I conducted the first two interviews while living in Munich, but the third one on a brief trip to Germany after having returned to the United States. He greeted me with his usual friendliness, but I noticed he was intent on making a point involving a copy of *Time* magazine that he held out in front of him. It was the issue in which a brief notice appeared concerning my research on Nazi doctors, stating that the work was bound to be very demanding for me as a Jew. Accompanying that notice was a frequently reproduced photograph of a uniformed German, identified as a Nazi doctor, leaning over a victim on whom he was conducting some form of harmful experiment. It turned out that S. liked to read the English edition of *Time* as a way of improving his language skills. Now he pointed to the picture, muttered something about the inaccuracies of journalism, and then declared triumphantly: "That is *not* a Nazi doctor!" He explained that the man in the picture was a Luftwaffe (air force) doctor who had "nothing to do with us [the administrative leaders of Nazi medicine]," and he went on to emphasize how separate he and his group were from military and other SS personnel in the camps.

Next came his response to my Jewishness, which he might have suspected before but was now made definite. In a newly unctuous tone he began to discuss "the whole Jewish question," and then made what would be my nomination for the understatement of the century: "There has been a tragic misunderstanding between your people and my people." As he further explained, "We were not anti-Semites" but merely "seeking to realize the *völkisch* ideal." He was saying in effect that the Nazis really had nothing against the Jews but simply had to get rid of them for the sake of consolidating the German "national body." And he added that the process was furthered by "advances in biological science." He admitted that there had been "excesses," but he wished me to understand the spiritual purposes motivating the Nazis, and that Hitler had the same goals as S. and was also "not really an anti-Semite." And in his fashion S. reached out to me by saying that, given the increasing Muslim threat (he had in mind especially the number of Turks in Germany), our two peoples should "join the same gemeinschaft." S.'s ideological narrative had been altered only by a shift in roles.

This time I felt less agitated by his obscene ideas and could experience them as useful for my research. I was not even troubled by the lunch invitation that I knew would be forthcoming. I noted later that, though I still found him "absolutely despicable," I was "a little more at ease" during the meal, though I "worried about this lest it show a kind of numbing and weakening of moral judgment on my part." Now I was more ready to break bread in the service of my research function.

There is a postscript. Something about this near-senile Nazi medical street fighter/visionary upset Matthias, more so than in any other situation I encountered involving a Nazi doctor and an interpreter. Matthias experienced uncomfortable family memories of his own, of conflict between his parents over their responses to the Nazi movement, and of his later disappointment in the behavior of postwar German political parties in relation to the Nazis. I wondered why these interviews in particular had that effect. S. himself gave me an important clue toward the end of our last session. He said that he enjoyed our interviews because they gave him a chance to reexamine in detail so much of what he had lived through. I realized that he had experienced what in psychiatric work with the elderly is called a "life review": an exploration of a person's past in quest of an overall sense of meaning, purpose, and integrity. And S.'s personal story was a kind of "life review" of the Nazi movement itself, revealing much about not only Nazi medicine but the overall National Socialist phenomenon with its bizarre pseudological narrative. S.'s personal and Nazi party life review made contact with Matthias's own family story.

I had a problem of a different kind with that issue. By offering S. an opportunity for a life review, was I not contributing to this highly objectionable man's affirmative integration of the details and sequence of his Nazi-centered experience? I had raised questions about Nazi mass murder, but he sloughed these off with his ideological rationalizations and falsehoods and held tenaciously to the "integrity" of his beliefs and actions. I knew this was characteristic for people enmeshed in totalistic ideologies and was aware that the life story he presented to me was already very much part of him. But I was not pleased by the idea that his airing that narrative to me might have strengthened it in his mind. Nor could I emerge from those episodes of breaking bread without a residual feeling of considerable uncleanliness. But looking back at our difficult interaction, I have no regrets.

Nazi Tears

Another elderly Nazi doctor, toward the end of our second and final interview, suddenly began to weep. For about thirty seconds the only sound in the room was that of his urgent sobbing. He then apologized and we completed the last few minutes of our exchange. What made him break down? And how did I react? To begin to answer these questions I need to say something about who he was and what he had done.

Dr. Johann G. had served a long prison sentence for his collaboration in human experiments in which camp inmates were infected with typhus microorganisms in order to test the efficacy of vaccines, with many resulting deaths. During our interviews he vigorously protested his innocence, as he had done publicly as well. Among physicians convicted of such crimes, he was one of the few of considerable professional distinction and international reputation. He was intent on making this clear to me and attempted to receive me as an overseas colleague who would understand his mistreatment.

Dr. G. came from a middle-class background, was wounded during his military service in World War I, and, like Dr. S., joined the Freikorps after the war ("I always tended to the extreme right"). More cosmopolitan and intellectually gifted than S., G. studied abroad, forged a career in the higher echelons of German academic medicine, and spent years in the Far East applying his knowledge of bacteriology and public health to contain epidemics. At the same time he embraced the Nazis early, rose quickly in the medical hierarchy, and became one of the leading consultants to the military, achieving the rank of brigadier general. He had an audience with

Hitler, who impressed him deeply, especially because of his willingness to listen to G.'s views on international medical questions.

G. presented his Nazi medical world to me as an environment of intelligent, thoughtful people concerned with making life-enhancing decisions. He spoke of "talking shop" with colleagues, suggesting an ordinary, medically constructive atmosphere. When something went wrong, it seemed always to surprise him. For instance, he told of heading a high-level civilian committee in charge of allocating pesticides, especially cyanide, to various groups within the regime. He favored a sizable amount for the SS, "knowing that they had bedbugs in their wooden barracks," and was "later horrified to discover that the cyanide had been used to kill human beings." He said that was "like a man who sells a gun to another person and then discovers that the person used it for murder." My thought was that a more accurate version of that analogy would be a man presenting a gun to a group of murderers he was unable or disinclined to recognize as such because he was a member of that group. But I did not say that.

When, after the war, doctors in camps or killing centers were clearly revealed to have injected people with deadly substances, he treated the information as isolated examples of "morally insane" people, insisting that "the political system had nothing to do with it." I also noted that he sanitized the Buchenwald concentration camp by an Orwellian reference to its chief Nazi doctor as "medical superintendent." His overall personal narrative was one of steady, high-minded behavior in constant opposition to the scoundrels one might encounter anywhere. What he could never touch was the deep corruption and murderousness of the regime itself and the pivotal role of people like him in that corruption and killing.

Unsurprisingly, his relationship to the typhus experiments was a convoluted one. His need to see himself as upholding high professional standards led him to speak out at an early military medical conference *against* doctors' participation in unethical human experiments, an act that required some courage. He was then called in by the highest-ranking Nazi medical administrator, who, according to G., explained in a low-key "reasonable" fashion that he did not like the experiments, either, but because typhus epidemics threatened military personnel, it was crucial to find the best vaccine with which to protect the precious lives of German soldiers. In the exchange G. was treated with the respect due a high-ranking professional and party colleague. He found the argument completely convincing. So much so that he participated, at least tangentially, in the experiments, and the actions for which he was later convicted included providing the necessary vaccine and bringing his special expertise to high-level discussions about the results. During his trial G. disputed these accusations, emphasizing then, and later to me, that he had no part in the actual injection of contaminated blood into the bodies of the experimental victims. His conviction resulted not only in a decade of imprisonment but in lifelong professional dishonor.

Most doctors I spoke to sought in various ways to justify their behavior under the Nazis. But G. went much further. He was the only Nazi doctor who tried to make use of his encounter with me to restore his professional standing and rehabilitate himself in the eyes of the world. He wanted me, as an American academic physician, to bear witness to his high intellectual and moral qualities as a healer and teacher in our joint profession. He persisted in this hope despite my clear rejection of his ethical claims for Nazi medicine and for himself. He pleaded with me to take concrete steps on behalf of his rehabilitation. First he asked me to use my influence to bring about a reversal of his criminal conviction so that he could be declared legally innocent. When I refused, he suggested an alternative: that I arrange to invite him to give a prestigious lecture at Yale Medical School as a way of restoring his international reputation. I repeatedly made it clear that I would sponsor no such invitation. I did that once more during what we both knew were the last moments of our final interview, and it was then that he broke down and wept.

He wept because it was now clear that he would die without ever having cleared his name. But I believe there was a deeper reason as well. It had to do with loss of conviction in his own mind concerning his claim to honorable behavior in relation to the Nazi medical system, and the resulting collapse of the sense of self built around that conviction. In his case, the "life review" in our interviews had undermined rather than sustained his positive Nazi narrative.

My response to his tears said something about me. My initial feeling was one of surprise—he had been fluid and articulate, even in his self-deceptions—and I was unprepared for this kind of dramatic interruption. I then felt a twinge of pathos (not quite pity) in seeing this old man reduced to childlike humiliation. But as I sensed what the tears meant, that initial feeling was quickly replaced by a certain satisfaction in the collapse of his offensive narrative. I had a third, more self-interested reaction: a concern that, should he have some kind of breakdown, I could be accused of having violated my commitment to avoid harming those I interviewed (as stated in my research protocol approved by the Yale Committee on Research with Human Subjects as well as in the consent form that G. and I both signed). I didn't believe I had acted in a way that was harmful, but with a man of that fragility—physical, ethical, and psychological—who could say?

So what did I do? Essentially nothing. I did not reassure him in any way, nor did I make any comment or interpretation. I simply remained silent until the tears stopped, he made his apology, and we went on to finish the interview. By then I was intent on viewing the episode in terms of its significance for my research. I was relieved to see him able to function again and very aware that something important—and perhaps appropriate—had happened between us.

16

Historical Encounters

Nazi Nobel Laureate—Friend of My Friends

In my work, Konrad Lorenz formed a category of his own. He was not a clear-cut "research subject." But he was a Nazi doctor. Though better known as a biologist and ethologist, he was trained as a physician and had certainly been involved in the Nazi movement. Indeed, I had come across an astounding paragraph he had written in 1940, which suggested the most shocking kind of involvement:

> It must be the duty of racial hygiene to be attentive to a more severe elimination of morally inferior human beings than is the case today. . . . We should literally replace all factors responsible for selection in a natural and free life. . . . In prehistoric times of humanity, selection for endurance, heroism, social usefulness, etc. was made solely by *hostile* outside factors. This role must be assumed by a human organization; otherwise, humanity will, for lack of selective factors, be annihilated by the degenerative phenomena that accompany domestication.

I encountered no statement that provided better biological justification for the Nazi principle of destroying what was called "life unworthy of life."

Yet I had been introduced to this man by two mutual friends, each of whom had special meaning in my life. One was Fritz Redlich, who told me that Lorenz had actually saved his life. As a young Viennese doctor, Fritz had found himself in deep trouble with Nazi authorities, both because he had been a left-wing student activist and because his parents had been relatively recent converts from Judaism to Catholicism. Fritz turned to Lorenz, a family friend who had embraced the Nazis, to make use of influence with the regime to enable him to leave the country. The second mutual friend, Erik Erikson, spoke to me enthusiastically about having spent two weeks with Lorenz at his institute exploring the potential insights of ethology (the relatively new science of animal behavior in natural settings, which Lorenz helped pioneer) for human beings.

I had met Lorenz briefly at an interdisciplinary Josiah Macy, Jr. Foundation meeting in Princeton, New Jersey, twenty years earlier and had mixed feelings toward him then—admiring his work, aware vaguely of past Nazi affiliations, and having the impression that he overdid his charm. By the time of my 1979 visit he had become world famous, as an ethologist and corecipient of the 1973 Nobel Prize in medicine, and as an author of highly popular books for the general public. He had also emerged as an environmentalist and opponent of nuclear power who was now much admired by the Austrian political left. I encountered what I called a "mythic figure"—tall, erect, substantial in build, long hair and carefully trimmed beard, everything white—"in the full glory of [the] persona . . . of the grand old man." He received me in his elegant country home and research center, about an hour's drive from Vienna, which I described as "an imposing yet modest castle." Contributing to his aura was the presence of two women, his wife (who looked considerably older than he) and his daughter (middle-aged and lively), both of whom fawned over him and at the same time functioned as protectors.

I came without tape recorder or consent form, as my visit had been constructed as social and informally professional. But I felt myself to be still the researcher who could not separate Lorenz from that notorious Nazi paragraph, or from the phrase uttered to me by Dr. S. when explaining how the Nazi medical leadership spread its influence: "We gave Lorenz a professorship at Königsberg." Yet I did first seek common ground, as we briefly discussed the Josiah Macy meetings, issues of thought reform and totalism (I presented him with my book on the subject), and his active involvement in the Austrian movement opposing nuclear energy. When I sought to guide the discussion toward the Nazi era, Lorenz deflected things by launching into what I called "an interminable series of stories" on his incarceration as a prisoner of war in Soviet camps, where he could function as a physician. He took pride in presenting himself as a survivor and a healer, saving people from starvation by means of frequent small feedings of natural plants and developing psychological skills to induce those who refused food to begin to eat.

He did not even wish to talk about having saved Fritz Redlich's life because that was a reminder of his Nazi influence at the time, and much preferred to dwell on our mutual friendship with Erik Erikson ("Any friend of Erik Erikson is very welcome here"), with whom he had no such history. When I pressed matters by bringing up my work on Nazi doctors, I noted that Lorenz, who had been voluble, "suddenly became taciturn," and that the facial expressions of the two women changed from welcoming to disapproving. When I persevered by questioning him about Nazi manipulation of scientists and the degree to which they had been corrupted, he was at first evasive about what he called "a very difficult subject," but gradually began to talk about his own experience. He said that in such an environment compromises were necessary, that he "had to use Nazi language" when referring to evolutionary causes for the disappearance of desirable Nordic traits. I had the impression that he was attempting to explain away that notorious paragraph about the necessity of intervening to ensure the "elimination of morally inferior human beings"—all the more so when he insisted, against all evidence, that he always maintained his personal and scientific integrity.

I was surprised when he told me that he had just read *Mein Kampf* "for the first time," suggesting that he was still struggling with his Nazi experience. He marveled at Hitler's grasp of group psychology and stressed the idealism of young Nazis, adding that "I believed in it too." He then made the odd claim that when the young are drawn to any such ideological movement—whether Nazi, communist, or Christian—"it is the best people genetically who are the most affected" because they are the ones who have "the inborn capacity for profound emotional response." He bemoaned what he took to be the biological, even evolutionary vulnerability of the young toward such conversion, and admitted that in his own case it provided him with "a sense of great freedom and happiness."

Even as we discussed these matters, I was being treated as a guest, the two women serving tea and cakes, which made me worry that my "guest self" would dull my "research self" and attenuate my probing of painful questions. That worry increased when Lorenz took me to "feed the fish" and also invited me to "have pot luck with us" and stay for dinner. I was not prepared for the power of the fish scene, which encompassed two large rooms each made up entirely of enormous tanks containing (as I noted) "fish that were exquisite, compelling, and caused me to feel I did not want to leave that room." Lorenz held forth about the different species and their "most extraordinary sociology," demonstrating with great excitement a particular fish that actually walked on the bottom of the tank and then engaged in a courting display. I had the sense I was witnessing a remarkable combination of beauty and science, making it easy to forget that this was the same man who paved the way biologically for Nazi extermination policies.

At dinner Lorenz displayed a new book of exquisite photographs taken at his Max Planck ethology institute in Germany, about two hundred miles away. They included Lorenz himself elegantly stretched out among the geese, and a young woman coworker looking ravishing in her bikini. I found the photographs to be both striking and a little troubling in reminding me of the work of Leni Riefenstahl, the talented filmmaker and photographer who was close to Hitler and did much to mythologize the Nazi movement. There was a similarly romantic worship of nature and of animal and human bodies, sharply contrasting (in Susan Sontag's words) "the clean and the impure, the incorruptible and the defiled," an approach Riefenstahl described as a quest for "perfect harmony," and that Sontag called "fascist aesthetics." Looking at the photographs I also felt a certain envy toward Lorenz for being able to do his work in situations of paradise, whether on land among beautiful creatures or the underwater paradise of the fish tanks. I contrasted the ugliness of my professional subjects—Nazi killing, Vietnam massacres, the atomic bomb—even if I sought the paradise of Wellfleet as an antidote.

We then went into a freewheeling intellectual discussion that was the most enjoyable part of the visit. He talked about his lifelong concern with the problem of aggression and with "ways of restraining aggression." I had read some of that work and found him to be too quick to anthropomorphize animal findings. That tendency continued when he spoke of his fish as "happy" because "swimming and playing and courting," I asked whether we could not see them as neither happy nor unhappy but simply carrying out their natural functions. When I suggested that unhappiness was the price of the human evolutionary leap, and he added that the knowledge of death was another, my notes record that "I said the obvious—it was the same thing." He then spoke eloquently about how the scientist's all-important observations lost their elegance and nuance as soon as he wrote them down, how intuition was crucial but at times had to be suppressed in favor of observation. That perspective seemed consistent with thoughts I'd had about theoretical concepts or interpretations of one's work bringing an end to the flow of experience, though, paradoxically, necessary if one is to make any observations at all.

Toward the end of my stay, Erik Erikson resurfaced (one could say that he had been there all along) when Lorenz suddenly declared: "You know, he is a caricature of me." What immediately went through my mind was the silent thought: "No, you have it reversed—*you* are the caricature of *him.*" Erik had in fact once told me that their appearance was sufficiently similar for them to have been mistaken for one another, to which I would add parallels in their imaginative minds and in the south German charm with which they spoke and acted. They were doppelgängers with a difference: Erik, though fearful and full of doubt, never without humor, maintaining the integrity of his work and producing a humane opus; Lorenz, bolder, more pompous, and less humorous, drawn to the absolute and deeply corrupted by it in his work and his life, able to reconstitute himself while retaining inwardly the shadow of his transgressions. By the end of my stay I was aware of the ambiguity of some of my responses—there were moments when I quite liked the man—but those Nazi transgressions continued to define him for me more than anything else. Nor did I feel he had freed himself from his past, since, as I noted, "Nazi ghosts are most difficult to exorcise."

After the visit I probed further into Lorenz's Nazi involvements, which turned out to be even more flagrant than I had imagined. He had joined the Nazi Party in June 1938, almost as soon as it was legally possible in

Austria to do that, and quickly became a member of the party's Office of Race Policy. In September 1940 he was appointed professor and director of the Institute for Comparative Psychology at the University of Königsberg. The chair was arranged by the notorious Nazi education and culture minister Bernhard Rust, who overruled faculty objections and more generally, as one historian put it, "presided over the sabotage of Germany's intellectual life in the name of racial purity." Lorenz then engaged in what a commentator called "a process of reciprocal legitimation, whereby the Nazis lent political power to ideas which were already part of Lorenz's worldview." He actively contributed to Nazi policies of repopulation and ethnic cleansing in Poland, wrote that a "people's doctor" could readily identify "inferior forms" because "a good man . . . knows full well whether the other person is a scoundrel" (a caricature on a grand scale of the principle of intuition), and more broadly declared that "the racial idea is the foundation of our form of government."

Lorenz's postwar washing away of his Nazi past is no less striking. Minimizing rather than denying that past, he could be effectively rehabilitated in Germany because of support he received from prominent scientists like Otto Hahn and by non-German ethological colleagues (notably Niko Tinbergen, who worked closely with Lorenz, though he himself was a Dutch anti-Nazi) because they admired Lorenz's scientific work. Americans played no small part in that cleansing of his past, undoubtedly affected by his prodigious charm, as I could witness in the adulation he received at that early Josiah Macy conference. Significantly, a 1993 edition of the *Columbia Encyclopedia* includes a dense paragraph on Lorenz mentioning his many scientific achievements and honors but making no reference at all to his Nazi background. Nor was that background a barrier to his receiving the Nobel Prize in 1973, protested by just a few scientists with memories in Germany and America. The award helped cast aside Lorenz's Nazi involvements and early scientific corruption and enabled him to move readily into the persona of the wise old man.

It is possible that Lorenz drew on his Nazi past even in his later embrace of environmentalism, as the Nazi movement tended to revere the natural environment in its focus on the purity of rural life and the struggle against chemical pollutants. Whatever the case, I noted that a number of former Nazi doctors I interviewed prominently displayed books by

Lorenz on their shelves, apparently finding in him a link between the Nazi and postwar worlds—a prominent Nazi intellectual given worldly recognition despite the collapse of the movement and holding to relatively familiar versions of instinctualism and environmental purity. As for me, whatever the contradictions in my response and the vibrations of his friendships with Redlich and Erikson, my research self—my unyielding awareness of Lorenz's participation in the Nazi biomedical vision—clearly prevailed.

Family Support for Auschwitz Killing

About halfway through my work I found myself in Hamburg interviewing a forty-year-old woman who was neither a doctor nor a Nazi. She had the concerns of the housewife she was, scheduling the interview at a time that would permit her to pick up her young children at school, and would have been quite unremarkable except for one thing. She was the daughter of Eduard Wirths, chief doctor at Auschwitz during the camp's most efficient phase and architect of its structure of medicalized killing.

I could not interview her father because he had hanged himself soon after being taken into British custody. He was nonetheless a continuous presence in my research, talked about with considerable feeling by other Nazi doctors and by survivors as well. Learning that Wirths had been a dedicated family man, I sought to find out all I could about him from family members he had been close to: the daughter I was interviewing, his younger brother, Helmut, whom I was also able to talk to, his widow (who would not see me but eventually made available to me a revealing series of letters Wirths had written to her from Auschwitz), his father (who was dead but had made a number of public statements, and whose influence Helmut could decribe to me), and his son (who conveyed some of his feelings through his sister, the woman I was talking to).

The daughter had been told by her mother from an early age that her father "had died in the war," saying little about him other than that "he was a good man and a really good father." That description seemed consistent with the daughter's memories of the kind man who had played with her and bounced her on his knee. Only later did she discover that much of the bouncing had occurred in Auschwitz during periods when the family stayed there with Wirths. Her mother never wanted to talk to her about what went on in Auschwitz and she went along with the avoidance. But inevitably she began to hear more about that dreadful camp, and the situation came to a head when a Dutch film crew succeeded in enlisting the family's help in a documentary about Wirths's life, which was eventually shown in 1975. Now her mother began to tell her much more, but still defended her husband as a man deeply troubled by Auschwitz who remained there "in order to prevent an even worse situation." As the daughter began to read on her own about the camp, however, she found that, as she put it to me, "all of a sudden there is a completely different picture [of him]," and he became "a totally different [person]." She found what she read to be "difficult to believe," and had conflicting emotions of wishing to "apologize for him . . . to understand him . . . to find justification."

She had long talks with her younger brother, who shared her pain and confusion. They recognized the terrible events their father had been part of but concluded that "we cannot condemn him, *him* himself." She seemed to appreciate the opportunity to explore these feelings with me, but remained anguished by this basic contradiction about her father. At the end of our interview, she summed up her dilemma by asking me, as one who "studies these matters," a terse question: "Can a good man do bad things?'" I did not have a simple answer for her, and there was not time for a more complicated one. What I did say was "Yes, but he's then no longer a good man." But I knew that the question had great relevance for my overall work with Nazi doctors, and for human behavior in general.

Wirths had been considered by most to be a good man until he came to Auschwitz. His father, a successful stoneworks owner, had been a medical corpsman in World War I, from which he emerged with symptoms of depression and pacifist leanings. He had much to do with "making doctors" (as Helmut Wirths put it) of two of his sons (the third died in childhood). Eduard, greatly influenced by his father, was an ideal older son—meticulous, obedient, and unusually conscientious and reliable. He neither smoked nor drank, and married the only woman with whom he was ever involved. Always a good student, he became by all accounts a very good doctor.

But during his student days he was deeply drawn to prevailing currents of extreme nationalism and accompanying *völkisch* ideas. He joined the Nazi Party and the SA in 1933 and applied successfully for admission to the SS the following year. He extended this enthusiasm to Nazi views on "racial hygiene" and "applied biology," though his early attitude toward Jews was strikingly contradictory. He continued to treat his Jewish patients even after it had become illegal for Aryan doctors to do so, sometimes sneaking them into his consulting room at night. At the same time he embraced Nazi ideology that held the Jews to be a grave danger to Germany and the world. While in private practice he contributed to various Nazi medical projects including the resettling of ethnic Germans from the east, and later volunteered for active military service and saw two years of combat with the Waffen SS in the invasion of Norway and on the Russian front. Then judged medically unfit for combat because of a cardiac ailment, he had short assignments to Dachau and Neuengamme (concentration camps in Germany) before being appointed chief doctor at Auschwitz in September 1942. Considered by his superior to be "the best physician in all the concentration camps," he was sent there because other doctors had failed to stop deadly typhus epidemics in the camp. He succeeded in that, but his position as chief camp doctor, along with his own organizational impulses, took him deeply into the Auschwitz killing function.

Survivor doctors described him to me as relatively pleasant, or at least "correct," in his interactions with them, and as having saved a number of their lives by helping them or their patients avoid selections. One of them called him "a Nazi ideologist . . . who did not like the methods of the gas chamber." So what Wirths did was to try to *improve* those methods. He insisted that *doctors* perform and control selections, in that way giving a medical structure to the killing of Jews and adhering to an SS version of racial hygiene. In doing so he consolidated his own power in the camp, while creating the Auschwitz system of efficient mass murder. Never one to shirk responsibility, he took overall charge of selections, guided other doctors through this "difficult assignment," and insisted upon doing them himself as well. He collaborated with other SS leaders in "balancing" the camp's slave labor function (keeping a certain number of Jews alive) with the danger of epidemics through overcrowding (limiting the number of Jews kept alive), without interfering with the camp's raison d'être of killing as many Jews as possible. So even as he saw himself taking a "humane" stand—showing a certain amount of civility to those around him, saving a few lives, and combating the more vicious Gestapo leaders in Auschwitz—he did more than anyone else to lend medical authority to Auschwitz killing.

When I interviewed Helmut, he told me that his older brother had been "an extraordinarily misused person, a very good human being—the best father, a good doctor—who had the terrible misfortune to be brought into this situation." A trim, articulate, successful doctor in his late sixties, Helmut Wirths had been the family member most involved in the issue. He had read widely on the subject and had attended the Auschwitz trial in Frankfurt together with his son, also a doctor, with whom he was in painful dialogue about the whole Nazi era. Helmut's comments to me could be quite clear, even eloquent: "Sure, there are peoples who have hated each other for centuries. But that one kills people so systematically, with the help of physicians, only because they belong to another race, that is new in the world." Helmut's efforts, however, were complicated by his own involvements with his brother in relation to Auschwitz. When Eduard Wirths, horrified by what he found there, consulted with family members about whether to try to leave, both Helmut and their father argued that he should remain in Auschwitz because he could play a constructive role there. Helmut made clear to me that he now considered this a mistaken view, which he attributed to his own as well as his brother's youth and inexperience (they were in their early thirties at the time); had he been "a mature man able to judge things better," he would have realized that "the only thing to do in a situation like that is to say, 'No, I won't do it!'" He was telling me that the two young physician-brothers were all too susceptible to both their father's wrong advice and the overall influence of the Nazi regime.

Helmut had an even greater problem. He had collaborated with his brother on research, conducted in Auschwitz, on precancerous growths of the cervix, research that might have begun as genuine, but in that setting inevitably led to abuse, infections, and deaths. Biopsy materials were sent to Helmut's laboratory in Hamburg, and he made a number of visits to Auschwitz to work with his brother. In our discussion Helmut tried to minimize his collaboration, claiming that his visits to Auschwitz were more for the purpose of lending emotional support to his brother than for the research itself. But the collaboration gave him a more direct Auschwitz connection, which complicated his ethical struggles concerning his brother and himself.

Helmut related his brother's culpability to the "tragic guilt . . . inescapable guilt" of classical Greek drama. I felt that in our talk Helmut had two motivations, which were at odds with each other: that of defending his brother, himself, and the family name in general; and that of genuinely helping me probe his brother's psychology and behavior in Auschwitz. He made an additional contribution to my probing by convincing his sister-in-law, Eduard's widow, to make available to me the remarkable set of letters her husband wrote to her from Auschwitz.

The letters were written from the day after he arrived in Auschwitz (in September 1942) to the time of the approach of the Russian armies and his flight from the camp (in July 1945), except for the time that she and the three children lived with him there (from late 1943 through September 1944). Wirths makes clear in the letters that his bond with family members, especially his wife, gave him the capacity to do what he did in Auschwitz. In his first letter to her he reveals the shock and horror he experienced on arriving at the camp, from which he finds "protective inoculation" in their "immensely great love." But he sees the task of rebuilding camp structures as requiring "much German spirit, energy . . . the work of pioneers [that] must be done for our children, my angel, for our children." In subsequent letters, he conveys a similar sense of an immortalizing crusade, always for the benefit of his and others' future German descendants, and imbued with his immediate love for his wife and children. Indeed his expressions of endearment are infinite and transcendent ("beloved little treasure," "dear soul," "little birdie," and "Almighty One") and seem psychologically to serve both to counter Auschwitz horrors and to enable him to participate in them. He asks, "Is it a sin that I love you so much?" When Wirths and his wife were actually together in Auschwitz, there were problems between them because of her discomfort there. There is evidence that she wished to leave but was told by a confidant that she had better stay "if you want to save your husband," suggesting Wirths's rocky emotional state (he was described as frequently agitated and sometimes depressed) in the midst of his organizational efficiency.

When Wirths surrendered himself to the British at the end of the war, now in a state of extreme depression, he prepared what I viewed as a desperate autobiographical apologia that was a mixture of truths, half-truths, and gross distortions. Soon after that a British intelligence officer greeted him and declared, "Now I've shaken hands with a man who is responsible for the deaths of four million human beings." Wirths hung himself that night. One prisoner who had been sympathetic to Wirths said that he killed himself because he "had a conscience." The difficulty was that the conscience was bound up primarily with German and Nazi loyalty. His final despair had to do with the collapse and dishonoring of the whole Nazi project, with his sense that he had no future (he knew he would be executed and wanted to avoid the pain, for himself and his family, of a humiliating trial). He did undoubtedly have feelings of guilt in connection with his role in mass killing, but wrote that his "greatest guilt" was toward his family. One articulate prisoner-doctor, whose life Wirths had saved, remained grateful to him but also judged him "a criminal" and summed up her view by saying, "Anyhow, he did the decent thing. He killed himself."

In learning all this, I had the overall sense that his suicide came too late. He had, unfortunately, functioned sufficiently well to carry out his work in the camp. And it was the loving family support he received that enabled him to adapt to Auschwitz and set up its structure of medicalized killing. That family support strengthened his own deep loyalty to the Nazi project, wherever that project took him. It was through Wirths that I had my only encounter with close family members of a Nazi doctor involved in killing. What I learned was this: Though the love experienced in one's family can be the most precious, life-enhancing gift, such love can also provide the kind of strength that enables one to participate in mass murder. Much depends upon the prevailing morality of the larger community, and on individual family members' relation to that community.

To return to Wirths's daughter's question, "Can a good man do bad things," I would now answer this way: At the time you bounced on your father's knee in Auschwitz, he was surely not a good man. He may well have been a decent father and husband, but he was immersed in the practice of great evil. The human mind can be sufficiently complex to include these contradictory tendencies. He might have been a good man some years earlier, but had been profoundly corrupted by his embrace of a murderous ideology that then dominated his country. Ironically, the love of members of his family contributed greatly to the choices he made and to what he did. Since your father was not *innately* bad, you raise an important question when you ask how people like him can come to do "bad things."

The Psychiatrist and the Killer Troops

I knew that one of the main reasons for the Nazis' creation of death camps with their efficient gas chambers was the psychological toll on German soldiers from face-to-face shooting of large numbers of Jews. But I had given little thought to doctors who might somehow be involved in that earlier operation. Then, about halfway through an interview with Dr. Hans K., he mentioned to me that he had been a neuropsychiatrist assigned to what he called "killer troops," members of the notorious SS Einsatzgruppen responsible for the murder of 1,400,000 Jews in Eastern Europe. That came as a surprise, as K. had been introduced to me simply as a Nazi doctor who held a high position in the military. I was extremely interested in hearing about this assignment because I realized that he had been at an intersection of psychiatric work with a dreadfully significant historical shift in Nazi killing methods.

Dr. K. had been described to me as "a nice man," and during our talks he was responsive and intent on conveying useful information to me. It turned out that he had known Fritz Redlich when the two were students in Vienna and he had even written a brief, early paper with him. But like many Austrians, K.'s ardent pan-German nationalism at the time of the Anschluss in 1938 led to an embrace of the Nazi movement. He told me that, before long, he became troubled by what he began to hear about killings in the "euthanasia" project and the related fear that came to permeate much of German psychiatry. He described the decline of his enthusiasm for the Nazis as "like the sensation after amphetamines— three months happy and then depression." But he did join the German army, serving in France and Russia before being wounded and then sent back to Vienna, where he worked with brain injuries.

In late 1941 or early 1942, while he was assigned to Russia, two soldiers were sent to him for examination. He found them to be in profound "psychological shock" and was "startled to learn that they were reacting not to combat but to massive 'Jew killing' taking place far from any battle lines." They described to him how Jews would be taken into custody and "herded together and told that they would be deported, then brought to a ditch where they were lined up until the SS got the order to shoot them. The children were screaming and the women were screaming." K. was struck by the complete absence of feeling in the SS men as they described these scenes ("just as if I were talking to you now and saying 'I traveled by automobile to Vienna'"). Finding the two men to be pale, trembling, and immobilized or what he called "finished," he considered them to have been "decompensated" or broken down by their experience. They asked him for "a medical statement that they had a nervous disease so that they could be transferred," which he provided, along with a recommendation that they be sent to Germany for treatment.

He told me that he had heard rumors of those mass killings and thought them "just not possible," but now had to believe what he had not wished to believe. He came to examine about fifty SS troops with such stories and symptoms, and in response to my questions described his psychological observations on them and on himself as well. He spoke of finding a consistent "killer response," even a "killer syndrome." The syndrome was similar to combat reactions, but much more severe. Troops sent to him from combat, he observed, were anxious, with high blood pressure and rapid pulse, insomnia, loss of appetite, and other bodily symptoms—all of which would greatly diminish or disappear within a day or two when the men were put into a quiet setting. With the "killer syndrome," after a slight delay the same set of symptoms would occur in more extreme form. The men would compulsively repeat all they had seen and done, while manifesting what K. called "neurological excitement" (increased reflexes and tremors) and also disturbing dreams in which the killer (the SS soldier) often became the victim who was being shot to death. And these symptoms tended to persist, without respite, for weeks and even months.

The most intense reactions came from murdering women and children, and especially "the mothers who had children in their arms." As K.

further explained: "They had to dig these trenches . . . and not all were dead. . . . Some of the children were still [alive]. . . . It affected them [the killer troops] most when the ones who weren't immediately killed screamed loudly or cried or prayed." K. went on to compare the "killer syndrome" in SS troops to the "concentration camp syndrome," the profound long-lasting symptomatology in many of those emerging from the camps. But he pointed out that the latter was incurred over months or years of trauma from incarceration, while the killer syndrome required "just one day" of carrying out the assignment of murdering helpless Jews. K. was trying to convey a clinical comparison to another physician, but whether or not it contained a kernel of truth, I found myself jarred by this rather casual juxtaposition of killers and victims.

K. stressed that any estimate of the percentage who reacted in that way was highly approximate but he put it this way: "Let's say, a hundred SS men shot 10,000 Jews, I don't know how many had that [syndrome] but I would say about twenty." Even if highly uncertain in its accuracy, that estimate of 20 percent suggests that a very considerable number of troops were strongly affected. He emphasized, however, that only about half of those with the syndrome had genuine moral qualms, felt that it was wrong to do what they did, or expressed some form of ethical or religious remorse. The others, without questioning the project, simply felt that the ordeal of carrying it out was too great and would ask, "How did I get such a shitty job?" Yet many of those (like Nazi doctors at Auschwitz) preferred to continue what they were doing rather than the alternative of being sent into combat. K. estimated that, whether or not experiencing the syndrome, as many as 60 percent of the men were "really unhappy about this activity." He found that the more sensitive the human being was, the more difficult the killing. In contrast, those closest to being psychopaths without emotional ties to others were best at it, and the SS strongly preferred this "cold killing type."

Of course, I was interested in how a fellow psychiatrist dealt with this pre-Auschwitz system of mass murder. What I learned was that, in essence, he adapted to it. K. told me of his sequence of response, from "first the shock of finding out that all one had been hearing [concerning Nazi killing] was true"; then "the reaction to help where possible [by providing medical certificates enabling individual men to be transferred], while of course aware of the fact that one can do nothing to change what was occurring"; and finally, resignation and compliance. It turned out that he provided medical certificates on only two or three occasions, as "that was noticed" and a psychiatrist providing too many could be viewed as a "saboteur." (According to K., he himself was so accused by a prosecutor when he gave testimony at a military trial to the effect that a man's desertion of his unit had been caused by traumatic effects of battle, testimony that saved the man from being hanged.)

Even when K. did have those very few men transferred back to Germany, he was uncertain about what awaited them there. He said vaguely that they could have been provided some form of recreation or rehabilitation, might have been discharged and sent home, or assigned light duty "guarding a railroad station" or be "sent to a concentration camp." What he mainly did with the great majority of men sent to him was to provide a little sedation and return them to active duty in the killing project. Here he deflected our discussion by contrasting the sympathy that he and other army doctors showed to the men "lucky enough to come to us" with the antagonistic stance of SS doctors who viewed their behavior as "cowardice" and would say: "Give that shithead a kick in the ass" or "I'll send that bastard to the front, where he'll really have to sweat it out." The ultimate disposition of the soldiers was probably the same in the two cases, but K. could find solace in his more "humane" approach.

He went on to describe how careful he had to be in what he said in his reports: "If I write that he is in psychological duress because of killing Jews, I would be the next [victim]. Therefore one had to write a false diagnosis . . . say that the nervous breakdown was caused by such things as demanding night duties and combat." His overall explanation of his behavior was that "the strongest desire in all of us was to survive." "All of us" clearly included both the killer troops and the psychiatrists. I noticed that, in talking about the troops he examined, K. often used the first person ("I can't sleep now because of this stupid activity"). He was being vivid, conveying the men's feelings from within; but he was also, I came to realize, identifying himself with the troops as sharing a mission and an entrapment.

There was an aspect of K. that was confessional. He spoke critically of his own passivity, though he did so as a somewhat detached, retrospective narrator: "The normal reaction would have been, 'It is a terrible thing. We must do something about it immediately.' The actual reaction was, 'It is an immensely terrible thing. But we cannot do anything.'" I again thought of the Camus character who insisted, "Authors of confessions write especially to avoid confessing, to tell nothing of what they know." K. was actually telling *something* of what he knew, but in a dissociated fashion characterized by a grotesque objectivity, which covered over what he could not or would not say. So he equated his behavior with that of all Germans and, generalizing still further, to that of all human beings ("Man is horrible"). He did acknowledge that psychiatrists underwent "mind anesthesia," and recognized that helping a few of the killer troops to be transferred was a form of "expiation" or "penitence"—a feeling of "Let's at least send this poor devil back home so he doesn't have to do that anymore." And K. kept repeating, almost rotely, "I'm so sorry."

When exploring with him soldiers' dreams and nightmares, I asked whether he himself had any dreams related to those experiences. He first answered in the negative, that he did not have the kind of dreams the soldiers had because "I never killed anybody." But he admitted that he did have what he called "Russian dreams . . . dreams that we couldn't help somebody or other." And he associated those dreams with the "passivity" he had previously mentioned. I thought of Alexander Mitscherlich's point about former Nazis being unable to cope psychologically with the evil they had been part of, and instead seeing themselves as victims. K. did that to an extent, feeling himself to be caught in his assignment. But Mitscherlich's observation needed modification as well: K.'s sense of being victimized did not completely replace his feelings of self-condemnation. Like Lorenz (and like Albert Speer, as we shall see), K. maintained a delicate balance between touching and avoiding the genuine guilt of his behavior.

But these interviews raised a larger question about Nazi mass killing. There is a real sense in which doctors—in this case psychiatrists—shared an atrocity-producing situation with those who performed the actual killing. The latter, like soldiers in Vietnam, were thrust into Camus's two undesirable roles, but with staggeringly greater consequences. They were clearly executioners. But they were also pressed by the environment to which they were assigned toward psychiatric collusion in atrocity, and in that sense were victims. Himmler was probably right in his belief that face-to-face murder was too much of an ordeal for German soldiers (although he praised the nobility of those who managed the ordeal). Reports he and other Nazi leaders received from psychiatrists like K., even if often falsified for self-protective reasons, undoubtedly contributed to the momentous Nazi decision to find a method of mass murder that was easier on the murderers.

In that way psychiatrists not only facilitated genocide (as they also did in connection with the "euthanasia" project and its extension to the death camps), but also became historical actors in the bureaucratic policy decision in favor of gas chambers. No wonder that these two interviews with K. aroused in me a particularly intense combination of fascination and revulsion. I had read about Jews of all ages being murdered next to ditches by Einsatzgruppen killer troops, but now I was hearing such scenes described by a member of my own profession who had served the project. K. was, moreover, a "nice man" who fell into the category of the "decent Nazi"—surely a warning of what psychiatrists and other professionals are capable of doing when serving evil projects. In writing about this decades later, I have the added feeling: what a monstrous research project I had taken on!

The Quiet Life at the Chancellery

The most intriguing response I received from a Nazi doctor to our first letter (sent by Paul Matussek on my behalf) was that of an elderly surgeon, Dr. Warner L., who wrote that he was quite willing to meet me but would probably have little to tell me because during most of the war he worked in Hitler's chancellery, where there was "very little stress." (He was responding literally to our euphemism of physicians' "stress under National Socialism.") He was taciturn during our interview, as he had predicted, but managed to convey to me what it was like for a doctor to be in close contact with the Führer on a day-to-day basis as well as in a moment of crisis. In both situations I could be there in the chancellery together with the two men.

L. looked like the prototype of the wizened retiree, appearing to be much older than his seventy-five years and working on his stamp collection when I arrived. He responded to me with a mixture of naïveté and slyness. He told me of having been chosen for his position at the chancellery "probably because I was a good surgeon and of course you had to be a National Socialist." He was in fact a dedicated Nazi and had also spent several years in the military close to combat in Eastern Europe and France. Life was indeed quiet at the chancellery so he busied himself reading up on professional issues and writing articles for surgical journals, while finding himself very taken with his Führer:

> Hitler made a profound impression on me. He had the demeanor of a great personality. He was very intelligent, had a great deal of information, a very good memory, and was also interested in medical questions.

Those medical questions of course had to do with race: "He preferred the Nordic race, felt that it was especially industrious compared to the southern Europeans, to say nothing of blacks and Chinese. And doctors were to do everything possible to help the propagation of the Nordic race." L. claimed that doctors did so in humane ways, not forcing anything but simply encouraging couples "who had the proper racial characteristics" to marry and have children.

He went on to reminisce about Hitler's idiosyncratic eating and drinking habits, his refusal of alcohol "except for a nip now and then," and especially about his vegetarianism and conviction that "meat was not good for the human body, that it made him sluggish." L. chuckled affectionately as he recalled how "he always called us flesh eaters," but added that the Führer would "once in a while eat a liver dumpling." L. was briefly including me in Hitler's everyday domestic life, details of which he sympathetically attributed to the quirks of a great man.

But L. mostly continued to speak in phlegmatic tones, offering almost nothing spontaneously. He generally seemed a bit fatigued—at one point he actually dozed off for a few seconds—until he suddenly declared: "I had a true stress situation on the 20th of July, 1944." That was the date of the attempted assassination of Hitler, and L. did not need much encouragement from me to plunge into his story. Indeed, he had come to his great moment, both in the interview and in his life. Now he became suddenly animated and launched into a spirited soliloquy in which he could hardly get the words out fast enough. He said that it was fortunate that he had not gone swimming that day, as he frequently did, and that he heard the detonation of the device placed in a briefcase but didn't think anything of it because wild animals often stepped on mines implanted in the area. But then:

> I received a telephone call telling me I should come immediately to the *Führerbunker* (in Hitler's Eastern Front headquarters) and treat the wounded Hitler. He had a contusion on his right elbow . . . a light wound on the left arm . . . and superficial burns on both legs and the back of his head. He had two ruptured ear drums—everyone in the room had ruptured ear drums. . . . Hitler certainly would have been killed if [Colonel Heinz] Brandt (a prominent figure in Hitler's military entourage), had not moved the briefcase [which held the bomb] from one side of the table to the other. . . . Hitler was thrown to the ground but was not unconscious.

Hitler's immediate behavior, before even being attended to medically, was L.'s most interesting observation: "He was very excited, hitting himself repeatedly on the thighs and laughing. He said, 'Now I have this clique and we can exterminate them. It will be a severe judgment, no exceptions.'" L. thought Hitler to be "psychologically deranged," which he considered "natural" under the circumstances, but not seriously injured, which he thought "very fortunate." L. suggested something close to supernatural intervention in Hitler's survival, claiming that one of the conspirators later said he could have shot Hitler at point-blank range but felt himself unable to do so and instead congratulated the Führer for his amazing deliverance, a sequence L. considered "awe-inspiring."

In the aftermath of the assassination attempt, the Führer would accompany L. when he went to examine some of the injured, and would take an active interest in their condition: "Hitler and I talked about the wounds, how we could treat them, and whether we could get the splinters out." I imagined myself accompanying the two men on these "rounds," L. both the "attending physician" explaining everything to his less knowledgeable "colleague," while also the worshipful acolyte of that colleague. However bizarre the scene, it had enormous seriousness for each of the two men.

When I asked L. whether Hitler ever said anything about the Jews, he said that he did at times "in the evening by the fireplace," bringing me into a tableau in a cozy setting in which the Führer would reflect to his followers on how the Jews "were the scourge of mankind" and how he was making plans "to do away with them." L. was characteristically disingenuous when asked about his own feelings concerning these sentiments. First he responded in exclusively technical terms: "I thought only that it would be impossible to carry out a program like that." And then he added that Hitler's words were not too significant anyway because they were "exactly the same thing he wrote in *Mein Kampf*." As if to defend his own innocence, he emphasized that Hitler "never talked about Auschwitz or anything like that." His account suggested that the idea of large-scale killing of Jews was openly expressed within the Hitler circle but without concrete details about the place or process of mass murder.

L. did observe increasingly unbalanced behavior in Hitler, "breaking down both physically and mentally" and "doing a lot of crazy things." But he tried to explain this behavior away by attributing it to medical mistreatment. He described how Theodor Morell, Hitler's personal doctor, used a variety of dubious medications, including not only injections of glucose but prescriptions of pills that contained strychnine. By all accounts Morell was a charlatan who did use treatments that could have been harmful, but here L. was colluding in a medical exculpation of his beloved Führer: the argument made by some Nazis that the Führer was a beneficent and heroic leader until his health was undermined by a quack doctor, and that any excessive behavior on his part resulted only from that medical mistreatment. L. attempted to combat Morell's influence with Hitler, together with Karl Brandt, the extremely high-ranking Nazi doctor (sentenced to death at the Nuremberg medical trial for having headed the "euthanasia" project) who had brought L. to the chancellery as his assistant. But they could not succeed in breaking Morell's hold on Hitler. L. himself was eventually forced out ("One man poisons the head of state, another man discovers the poisoning, and the one who poisons stays and the one who discovers it is sent away"). But even here he could not be critical of Hitler for making this decision, explaining that "he did not want doctors countervailing each other's orders."

L. presented himself as a man of the highest medical integrity, and was irate when after the surrender he was put in the category of "war criminal," insisting (like Dr. K. and a number of others) that "I never killed anyone." He managed to be removed from that category by resorting to his usual pattern of "having nothing to say."

When I look back on the interview I am struck by L.'s version of Hitler as a combination of the benign "Uncle Adolf" and a godlike savior. In that high moment of responding to the assassination attempt, L. could tend to the kindly uncle and contribute to "saving the savior" and then collaborate with him in the medical healing of others. Listening to his description of the explosion and its effects provided an interesting moment for me as well, though in a very different way. In previous experiences over the years of hearing accounts of violence and suffering, I would often find myself attempting in my mind to interrupt that course of painful events and imagine history reversed to permit less violence and less suffering. But in this case I found myself wishing for the opposite kind of historical reversal: I wanted Hitler to be killed, his headquarters pulverized, and the Nazi movement destroyed. Though I knew that the actual historical outcome was otherwise, I still experienced a letdown upon hearing that the damage had been so limited and that Hitler had sustained only minor injuries—and that I had to return to the monosyllabic evasions of the old man before me. I knew that when I left he would happily return to his stamp collection and his gardening and continue to have "nothing to say" (meaning "nothing to feel") about Nazi truths.

But it turned out that he had something additional to say after all. As my assistant and I were leaving and L. was remarking on his good fortune about having survived the war, he added what was probably a half-consciously meant parting shot: "I'm lucky I was not in Hiroshima." He was retaliating to my probing of his ethical behavior by invoking what many (including myself) have considered an American war crime, and which was mentioned as such by a German defense counsel at Nuremberg. As he said that, I imagined him in Hiroshima when the bomb was dropped, and then I imagined a still more vast and terrible scene of destruction that I knew to be a combination of Hiroshima, Auschwitz, and bombed-out

Germany. There seemed to be no end of horror that could be associated in my mind with this seemingly innocuous, permanently numbed Nazi doctor.

Speer and Hitler—Architectural Folie à Deux

I interviewed another man who was much closer to Hitler, for a period of time in fact his most intimate associate and even his possible successor. Albert Speer was an architect and not a physician. But I sought him out as one of a group of prominent nonmedical professionals, with whom I probed the experience of professionals in general under the Nazis while also seeking their observations on physicians. Few were better positioned in the regime to make such observations. Speer had been convicted at Nuremberg of "war crimes" and "crimes against humanity," mostly on the basis of his participation in the forced labor program, and had served twenty years in Spandau prison in West Berlin. This relatively light sentence (all other leaders of his high standing were sentenced to death) had to do with his cooperation with Allied authorities in turning against the Nazi regime. He was later to reveal much about the regime's function in two highly influential books, many articles and public statements, and frequent meetings with researchers like me. While many applauded his behavior, others saw him as a clever, self-serving manipulator.

Speer was introduced to me by the Mitscherlichs, who spoke of him with considerable sympathy—Alexander said that twenty years in jail "was enough" and that "we should not isolate people like him"—and asked me to convey their personal greetings to him. But I had also read a couple of more skeptical pieces on Speer by Kenneth Galbraith (who had considerable contact with him at the end of World War II), in which he spoke of the architect's self-serving "survival strategy" and deemed him "a very intelligent escapist from the truth." Despite my friendship with the Mitscherlichs, I felt myself more inclined to the Galbraith view. I would waver considerably over the course of my four memorable interviews with Speer, after which I achieved greater clarity in my mind about him—but to what degree, I'm still not sure. What I am sure of is that in the process I learned much about the "friendship" between Speer and

Hitler and about the psychological atmosphere of the Nazi regime as it affected everyone, medical or otherwise, working within it.

Three of our four meetings took place at his home on the outskirts of Heidelberg, and the fourth at his isolated retreat in southern Bavaria. His Heidelberg home seemed isolated enough, high in the hills behind the city's famous castle. I remember the house seeming cavernous, its furnishings neither attractive nor cozy. Speer himself was welcoming but I was struck by how old he looked (he was then seventy-three), by the awkwardness of his movements (he had considerable difficulty getting up and sitting down, leading me to wonder whether he had Parkinson's disease), and by his "thousand-mile stare" (the term we used to describe the psychological remoteness in repatriated American prisoners of war in Korea in 1953). The word I used to characterize his general demeanor was *weary* (though I should add that a little more than a year later he was to be enlivened by a passionate love affair with a younger woman).

Speer was interested in talking to me, and made clear that nothing he said was confidential. But he quickly suggested an agenda of his own centered on his bond with Hitler. He told me how he had heard the Nazi leader speak at his university in Berlin in 1930, was "really spellbound" at the time and remained so for the next fifteen years covering the entire Nazi era. His question for me was how, in retrospect, he could have been so enthralled by such a man. He then made a startling proposal: that he undergo psychotherapy with me in order to better understand how that had happened. The strong implication was that the relationship still had a hold on him, from which he wanted to extricate himself. I was much interested in hearing more about his conflict but had no wish to take on responsibility for his psyche. I needed my freedom as a researcher and did not see my task as one of easing the pain of a prominent former Nazi. Nor did I wish to have our meetings structured around his way of framing his problem. So I suggested instead that we explore in some detail his relationship with Hitler without my becoming his therapist. Speer agreed and we did so, but we were able to explore much else that enabled me to relate this strange bond to larger questions of evil and knowledge of evil, and of death and immortality.

Speer explained that the speech that had so moved him was Hitler's relatively intellectual and historical treatment of German history, as opposed to his more demagogic, rabble-rousing street version. The narrative was one of revitalization: now Germany is weak and everything seems hopeless but by uniting behind Hitler and the National Socialist movement—and above all renouncing the guilt for World War I assigned by the Versailles Treaty—Germany and its people can once again be strong. Speer was then a twenty-five-year-old instructor in architecture in a collapsed economy and he and others around him were experiencing only despair about their future. Images of wounded and humiliated German troops returning from World War I twelve years earlier were still fresh in his mind, as were postwar scenes of every kind of social chaos. Hitler's words were for him transformative, a message of new hope and a promise, as he put it, that "all can be changed" and "everything is possible." Feeling "drunk from the talk," Speer walked for hours through the woods outside Berlin, seeking to absorb what he had heard. He was in the process of experiencing a secular form of a classical religious conversion, described by William James as "perceiving truths not known before" that enable a "sick soul" to "give itself over to a new life." Intense "self-surrender" is accompanied by new spiritual strength. Speer demonstrated the energizing power of the combination of *national and personal revitalization*, which I came to see as the psychological core of Nazi appeal throughout the German population.

Speer joined the Nazi Party soon after that speech and told me of his rapid rise within its circles, first as an enthusiastic party worker and then as an architect. From his sensational early success in designing the light and space for the large Nuremberg rallies, beginning in 1933 (as depicted by Leni Riefenstahl in her film of the 1934 rally, *Triumph of the Will*), he progressed to the planning of vast buildings, even cities, to extol the omnipotent Nazi regime and, above all, its Führer. He emphasized how, in becoming "Hitler's architect," he was drawn toward a vision of personal immortalization, of "having a place in future history books," "building for eternity," and becoming in that way "someone who is surviving his own life." The sense of immortality, which I emphasize in my work, intoxicated Speer to the point of becoming something close to a promise of literally living forever. So grandiose were the projections he and Hitler made together that some of the buildings were to hold as many as 150,000 people on vast balconies in a new Berlin that would become the center of the world, dwarfing the grandeur of Paris and the Champs-Élysées. Few of the structures were actually built but many were imagined, as part of what Speer called "a daydream that was a very serious daydream."

On one of my visits to his Heidelberg home, he showed me a large glossy book that had just been published, titled *Architecture of the Third Reich*. It contained gaudy photographs of buildings I noted to be "profoundly vulgar" and "totalitarian," and Speer seemed initially to share that judgment: "I admit that the proportions are all wrong," he said, and "I criticize the grandiose side." Then, without the slightest trace of irony, he added, "But of course it was what the client wanted." He attributed all excess to that "client," but he could hardly dissociate himself from the grandiosity involved. Indeed, his pride in the volume was clear enough as he clutched it affectionately and pointed also to pictures of rally sites he had designed: "I was one of the first to use light in nighttime as a device for creating space. The searchlights came so high that when you were standing inside you saw it as being in the stratosphere." He did not say that his innovative lighting enabled the Führer to be seen as descending from the heavens. I thought of Speer's overall contribution to the mystical appeal of the Nazi movement, converting Nazi darkness into a manipulated sense of illumination. Witnessing his enthusiasm for that early work and his nostalgic pride in projections of architectural world domination, I felt that whatever sympathy I had for Speer was dissolving. It occurred to me that Nazi architectural hubris had a certain parallel to its biological hubris: apocalyptic architecture followed upon apocalyptic biology.

Speer made it clear that Hitler was more than a mere client: he was the closest of collaborators. Hitler was not only a constant critic and appreciator of Speer's architectural suggestions; the Führer became himself an architect and even provided sketches of his own. As they imagined the unprecedented grandeur of buildings, highways, archways, and cities, their thoughts blended to the degree that it became unclear who had provided the original idea. The two men shared this descent into a version of apocalyptic fantasy: they were re-creating a perfect Nazi world from the ruins of what they were destroying. It is this merger in fantasy that constituted their architectural folie à deux.

Yet however superior Speer's knowledge of architecture, Hitler remained the guru. As Speer put it, "I was so much in that ambience that I was infiltrated with [Hitler's] ideas without realizing how much I was infiltrated." He said that even now, when working on his writing, he frequently has the experience in which "I see that it's an idea Hitler had in some way" and "I'm quite astonished." In their particular fashion, the two men formed a close personal relationship. Speer would later write that if Hitler were capable of having a friend, he, Speer, would have been that friend. But gurus, especially the most paranoid and destructive among them, do not have friends; they have only disciples. Speer believed that Hitler was drawn to him as a fellow artist, and that appreciation worked both ways: "For an artist to see somebody at the head of the state who is something of an artist too . . . has a gift of excitement. Being overwhelmed by . . . a Wagner performance or a ballet in Nuremberg, this for me was a strong, positive influence." They also shared an intense theatricality—Speer with his dazzling night-lighting of rallies, and Hitler, whose "whole life," Speer told me, "was acting, performance, theatre."

Speer's merging with Hitler resembled the kind of fusion of guru and disciple that I encountered in studying fanatical religious cults, notably Aum Shinrikyo in Japan in the nineties. But with Speer and Hitler the fusion involved the shared hubris of a perceived artistic and structural project to transform the world. In that way Speer was probably, at least for a period of time, the disciple most important to Hitler in affirming his omnipotent guruism. But Speer also provides for us a kind of window to more ordinary German people who also experienced fusion with a guru/leader rendered godlike. As Speer poured out details of his interaction with the Führer, I could be there with the two men at various levels: observing them pore over their architectural plans as "friends" and "colleagues"; and imagining their fusion in a version of architectural madness perceived as an all-consuming gift to the world. And here was this man sitting opposite me describing quite rationally and methodically this most bizarre expression of evil from his past—wishing to separate himself from it and renounce it, but not entirely. No wonder that Speer was so difficult for me to grasp.

An important clue to his psychology was the anxiety he began to develop in connection with his projections of grandiose building. As he explained to me, he found himself as a young architect with little experience thrust into a situation without rules or boundaries, one in which "nothing is fixed." He had no clear tradition or architectural group that could guide and constrain him, so that professionally "I could do what I wanted," and despite Hitler's support, "I was alone." The Führer's involvement, far from a steadying influence, obliterated limits and took the fused duo more deeply into unmanageable architectural fantasy. At some level of his mind, Speer perceived this gap between the grandiosity of the shared vision and what could be called architectural reality. He also had inner doubts about the quality of the architecture, "fear as to whether it would stand [the judgment] of the times, of how it would be acknowledged in future times." Related to that fear was his discomfort, as a highly educated upper-middle-class intellectual, among the mostly crude members of the Nazi inner circle.

He told me about experiencing two kinds of symptoms. The first took the form of claustrophobia: in certain enclosed spaces, particularly when on trains, he would feel anxious and would nearly pass out. On one occasion the symptoms were sufficiently severe that there was talk of stopping the train in order to get him to a hospital. The second set of symptoms required no particular locale, and were those of acute anxiety (or panic attack): he would experience a feeling of great pressure in his chest and a terrified sense that he was dying. These two sets of symptoms occurred only during his time of intense, unlimited architectural dialogue with Hitler and what he called his accompanying "burden." In my work I have related such symptoms both to feeling too much (the overwhelming anxiety) and too little (the numbing toward what one could not allow oneself to be consciously aware of). Speer was fending off his conflicts not only about his illegitimate architectural freedom, but about his overall role in the Nazi regime. Something in him began to doubt the Hitlerian vision of brutally remaking the world.

In our discussions he tried to explain—or explain away—his problem mainly in terms of his susceptibility to Hitler's charisma. That charisma was real enough but Speer would seem at times to hide behind it in order to avoid the probing of still more difficult questions of his own ethical responsibility. What I believe was involved in these symptoms was his struggle against the realization of the fraudulence of the Führer's larger vision, and of his own corruption personally and professionally. His architectural folie à deux with the Führer epitomized the problem. As in the case of doctors at Auschwitz, Speer could adapt sufficiently to diminish his anxiety and serve the regime, in his case with high energy and intelligence. His symptoms contributed to that adaptation by covering over existential truths, and then disappeared when he ceased to be "Hitler's architect" and became instead minister for armaments. Nor did they reappear during his imprisonment or the years following his release.

I knew that Speer had been friendly with Karl Brandt, the high-ranking Nazi physician who was also close to Hitler, a friendship that took us back to my medical theme. Brandt had certain parallels to Speer as a well-educated younger professional who had undergone a powerful conversion to Nazism and possessed skills Hitler could utilize. The two men were characterized by one Nazi doctor I interviewed as "son figures," referring to their discipleship and their respectable position in society (which Hitler himself lacked) no less than their age. Speer told me with some feeling how the Führer eventually turned on both men, and each was able to save the other's life. Speer's ordeal occurred when he found himself being medically mistreated by Karl Gebhardt, a notorious SS physician, for what was apparently a life-threatening pulmonary embolism. Speer told me that Gebhardt was in daily contact with Heimrich Himmler, who viewed the architect as a dangerous rival for being chosen by Hitler as his successor, and therefore "wanted to kill me." He survived only by getting in touch with his friend Brandt, who was able to arrange for genuine medical care that brought about his recovery. Speer was intent on gaining historical recognition for this incident and attempted to involve me in that effort. He had assembled an array of documents to support his version of what had happened and asked me, as a physician, to review the evidence and certify in writing to the gross violation of medical ethics. While I had no reason to doubt his case, it was another request that I politely refused.

Speer was able to return the favor to his friend when, toward the end of the war, Hitler accused Brandt of "defeatism" and "betrayal," which could have resulted in his execution, for arranging to send his wife and child to the American zone rather than have them participate in the mass suicide of loyal Nazis and their families. Speer was able to find safe hiding places for Brandt during his successful flight. Speer himself had turned against the Führer by this time, reversing orders for a "scorched earth" throughout Germany that would have resulted in mass starvation. Yet he did feel the need to make a final dangerous trip to Hitler's Berlin bunker just before the Führer's suicide for a final good-bye. Though according to his account he told Hitler of having failed to comply with his orders, the Führer, still possessing the last vestiges of power, refrained from taking any action against him.

In rendering these accounts involving Brandt and himself, Speer was attempting to salvage something ethically from the Nazi experience, to demonstrate that "good men" ("decent Nazis") could function with integrity within the regime, at least until finally being turned upon by it. But Speer also knew that what happened to Brandt and him was inevitable, "the risk you take if you are living in such a system." That risk, as I learned from later studies of extreme guruism, is that of the rage and revenge of the half-mad guru when rejected by his most valued disciples, those who had been crucial to his own affirmation of the validity of his guruism.

In keeping with my concerns about different forms of participation in evil, I focused much of our discussion on Speer's relationship to the "Final Solution," the Nazi program of systematic mass murder of the Jews. Over the years he had claimed ignorance and uninvolvement, a claim that seemed increasingly untenable, and toward the latter part of his life he backtracked and admitted having sensed that "something was happening to the Jews," without having wished to learn any more about what that was. As evidence mounted against his earlier claims, many who had been sympathetic to him became critical, including one of his biographers Gitta Sereny, who concluded that he was "living a lie." In order to explore the matter with him I pressed him on the sequence of his attitude toward Jews and encounters with their suffering.

He made clear to me that he was by no means immune to the anti-Semitism of the time, resonated to it in Hitler's early speech, resented "rich Jews in furs" during times of economic deprivation, was critical of the Jewish domination of the medical profession, and, more to the point, of what he took to be the inordinate Jewish influence on German architecture in determining who received commissions for buildings. As he rose in the regime, Speer did not emphasize anti-Jewish ideas in speeches or writings but blended with the existing ambiance, with an anti-Semitism that was, as he put it, "standard" and "legalized" so that "one felt at home in it." He was aware of Hitler's rage toward the Jews, but the two men did not talk about the subject during their architectural meditations, or later when they were preoccupied with armaments. But he recalled (in an account similar to that of the chancellery doctor, L.) how the Führer would, in small groups of his inner circle, "speak in that cold, slow voice in which he revealed terrible decisions" and declare that he would "destroy the Jews." Speer even came to realize that doing so was a central motivation, Hitler's "engine." The murderous "engine," that is, did not interfere with Speer's fusion with his guru; indeed one could say that the fusion required that he himself connect in some way with the engine.

Speer admitted to me that he encountered considerable evidence of Nazi brutality and Jewish pain: the suicide of a distinguished scientist his family knew at the University of Heidelberg, a scene at a railroad station in which a few hundred "miserable looking people" he knew to be Jews were "loaded on trains to be taken from Germany," and selective tours of Nazi concentration camps in which he claimed to be convinced by his manipulative hosts that the inmates were in reasonably good shape. More damning, he told me of providing certain materials for the work camp at Auschwitz in 1943 and having at the time "some insight into the bad conditions of such camps." But he insisted that the construction materials were only for improving the facilities, and when I asked about his knowledge of the rest of Auschwitz and its role in extermination, he insisted sharply that "I knew nothing of the other." I had never before heard anyone claim in this way close knowledge of the slave labor function of Auschwitz and ignorance of its function as a death camp. (Nor did we discuss Speer's early participation in removing Jews from their Berlin homes and later suppression of that episode, or his providing, as minister of armaments, slave labor to German industry.)

Speer told me how he "pushed aside very quickly" all such matters, sensing that dreadful things were happening to Jews but stopping short of fully realizing what they were because "I didn't want to know. I didn't want to see it." Very much at issue was his sense that confronting the truth would have undermined his entire Nazi worldview and deepest life commitments and required him "to admit that all this was for nothing, that it wasn't right." At the end of our third interview I noted that one had two choices with Speer: either one could believe that he was consciously lying all along, or one could see him as involved in a sustained inner struggle around the psychology of knowing and not knowing. I favored the latter view. I thought he was "living a lie" but that he had not experienced it as a lie. Because of his extreme psychic numbing, he had ceased to *feel* almost anything of the abuse and suffering of Jews. And because of his "derealization" (emphasized by Mitscherlich in connection with Nazi behavior), he could avoid experiencing his participation in the Holocaust as actual or real. Speer could explore his participation in a regime he now condemned but could never allow himself to experience the dimension of guilt associated with its mass killing. Therefore, he could never allow himself fully "to know." His wish to focus exclusively on his emotional bondage to Hitler—and with my help find a "cure" for it—was an effort to psychologize his Nazi behavior in a way that avoided ethical truths. None of this makes him any less culpable for what he did and did not do, but it does help explain his contradictory statements about what he knew.

Throughout, I had been more critical of Speer and more reserved about his "repentance" than had such people as Alexander Mitscherlich, George Mosse (a scholar whom I knew and greatly respected), and Erich Fromm (the well-known psychoanalyst who befriended Speer and expressed great enthusiasm for his change). Still, I had conversed with him in a civil, even friendly fashion, finding him at least at moments likable, and had been impressed by the fact that someone so high in the regime was making this kind of articulate turnabout—even if Hitler was always there with us. I concluded that our interviews had revealed extraordinary dimensions of enthusiasm and corruption, of complex immersion in evil—and that to learn about all this I had no choice but to sit in that room with him and his Führer.

I have one more memory of Speer in connection with our third interview, which took place at his very isolated Bavarian retreat. He met me at the train and drove me in his small car up into the mountain. It was about a thirty-minute trip but there was a heavy fog, not much visibility, and the drive seemed endless. He made it clear to me that this was his sanctuary, that he was making an exception in inviting me to it (though when he mentioned that Japanese TV had been there the previous day, I wondered how many other exceptions he made). After we settled into his modest cottage, he told me that he was working less—only an hour or two a day—and spent the rest of the time taking short walks or "just staring into space." We talked of many things, including that early Hitler speech, and then he looked distantly at me and said that his entire fifteen-year Nazi experience now seemed "like a dream." Here was a man, worldly as he had become, expressing, in the most isolated of settings, the unreality of his vast service to an evil regime, and, by implication, of his life in general. As I sat there I could share his sense of unreality, but only for a moment, because however remote the setting—and for that matter, the man himself—the consequences of his behavior were all too real.

17

Annihilated by Europe

A FTER SEVERAL MONTHS of the research, while BJ and Karen were still with me in Munich, we decided to make a trip to Paris. Paris was an important city for my work, as I could arrange to meet there with a number of Jewish physicians who were Auschwitz survivors as well as several notable Holocaust writers and archivists. But the trip was also an opportunity to enjoy a city that BJ and I had not returned to in a while and Karen had never seen, and for the three of us to spend a little time together outside Germany. We also looked forward to seeing a good friend of ours, whom I'll call Jackie (I'm using pseudonyms for the three participants in this incident), a writer then living in Paris. But that city has always had surprises for us, which have not necessarily been pleasant.

The story went like this. Jackie had become involved with a member of a prominent Parisian family, named David, and on the night of our arrival we were invited to a large dinner he hosted in an elegant restaurant, at which their relationship was on display. We were just finishing the pâté of our first course when the dinner was interrupted by the sudden appearance of an uninvited guest. She was an attractive young woman named Suzanne, the daughter of an ambassador, and apparently another girlfriend of David's. She was clearly upset about the whole event, and David looked less than delighted to see her, but took her coat in a courtly manner and invited her to join his table. At the end of the dinner David retrieved Suzanne's coat and in the process of helping her on with it gave her a warm hug, as if to say that things were still okay between them. Suzanne's mood was immediately transformed—her smile was not less than euphoric—and at that point David introduced us to her as someone who could drive us back to our hotel on the Left Bank since it was not far from where she lived. Though that left David and Jackie free to go off together, Suzanne retained her euphoric expression as we walked out of the restaurant with her.

As I sat down in the front seat of her dilapidated Volkswagen Beetle (Karen and BJ sat in the back) I reached for the seat belt and discovered that it no longer existed. I was not too troubled—in those days we looked upon seat belts as a good idea but not absolutely necessary—and made small talk with Suzanne as we drove along. But I soon began to notice that she was going a bit fast and was thinking of saying something to her about it when she ran a red light; we were then blindsided by a car that apparently did the same from a perpendicular street and slammed into my door, throwing me out of our car. I seemed to lose consciousness, but very briefly, and remember my mind going into a not unpleasant slow motion in which everything was deliberate—traffic passing by, voices of anonymous people, everything taking its course. Then I tried to grasp what had happened, and expressed semicoherent concern about Karen and BJ and then Suzanne. Next there was a jumble of ambulances, police cars, and, amazingly, the appearance of David and Jackie, who had been driving not far behind us and came upon the accident. When things were sorted out, it became clear that I had fractures of my right arm and left leg, BJ had fractures of her clavicle and of several ribs, while both Karen and Suzanne were physically untouched. BJ and I needed hospitalization, so Jackie immediately took over responsibility for Karen, who was trying to be brave but was a very frightened thirteen-year-old.

The hospital where BJ and I would spend two nights was the Hôtel-Dieu, said to be one of the oldest hospitals in Europe, and it looked it. It had that aura of Old World deterioration that can be appealing in a cathedral or a castle but much less so in a hospital. Actually we were reasonably cared for but separated from each other and anxious about the alien setting and our difficulty communicating with the people trying to help us. I underwent X-rays, and casts were appropriately applied to my arm and leg, but I was unsuccessful in my pleas to the doctors to provide relief from the severe pain I was experiencing, because they seemed to feel that a painkiller would interfere with the accurate information they needed for treating me. BJ's injuries required no casts but she experienced similar difficulties.

Happily, Jackie prevailed upon David to use his influence to arrange for us to be transferred to the American Hospital in Paris, where everyone was bilingual and the style of medicine was closer to what BJ and I were used to. The hospital bent its rules to allow us to stay in the same room, and Karen and Jackie could have long visits with us. We became comfortable and relaxed, at times even giddy, which led to a new problem: BJ's rib and clavicle fractures caused her pain when she laughed, and there was no restraining my humorous asides and bad jokes. BJ's injuries, in fact, caused more sustained pain than mine but were invisible as opposed to the outsized arm and leg casts that made me look like a wounded war hero. Add to that a bit of male chauvinism on the part of French doctors and I seemed to get most of the medical attention. The two of us became a kind of spectacle in the hospital, and I remember a large nurse who got into the spirit of things by declaring to me in her French English: "You come to Paris to see the sights and all that is seen is your rear end!" (The comment seemed hilarious at the time.)

But in recovering we were faced with another problem. After about ten days the doctors told us that they had completed the treatment of our fractures and that it was now time for us to leave the hospital. Yet it was clear to everyone that we could not yet manage by ourselves, and I was horrified to hear muttering about our entering a "rest home." Desperate for a solution, I had the idea of seeking advice from Donna Hartman, whom we had met years before and who was now the wife of the American ambassador Arthur Hartman. Donna staggered me by suggesting that BJ and I immediately move to the embassy living quarters, and she and Arthur did not wince when that included hoisting the large hospital bed I required for my fractures through a second-story window. Donna and Arthur were the most generous of hosts and included us in a dinner they gave the next night for American ambassadors to countries in Western Europe (at which BJ and I would have our reunion with Kingman and Mary Brewster). I confess that I enjoyed the sympathetic attention resulting from my wheelchair and casts (I did have very slight feelings of guilt but not enough to be troubling), and BJ and I agreed that we had come a long way since those first nights at the Hôtel-Dieu.

During a three-week stay at the embassy, I was even able to resume my research interviews. I was provided with a quiet, comfortable room, in which I could meet with a series of Jewish physician-survivors who had much to say about Auschwitz. As my wheelchair and casts could not be ignored, I told them about my accident. Some of them, as doctors, requested more information about my physical condition, and all of them expressed concern about me. I felt strange, even fraudulent, that *they*, Auschwitz survivors, were feeling sorry for *me*.

By the time we left our restorative stay at the embassy, my leg cast was off and I was able to walk reasonably well, and BJ too had mostly recovered. We could rejoin Karen in Munich (she had returned a bit earlier to meet her school schedule, cared for by another friend). I could resume my research trips to German and Austrian cities, still with the cast on my arm, for a while making use of wheelchairs at airports. In general BJ and I were pleased at how well we had come through the whole thing. I even found a whimsical (but pertinent) moral to the story: "Don't get into a car whose driver is euphoric."

But I had two dreams that suggested more psychological trauma than I had suspected. The first dream occurred just after the accident, during one of my nights at the Hôtel-Dieu. In the dream I am playing tennis in a "European stadium." My opponent "is pulverizing me, leading four games to love. It is clear that he will win that set. I am eager to start the second set with a clean slate. But I wonder whether I can win it." In my notes I associate being pulverized in a European stadium with being "annihilated by Europe." The tennis metaphor was natural for me, given my intense involvement in the game and fierce competitiveness on the court. But I also observed that the tennis imagery enabled me to depict defeat while "slightly softening the whole experience." In fact tennis had long been a barometer of my physical and spiritual health, so that over the years when I would have back symptoms from chronic disc problems, my treatment goal would be getting back on the court. And in the ambulance carrying BJ and me to the Hôtel-Dieu, I told the paramedic, in a feeble effort at both humor and French conversation, "Je veux jouer á tennis." While in the dream I could not be certain of prevailing in that "second set," it suggested an effort at resurgent energy, a second wind in my research. It was a death-and-rebirth dream in a tennis idiom, with uncertainty about the rebirth.

In another dream about three months later I still have my broken bones—casts on my right arm and left leg—but at the same time "I seem over that situation." I am in fact instructing another person with similar fractures but one who "did not know how to use his strength," in the process demonstrating how to use one's good left arm and right leg "as I did . . . [and] going through the motions of showing how I use them." I noted that in the dream "there was a certain amount of anxiety . . . but also a sense of pushing forward." Recognizing that all characters represent aspects of the dreamer, I was struggling with calling forth strength to overcome incapacity and weakness. But whatever the dream's bravado, it also suggested psychic wounds. It occurred less than a month after BJ's decision to stay in Israel with Karen, a decision we later recognized to have been considerably affected by the accident. I also concluded that the accident had tested each of the four people who had been in that car. BJ, Karen, and I, while vulnerable to its trauma, managed to find ways to keep going. (Suzanne met the test by disappearing altogether, as she and her family decided that she should have nothing more to do with us because there might be some kind of future litigation.)

In a broader sense, the dreams portrayed the accident as symbolizing the ordeal of the entire study. They revealed my anxiety over conducting it in an area devoid of American moorings. As in those two days and nights in the Hôtel-Dieu, I was being exposed to ancient forces on profoundly unfamiliar terrain. Being "annihilated by Europe" was part of the scheme of things. As a friend put it with a Jewish question-comment (along with a Celtic component), "Did you expect to get out of that study scot-free?"

Inmate Doctors—Remaining Healers

Among the eighty Auschwitz survivors I interviewed, more than half were doctors, most of them Jewish. Painful as their stories were, the gemütlich atmosphere in the interviews could serve as an antidote to my strained interactions with Nazi doctors. As I sat with those Jewish doctors, I was always aware that only accidents of history (my grandparents' decisions to make their way from their Russian shtetls to the United States in the late nineteenth century, and the interviewees' or their families' having instead remained in Europe) prevented our positions from being reversed: I could well have been telling him or her about my experience in Auschwitz. Still, I remained the researcher and tried to go about the interviews as systematically as possible.

There were two inmate-doctors with whom I became particularly close, both of them, as it happened, originally from Czechoslovakia. Each was remarkable in coping with his own suffering and in helping fellow prisoners medically and otherwise, making good use in the camp of the knowledge of German language and culture possessed by many Czech Jews.

Karol V.'s story was that of a man who, after remaining a healer in the camp, had to face formidable post-Auschwitz struggles, psychological and political. I had heard that he had been a prominent physician and teacher in Czechoslovakia, and was surprised to locate him in a small German spa town attending to people who went there to bathe in the mineral waters. A friendly, responsive man who told me that he was about to turn sixty-three, he seemed both younger (in his high energy and quick movements) and older (in the heavy lines in his face and his completely white hair) than that age. When we exchanged name cards he asked me two questions. The first was one often put to me by survivors: was I Jewish? When I told him I was, he rather shrewdly inquired about the origin of my middle name "Jay." With my explanation that it was an Anglicization of Chaim Jacov, the name of a great-grandfather in a Russian shtetl, we quickly achieved a measure of Jewish brotherhood.

Karol V. told me that he had been sent to Auschwitz both because he was Jewish and because he had been a member of the communist youth movement in Czechoslovakia. Four younger brothers sent there at the same time died in the camp within two months. To cope with those deaths and other horrors, including witnessing deadly phenol injections to the heart, he developed what he called "a psychic immune reaction," which he likened to "wearing an asbestos jacket." It was his way of talking about the extreme psychic numbing that inmates required for survival. As a lover of literature he thought constantly of Dante, but as an "always optimistically minded" person he was determined "to live to be a witness."

He was well aware of his relatively privileged position among inmates as a doctor assigned to a medical block, "without which I would be dead too." He used that status to do everything possible to help others to survive, whether doling out the few sulfa tablets he could obtain or encouraging them psychologically to maintain a will to live and avoid lapsing into a *Muselmänner* state of living death. He told me how he succeeded in doing that with another Jewish doctor whose despair had brought him close to offering himself for the gas chamber, and how years later that same man, when working with him at a hospital in Czechoslovakia, became mortally ill and pleaded with V., "Please save my life as you did in Auschwitz!" He shook his head sadly in telling me he had been unable to do so, and then commented (as if newly realizing the strangeness of it all), "This is material for a novelist."

The most wrenching conflicts he experienced would occur when an SS doctor visited his medical block and declared that he would return at a specific time to select, say, fifty patients for the gas chamber. Like other inmate doctors in that situation, V. was horrified by the idea of helping a Nazi doctor and becoming part of the SS machinery for killing. But he also realized that if he withdrew from the process completely, the SS doctor would include in his selections not only moribund patients but some who were strong enough to survive. So he consulted with other inmate doctors about achieving a compromise by conversing limitedly with the SS doctor to try to protect those patients with a chance for survival. Such stories made me realize that there is such a thing as an evil situation in which no "good" decision is possible.

V.'s wife was also in Auschwitz and he could occasionally make the complicated arrangements to meet with her either at his hospital block or in the women's camp. Though he was punished for doing so on a couple of occasions (once by being beaten and another time by being reassigned to a more undesirable part of the camp), he felt inwardly strengthened by those visits. They could also exchange letters, in which he quoted passages from a volume of *Les Fleurs du Mal* that he had found among the remains of a French prisoner. He set for himself the task of gradually translating the Baudelaire poems into Czech, about one per week, over the course of his stay in Auschwitz—a translation project he thought of as "soul preservation."

After the ordeal of the "death march" from Auschwitz to Buchenwald, V. escaped with a group of prisoners as the war ended and made his way back to Czechoslovakia. He was soon reunited with his wife and gained distinction in Czech academic medicine. Disenchanted with Soviet-style communism, he threw himself into the 1968 Prague Spring reformist movement. When the movement was crushed and a warrant was put out for his arrest, he and his wife fled to London. He adapted to the new country and quickly found medical work. But his wife became depressed and reclusive, felt British culture to be painfully alien, and rarely left her room.

The couple came to an unusual solution. They moved to Germany, where they could be in a culture with which she was more familiar, whatever their ambivalence about living in that country. He accepted the relatively lowly position of a spa doctor, and she trained in medical technology to work as his assistant. Though not without restlessness, V. showed his usual resilience and told me with some pride how he and a German former SS doctor had become close colleagues who were able to talk extensively to each other about their experiences.

After the interview V. insisted upon taking me to dinner at the best restaurant in town, and then took me back to his home to meet his wife. She greeted me warmly, expressed enthusiasm about my study, but asked, "Why did it take you so long to do it?"—to which I had no good answer. Mostly she asked me questions about my family, and urged me to return with my wife and children for a visit with her husband and herself. I said I would try to do that, knowing that it was unlikely.

The encounter left me with a number of strong feelings. The first had to do with compassion and admiration for V. and his wife: for coping with the ordeal in Auschwitz and his having remained a healer there; and for their idiosyncratic resolution as a couple of difficult post-Auschwitz problems, including that of survivors' extreme vulnerability to a second trauma. The other feeling I had, one that occurred frequently in this study, was how privileged my life as a Jew in the twentieth century has been.

I originally met Dr. Viktor T. at a conference in New York City in the mid-seventies, at which I compared Hiroshima survivors with those of Nazi death camps; and he, himself a former Auschwitz inmate, discussed psychiatric studies he had made of Holocaust survivors of different nationalities. A couple of years later, after I had decided to do my study of Nazi doctors, I found myself sitting at a table with him in a coffee shop in Copenhagen, a city in which neither of us lived but which happened to be the most convenient place to meet at that time. Dr. T. seemed elderly and worn (he was just sixty-five years old), his manner suggesting deep seriousness, quiet energy, and a certain amount of melancholy. But at moments he brightened and, as I noted, "I've never seen a smile have so great an impact on a face."

T. completed his medical training in Czechoslovakia but, after the Nazi occupation, fled to Norway, where he lived in a small town working intermittently as a doctor and a logger. Soon after the Nazis invaded that country he was arrested and sent to Auschwitz in a transport group of two hundred and fifty people, 90 percent of whom were immediately selected for the gas chamber. T. was permitted to enter the work camp "because I was young—just thirty—and reasonably strong." He told me of the horrors of his first days of Auschwitz—the grotesque dying everywhere and prisoners being "depleted of everything, including the hair on your body (routine shaving of the head, pubis, underarms, etc., to prevent lice infestations but also to humiliate prisoners)—so that "there was absolutely nothing left from life on the outside except your spectacles" (which he still "cherished" as his only personal link at that time to non-Auschwitz existence). I noted that it was painful for me to imagine "this gentle, dignified, elderly man sitting before me" being subjected to such humiliation.

One way he coped with the situation was to view it as a kind of fictional narrative that "you weren't really experiencing." Such "derealization," for Nazis a means of distancing themselves from their cruel behavior, could in this way be a useful defense mechanism on the part of prisoners: horrific experience became dissociated narrative. At the same time T. took advantage of his position on the medical block to find ways to help other Jews survive. Sometimes that meant falsifying diagnoses—using terms like "mild influenza" or "upper respiratory infection" for actual cases of malaria or tuberculosis, since any prisoner diagnosed with either of these two conditions would be sent to the gas chamber. When lacking medicine to dispense in Auschwitz, his impulse to heal took the form of simple words of encouragement, which in some cases could be surprisingly effective. I found myself ending my book on Nazi doctors with his phrase: "I was impressed with how much one could do." I was aware that "how much" was still very little, but I also knew that the attempt mattered.

As was frequently the case with those who did most to help others, T. remained highly self-critical, "haunted by" certain things he did, such as kicking a fellow prisoner when trying to bring order to an overcrowded block for distributing the meager food supply. He considered that "my worst deed [because I] assumed the same attitude [as the Nazis]."

He could be bold in his maneuvers to survive: taking advantage of serving as a scribe by writing an order for his own transfer into a more desirable assignment and giving it the appearance of coming from a Nazi doctor; and also in the service of survival, signing his own death certificate and taking on the identity of a dead prisoner. He also stood up to other inmate-doctors who abused fellow prisoners: a Polish doctor who sought uncontrolled power, and a Jewish doctor who hoarded bread meant for patients.

At the time of liberation, he played a leading role in restraining those prisoners who sought vengeance by either killing SS men or subjecting them to "the torture they had done on us." An understated man, he told me with some feeling how he held on to "my right to be a human being, even if it was withheld by the Nazis." Yet whenever he spoke positively of his own behavior, he would feel it necessary to insist upon avoiding self-praise by adding a comment such as "But I must not make a holy person of myself."

T. also made clear that the effects of Auschwitz were still very much with him. He told me how, at the recent funeral of a close friend, his sadness was mixed with a sense of relief that he was once more able to cry. He also said that, despite decades of work on the Holocaust, he found himself in our conversation talking for the first time about many of these Auschwitz and Auschwitz-affected experiences.

After hours of sitting and talking he suggested that we go for a walk, during which he was careful to keep his good ear (the other ear had been permanently injured in a beating administered by a guard because T. had broken a camp rule to help a child) next to me. He examined shop windows and told me he was looking for a menorah for Hanukkah, that he had earlier rebelled against the religious orthodoxy of his childhood, but because of his camp experiences had become a "practicing Jew" and a leader in his small Jewish community. I told him of my sense of the oppressiveness of my grandparents' religious orthodoxy and of my secular Jewish identity, but also mentioned that my work on Nazi doctors had intensified my feelings of Jewishness and awareness of Jewish victimization and suffering over centuries. He then told me that, after reading *Death in Life*, he thought to himself: "Why doesn't a man like this do a study of the Holocaust?"—and I told him of my rabbi friend's related comment that Hiroshima was my path as a Jew to the Holocaust. I wondered whether, had he asked me that question years earlier, I might have taken less time to get there.

T. and I were becoming friends, but in a special way. He was aware of my admiration for his extraordinary human achievements, but I sensed that little would be gained by my reacting to him with either extensive praise or elaborate interpretation. Rather, I felt it more appropriate to remain a low-key, but increasingly close, partner in dialogue who was learning a great deal and at the same time providing mostly unspoken psychological support. As we corresponded actively and met in various countries over subsequent years, our conversation was increasingly about each other's work and lives, always converging on our shared concern about survivors. I know of no one who so combined personal death camp suffering with such a continuous immersion into the experience of fellow survivors and so great a dedication to finding ways to help them.

Of course it was T. who made the statement that, after forty years of involvement in the Holocaust, "I still can't believe that it really happened, that anyone could try to gather together all the Jews in Europe and take them to a place to kill them." I had that observation in mind during my two visits to Auschwitz, seeking to examine the camp's concrete topography as a way of connecting the specific physicality of the place with all that T. and others told me in our interviews. For T. also conveyed to me the necessity of deepening the reality of what occurred there. The image of T. that remains with me is that of a quietly persistent man sitting across from me telling me his painful yet always forward-looking story, a spiritual and psychological alchemist transmuting every humiliation into compassion and knowledge.

Inevitably, during talks with people like Dr. V. and Dr. T., I imagined myself in their situation in Auschwitz. It was uncomfortable for me to do so because I could not convince myself that I would have displayed the courage and resilience of either of them. But I was certain that they had revealed much to me about the mysterious human capacity for healing.

18

The Infernal Chorus

ON MARCH 30, 1979, after having lived in Munich for almost seven months, I hosted a small party to say good-bye to a few of my friends. At the gathering I told one of them that I was "tired of interviewing Nazis," and that I was not surprised but nonetheless troubled that not one of them had made a genuine moral confrontation of past behavior.

That night I had a dream in which I was part of a male singing group, a version of a barbershop quartet, and we were about to sing something. But I knew that it was no ordinary group, that it was an "infernal chorus," and was vaguely aware, even in the dream, that infernal meant the underworld, hell, death. I woke up with the phrase "infernal chorus" reverberating in my head, and quickly associated it with the voices of Nazi doctors. My interviews with them had made me part of the chorus, and I was expressing my discomfort at "singing" with such a group. I was feeling a strong need to sing my own song, detach myself from the infernal chorus, and have my say about it.

In one sense I was simply following my general pattern of returning from work in the field to the solitude of my American study to give structure and meaning to that work. What was different this time was my convoluted relationship with the country from which I was returning. I never forgot that, during their twelve-year Nazi binge, German leaders and large numbers of German people wanted to murder me along with all other Jews. At the same time I was aware of how much I valued the bonds I formed with individual Germans, many of whom were remarkable in their intelligence, sensibility, and dedication. Our shared confrontation of grotesque historical details infused our colleagueship with special intensity and our friendships with special affection.

I think of many warm dinners with Iring and Elisabeth Fetscher in Frankfurt. Iring, a political philosopher and leading German intellectual voice, contributed to my work at every level. He even appeared on a panel with me on Nazi doctors and, himself an authority on Marxism, defended my research against a Marxist critic who faulted me for a psychological rather than an economic emphasis. Elisabeth took loving care of me when I developed a gastrointestinal condition while staying at their home. Their son Sebastian, a physician who spent time in America, visited us at Wellfleet and became one of the German translators of my book. And their other son, Justus, a literary scholar, hosted us in Berlin and taught me much about German generational struggles in connection with the Nazi era. BJ and I had a memorable experience with the Fetschers as a family (two of their three adult children were present) in viewing together in early 1979 an episode of the German version of the American television series *Holocaust*. The original film was in many ways flawed, and had a mixed reception in the United States, but for many Germans it was an important historical event, evoking in a number of viewers confessional memories and expressions of guilt in connection with behavior at the time. The Fetschers had insisted that we rush through dinner to be able to see the film. We all watched it in silence, though Elisabeth sobbed during a portion depicting the killing of Jews, and no one had much to say afterward. But we knew we had experienced a moment of communion in confronting together what Germans had done to Jews.

Nazi Doctors on My Desk

Yet even when leaving Nazi doctors behind in Germany, I was far from rid of them. Facing my records of them, my thousands of pages of interviews and notes, was just as difficult as talking to them. I remember a revealing moment soon after my return when I walked into my Wellfleet study, perhaps my favorite room in the world, to find myself completely devoid of the pleasure I usually experienced when entering it. Great piles of folders on my large desk made me feel completely alone with Nazi doctors. Until then I had been somewhat protected from taking in fully what they had been part of and what they had done by the very activity required for arranging and carrying out the interviews. Now I had no such protection, and knew that I had no choice but to permit Nazi doctors to dominate my imagination so that I could interpret their behavior and compose what I had to say about them. Only by writing that book could I get them out of my study.

At the same time I was struggling psychologically with my whole German experience. As I wrote to Iring Fetscher, "BJ and I are still very much in transition spiritually. . . . I find that all kinds of things are working on me internally." Some of what was working on me came out in two kinds of dreams I was then having. One category was that of transition dreams involving European locales and activities as well as amorphous journeys. In one such dream I was in London uneasily seeking out two destinations: an open-air sports facility that somehow resembled a Nazi camp, and an obscure "massage parlor." I noted the next day the dream's unpleasant juxtaposition of "athletics, sex, and the Nazi death camps." In these transition dreams I could not seem to settle into, or even locate, a destination. I felt well-described by A. R. Ammons in his poem "Return," where he speaks of coming "a long way/without arriving" and of climbing a peak but finding "no foothold/higher than the ground."

The second category I called death dreams, and they were more eerie and disturbing. They involved people who had died but appeared as sometimes vigorous phantoms: my father, my mother, Robert Vas, Les Farber. Those dreams reminded me in turn of two earlier dreams: In one of them a friend notified me that my obituary had appeared in *The New York Times* and I checked and found it to be there. And in another dream, I observed someone spreading ashes, only to realize that the ashes being spread were my own. My psyche had long been accumulating macabre death imagery, and that process was greatly intensified by my exposure to Nazi doctors. I was surviving my travels among the dead, but not easily. Heinrich Böll's observation that "the artist carries his death within him like a good priest his breviary" extends, I believe, to the psychological witness of mass killing and dying.

I also seemed to require life-giving antidotes, some of which were expressed in other dreams I had that I related to healing. At about that time I had an additional dream that I still remember with some pleasure. It consisted solely of two neatly printed words, "Vatican grapes," surrounded by a vine of actual purple grapes to form an attractive tableau. It was clear to me even during the dream that the grapes were (as I wrote the next day) "associated with healing." While I have never been a particular fan of the Vatican, I thought of Pope John XXIII, the appealing ecumenical figure who, from 1958 to 1963, sought to heal the Catholic Church in its relationship to the world. I thought also of the healing encounters I had personally experienced with such Catholic figures as the Berrigans, Joe O'Rourke, and Bishop Barker. But the dream also seemed humorous, and when I told BJ about it we bantered about producing a healing elixir called "Vatican Grapes" that would make us rich, speculating on whether we would need permission from the pope for a patent, and on considering a brand of "Jewish Grapes" as well. And in my note I had a little fun with associations to "grapes"—"sour grapes, Grapes of Wrath, food, wine, Dionysus, orgies, languid sexual feeling." Maybe I was desperate for antidotes.

In working on the book and on articles and talks along the way, I was concerned—and not without cause, as it turned out—about how such emotionally freighted material would be received. When I spoke at medical schools and hospitals, physicians mostly raised thoughtful questions about potential American transgressions, such as giving lethal injections in carrying out executions, involvement in military violence as in Vietnam, or being socialized by their medical institutions to various forms of callous behavior. Psychiatrists and psychoanalysts tended to be fascinated by the psychological motivations of Nazi doctors and interested in my personal struggles over the course of the work. But there were notable exceptions, for instance doctors who were angered by suggestions of parallels of any kind with what American doctors did, insisting that Nazi behavior be seen as unique and unrelated to that of anyone else.

There were also more extreme reactions. I still have an image in my mind of the prominent psychoanalyst who stormed up to the podium after my presentation and screamed into the microphone: "I don't give a damn about what's in the mind of a Nazi doctor! I don't want to know what he's thinking or feeling!"—with a vehemence that temporarily disrupted the professional meeting. I responded by insisting on the importance of grasping motivations of Nazi doctors in order to combat the kind of behavior they represented and the kind of system they were part of. I was troubled by the incident because it threatened the rationale of my entire study. Together with a supportive colleague, I wrote a letter to the sponsoring psychoanalytic group, insisting on our profession's obligation to probe the most disturbing questions, in accordance with the Enlightenment principle "Dare to know!" I still believe strongly in that principle, but must confess a certain retrospective sympathy for the protesting psychoanalyst's simple outrage. I have frequently felt the same way myself.

My struggles in writing the book had to do not only with the extremity of the subject matter, but as always with structure, in this case with the kind of structure that could best encompass the full dimensions of what I had observed. Now the mosaic had to include the broad Nazi biomedical vision, leading from sterilization to "euthanasia" to the death camps, as well as detailed exploration of the psychology of Auschwitz as an institution and of individual Nazi doctors who served it. In the last section of the volume, I extended the mosaic to include a systematic grid of what I took to be the overall psychological steps of any genocide. I found getting this book written especially demanding, and the help of an astute editor crucial. The editor, to my good fortune, was my friend Jane Isay, who had edited several of my earlier books, had an unusual grasp of my work in general, and offered her counsel during trips to Wellfleet as well as in New York City. Were it not for her, those Nazi doctors might still be sitting on my desk.

More of the Infernal Chorus

The Nazi Doctors had more prepublication exposure than any of my other books. Largely through the strong interest of Abe Rosenthal, executive editor and dictator-in-chief of The New York Times, two chapters were adapted into full-length Times Magazine articles, one on Mengele and the other on the "euthanasia" program. My friendship with Abe was longstanding and ambivalent: I admired his early critical reporting in the late fifties from Poland and in the sixties from Japan (including sympathetic writings on Hiroshima survivors), where we were able to spend some time together. Unfortunately, he was to turn into a petulant reactionary, partly through backlash to the sixties, and came to alienate almost everyone around him. When he died in 2006 I had not seen him for almost two decades, but I am still grateful for the intensity with which he embraced my work on Nazi doctors and contributed to the launching of my book.

The Nazi Doctors received an anguished front-page Sunday *New York Times* review by Bruno Bettelheim, a psychoanalyst who was himself a survivor of Nazi camps but a controversial figure because of attacks on other survivors, including those of death camps, for alleged compromises they had made with Nazi jailers. In a similar vein he questioned my efforts to understand the motivations of Nazi doctors and ended his review with the enigmatic acknowledgment: "For this reason I may not have been able to do full justice to this book."

But I have come to realize that such a review, and a number of others as well, were a kind of extension of that "infernal chorus" from which I had to struggle to extricate myself. The moral insanity of the Nazi doctors reverberated in ways that could evoke a reaction that was itself caught up in the madness. My book was an attempt to expose that grotesque chorus, and in writing it I had to suppress my own rage, including sentiments not too different from those of Bettelheim. It would seem that any immersion into the world of Nazi doctors runs the risk of entering into that infernal chorus. Fortunately, the great majority of reviewers stepped back from it sufficiently to open themselves to what I was trying to do. I was especially pleased by the response of Neal Ascherson, the British journalist and historian, in *The New York Review of Books* because he affirmed what I most wished the book to convey: a way of grasping how Nazi doctors could do what they did, and a new and useful approach to the Nazi movement that was both psychological and historical. I had no idea that the work would have later relevance for American doctors and their collusion in torture during the Iraq War era (as I will discuss in the next section).

I began this section by saying there were moments when I could not believe I'd done any such work on Nazi doctors; the same was true about writing a book about them. My own work, I now realize, was a constant struggle to connect with the "separate planet" mentioned by both Nazi doctors and inmates, to make Auschwitz real to others and to myself.

While I knew there had to be a cost, I have never been much inclined to examine that cost, partly because of my awareness that whatever the study did to me pales before the suffering of actual victims and survivors. But I think there was also involved a certain research macho, pride in viewing myself as one who can deal with such painful matters.

BJ has always said that the Nazis turned my hair gray—it had been almost black—and if so, there was probably involved an element of survivors' despair concerning the human potential for such behavior. But the pain is inseparable from a sense that the work is a culmination of my life as a researcher. When the book was completed and published, I found myself saying that I could now better accept dying because something elemental in me had been realized. A friend once asked me whether, knowing what I know now, would I make the same decision to do the study—to which I replied that I would anticipate and share the dread of people close to me but would very likely go ahead with the project.

Part Five

Next Steps

19

―――――

Coming Home

A s I COMPLETE this manuscript in the summer of 2010, I am in the process of organizing our forty-fifth consecutive Wellfleet meeting on psychology and history. I usually invite about twenty or twenty-five participants, with their spouses or partners, to three days of discussions (the first few meetings were longer), and a number of them make prepared but informal presentations. We have always sought just enough structure to encourage a certain amount of focus as well as a free flow of responses. The meetings have fed my hunger for dialogue and enabled me to explore, together with thoughtful intellectual companions, many ideas emerging from my four studies and to extend those ideas by connecting them with more general human behavior. And it has all happened in an ambiance of openness and trust that has enabled us to find pleasure in confronting together the most demanding, even insoluble, matters. Freud (quoting the writer Romain Rolland) used the metaphor "oceanic feeling" to describe much-desired psychic states (such as those involving feelings of transcendence); in Wellfleet we have the real thing. I have no doubt that the ocean, visible as we talk and eat and drink, has a great deal to do with all we experience. But to explain the meetings, I need to say a little more about their meaning as part of Wellfleet for BJ and me.

In a nomadic existence, our Wellfleet house has been our longest place of dwelling, as we have lived in it for at least part of the year since 1966.

When I call Wellfleet my spiritual home I have in mind both the psychic power of the sea and dunes and the more prosaic pleasures of a quiet routine adjacent to them. To be sure, BJ and I have always required an urban counterpart with a university connection, whether New York, Cambridge, or New Haven—or, for that matter, Hong Kong, Tokyo, Kyoto, Hiroshima, London, Munich, or Jerusalem. And my New York sidewalk roots are so enduring that my mind never quite leaves that city no matter where I might be living. But in Wellfleet I feel closest to an elemental sense of my own being. So when I step into our Wellfleet house, and then into the special (sacred?) space of my study I feel myself, as nowhere else, to be home.

I've always had the sense that we willed that house into existence. BJ and I had been renting on the lower Cape (Wellfleet, Truro, Provincetown) since the late fifties. While staying at a place close to Newcomb Hollow Beach in 1964, we found ourselves deeply attracted to that area— mesmerized was closer to what I felt—and began to walk along the beach and the dunes looking for a place we might buy. We spotted a seemingly abandoned shack close to nearby Cahoon Hollow Beach and went to the main Realtor in town, a kind of local godfather, to ask him about a possible purchase. He dismissed the idea, pointing out that the shack and surrounding land were owned by a very prominent family who apparently had big plans for the place and would surely not sell it. I had no reason to doubt him but surprised myself by saying, "Call them anyway." When he did, we learned that the owner in question was not a person but a family trust, that the occupant planned to leave the Cape, and that the executors of the trust would be very interested in selling. The property was within the recently created Cape Cod National Seashore, whose director had to approve our plans for the house we wished to build. Such an agreement was feasible because the original shack contained a kitchen and a bathroom, and the policy of the National Seashore was to cooperate with the many private owners within their boundaries in making reasonable arrangements concerning size and harmony with the landscape.

That suited our talented architect, Olav Hammarstrom, who brought a combination of Scandinavian and Japanese influence (along with responsiveness to our own aesthetic and pragmatic needs) to the modern structure he created almost as an outgrowth of the dunes themselves. The only problem with Olav was that he carried over into the work his own Spartan living habits, which apparently did not require much in the way of closets (for which we had to wage a last-minute, only partly successful struggle). I had always envisioned a house combining dramatic proximity to the ocean with sufficient distance from it to provide a sense of solidity and seclusion for us and our children, our two studies, and our books. It all happened.

The everyday isolation our house provided could give way to lots of good talk with friends who stayed on various parts of the Cape. Erik and Joan Erikson had a place in Cotuit, about an hour away, and that became a family compound when their son and daughter-in-law, Kai and Joanna Erikson, bought a house nearby. My friendship with Kai had begun separately from that with his father in connection with related work with David Rioch back in the mid-fifties. Kai, just a few years younger than I, was to emerge as one of America's most original and eloquent sociologists. He and I were to collaborate closely on a number of projects, including work on several major disasters. Our bond seemed so natural that it did not occur to me until much later how unusual it was to have such intense personal and intellectual relationships with both father and son.

I also had sustained dialogues with artists and writers: with Budd Hopkins and Robert Motherwell, articulate painters who taught me much about twentieth-century art movements; and with the poet Stanley Kunitz, with whom I talked about survivors and rebels and who arranged two memorable encounters with his more unstable friend and fellow poet, Robert Lowell (in our experience, relaxed and curious about China and thought reform). One of those meetings included an unforgettable tennis doubles match in which Lowell's anticoordination was such that no leg or arm seemed related to any of the others but the owner of all four was sufficiently irrepressible to carry on as if he could play the game. I've had much warm exchange over the years with Larry Shainberg about writing and Zen, and with his brother David, until his death in 1993, about psychoanalysis and the world. And I've had many conversations with Howard Zinn and Noam Chomsky—and in recent years with Jim Carroll—about living, writing, and protesting.

Jim, a former priest and the son of a four-star Air Force general, became a dedicated anti–Vietnam War protestor; he made use of growing up around the Pentagon to write an incisive history of nuclear war planning in that building and has remained a rebellious practicing Catholic and historian of Christian anti-Semitism. In all these friendships, we talked about the same things people like us talked about elsewhere, but on the Cape, as I've sometimes put it, we seem to be better people, and everything seems more possible.

The Wellfleet Meetings

The Wellfleet meetings emerged from conversations with Erik Erikson, beginning as early as the late fifties. We talked about his work on relating individual psychology to history and sought a way to develop that emphasis by exploring it with both psychological colleagues and people from different backgrounds and disciplines. In that way the group had its source in Erik's ideas and my response to them, though the gatherings have taken us in many unanticipated directions. Those conversations with Erik could be backed up with concrete actions when BJ and I purchased our Wellfleet property and decided to renovate the original shack as my study. A small separate building, I saw it from the beginning as a place where such meetings could occur, and Erik enthusiastically agreed. In furnishing it with two huge oak tables I was quite aware that they were meant not only for my everyday use but for friends and colleagues who would sit around them and join Erik and me in conversation.

These meetings have been idiosyncratic and I find myself wondering whether they are professional conferences, salons, or communal ingatherings. I have no doubt that they have had aspects of all three. They are conferences with an academic tinge, both because most participants teach or have taught at universities and because they are scheduled meetings that take up specific subjects and ideas and discuss them with some rigor and nuance. But with most of the deliberations taking place in my own study, they have been conferences of a very personal kind. They have never been neutral about anything, with participants generally expressing passionate political and social convictions, though with an informality and easy quality of exchange. Their most startling feature of all may be the extent to which people listen to one another.

They have been salons in the sense of a gathering place for articulate people who share a certain sensibility, in this case a critical perspective toward political and professional arrangements, and intense feelings concerning war, nuclear weapons, and injustice. If a salon, then, it is one in which ideas exchanged tend to be associated with moral questions. Though there has been considerable divergence of thinking, the Wellfleet enterprise reflects my preference for sympathetic exploration of ideas and potential actions as opposed to the showy polemics of adversarial debate.

The communal dimension of Wellfleet has evolved over the forty-five years of meetings, despite and partly because of changes in participants. The community has formed largely from my relationships with people who come, and in that sense I have been at its center. But I have not been the leader of a movement on the order of Freud or of a rebellious surge within a movement on the order of the psychoanalyst Heinz Kohut, or for that matter a guru of any kind. Yet I would say that I have been more than a mere facilitator, perhaps a leader in providing a loose personal model that combines scholarship and committed dialogue with activism. At least that's what long-standing participants (we call them Wellfleetians) have told me. They have also implied that much goes on that I have little knowledge of in a kind of Wellfleet underbelly, exchanges of a more irreverent kind that take place in motels where many stay. There seems to be much fun involved.

In the first meetings Erik and I sought broader terrain for his mentorship and my discipleship. Although I have always done most of the organizing, during Erik's sixteen years in the group, I checked everything carefully with him. By the time we managed our first meeting in 1966, I was well along in writing up my Hiroshima work and my tie with Erik had changed, so that (as I later put it) "Erikson and I were seeking ways to further a relationship between a mentor who did not cultivate disciples but . . . was bent upon extending and consolidating his ideas, and a close student struggling to break sufficiently free of mentorship to explore directions that his own investigations seemed to suggest, if not demand." So fifteen or twenty interested scholars—psychologists, psychiatrists, social scientists, historians, literary critics—gathered in Wellfleet for that first meeting, most of which, as it turned out, I had to miss.

We were enjoying a welcoming dinner in Provincetown the night before our deliberations were to begin when I was called to the phone and told by my cousin Phyllis Brumberger that my father had died in the Yale–New Haven Hospital. I had driven him there the previous week, and the doctors had reassured me that he was recovering from an episode of heart failure, as he had the previous year in the same hospital. I returned to Wellfleet for the meetings while Phyllis, who lived in New Haven and was close to both my father and me, looked after him in the hospital. My father, who was sixty-nine years old, had had years of cardiac symptoms and I, like his doctors, overestimated the physical resilience of this most resilient of men. BJ helped me through a very difficult night, during which we talked endlessly about my father's fierce love and support throughout my life, his embrace of BJ as well, my feelings of guilt over having left his bedside, and of now being lost in the universe. BJ and I flew to New York City to do what we had to do through the blur of family arrangements and the funeral. That took six days, after which we returned to Wellfleet in time to participate in the last session of the conference, at which I presented the work on Hiroshima I had prepared. It was all rather strange but doing that permitted me to connect, and partly subsume, my personal grief to the grief and mourning of an entire city. My father's death, along with his nurturing energies, have not stopped reverberating in me.

The relatively academic ambiance of our first few Wellfleet meetings reflected our initial illusion, which it did not take us long to give up, that of creating an academic discipline of "psychohistory." As we came to know better, we could relax into the modest but still exciting task of approaching psychology and history in ways that newly combined the two. The early meetings were sponsored by the American Academy of Arts and Sciences. But grateful as we were for the support, we realized that it was contingent upon our becoming a more organized enterprise and, eventually, a training center for psychohistorical work. We were moving in precisely the opposite direction, toward presentations that were speculative, probing, and freewheeling. Our rejection of Academy support, about which I was especially adamant, was a crucial turning point for us, giving us the opportunity to create and re-create our group. Those early meetings included people who did much to help form the group (Ken Keniston and the historian Bruce Mazlish); others who stayed with the enterprise for some years (the psychologists Margaret Brenman and George Klein, as well as Kai Erikson, who in 2010 is still very much a participant); as well as others who were active early but for more limited periods of time (such as the sociologist Philip Rieff, the historian Frank Manuel, the literary critic Steven Marcus, and the psychiatrist Robert Coles).

Many of those I invited over the years were people I knew who had a lively interest in psychology and history and a generally critical perspective: sociologists Norman Birnbaum and Richard Sennett; the broadgauged humanist Peter Brooks; psychological feminists Judith Herman and Carol Gilligan, and the psychiatric authority on violence, Jim Gilligan; Harvey Cox and his wife, the historian of Russia Nina Tumarkin; the historian and psychoanalyst Chuck Strozier; and later, the Hindu scholar Wendy Doniger, the Indian scholars Ashis Nandy and Sudhir Kakar, the literary scholar and psychoanalytic historian Cathy Caruth, and the peace studies architect James Skelly.

Between Erik and myself, Wellfleet was an important bond that helped us to overcome our tensions with each other. Over time he came to recognize that my work had to take its own direction and could not be subsumed to his, but that in the process I, like others in the group, continued to learn much from him. BJ formed her own friendship with Erik, and their private conversation about the mysteries of his father (she had considerable exposure to such mysteries in her work on adoption) became something of a Wellfleet "backstory." Even as I steered our subject matter toward more contemporary issues—Vietnam, nuclear weapons, Nazi influences, and genocide—Erik remained the group's psychological wise man.

Concerning Erik's own presentations, there was usually a little ritual dance between us on the telephone that went something like this: "Erik, Wellfleet is coming around soon and I was wondering what you would like to talk about." "Nothing really, this year I think I'll just sit back and listen." "But Erik, others in the group would really like to hear from you." "Well, I can make a comment or two as we go along." "But let me ask you this, Erik. What sort of things have you been thinking about lately that you might just mention?" "Oh, not very much, Bob. I have been exploring parallels between Gandhi's militant nonviolence and psychoanalysis, but it's at a very early stage"—or "I've been taking a new look at adulthood in the life cycle but I haven't gotten too far." "But that would be wonderful to hear about, Erik, especially because you're just developing it. You could talk about it very informally." "Well, maybe I could—but I'd like to do it on the third day toward the end of the meetings, after I've had a chance to hear the others." "That would be great, Erik. We'll schedule it for the last session." Erik would then bring to the meeting his imaginative yet disciplined perspective on Gandhi, or the psychology of adulthood, his presentation carefully organized and at the same time highly digressive in his associations and speculations about whatever entered his mind.

We would later be witnesses to father–son dialogues between Erik and Kai, the only such intergenerational exchange the meetings have known. Kai had written fine books on the subjects of deviance and disaster. The two men affectionately (but not without intensity) exchanged views on those and other issues in which they spelled out their differences in expressing a sociohistorical, as opposed to a psychohistorical, viewpoint. Erik attended every Wellfleet meeting through 1981, after which his physical and mental state no longer enabled him to do so. Kai had become a central figure in the group long before that. Even now, when I look at Kai sitting at the table in our meetings, I cannot help thinking about those poignant father–son dialogues.

The Vietnam War made its way into the meetings early on. BJ and I returned directly to Wellfleet from our 1967 Vietnam visit to discuss with the group what we had learned there. The next year Richard Goodwin, advisor and speechwriter for a number of presidents and presidential candidates, made a dramatic entrance when he arrived at Wellfleet as an agitated and angry survivor of the Democratic convention that Norman Mailer was to term "the siege of Chicago." He told of the brutal police attacks on antiwar demonstrators outside the convention hall, orchestrated by Mayor Richard Daley, and of the equally disturbing manipulative actions within the hall against the antiwar delegates by the Hubert Humphrey forces. A few years later the historian and presidential scholar Doris Kearns, Goodwin's wife, brought to the meetings a memorable description of Lyndon Johnson's tragic personal sequence from high political and social achievement to hubris and self-destruction in pursuing the Vietnam War. This articulate and attractive young biographer had become close to Johnson, had clearly aroused erotic feelings in the benighted president, and highly sympathetic feelings in the members of the Wellfleet group.

The group had lively responses to my work with Vietnam veterans. But its members were somewhat puzzled when I told them I was undergoing a change in my way of functioning as a professional. I was referring to my efforts to combine psychiatric insight with strong political and antiwar advocacy, especially in my participation in rap groups with veterans. I think some of the confusion in the Wellfleet groups had to do with a lack of full clarity on my own part. But discussing that change in the friendly Wellfleet atmosphere helped make it happen, helped me to define and become the more committed psychiatrist I was talking about.

Nuclear Emanations

From that presentation on Hiroshima at the first meeting, I continued over the years to discuss my work on nuclear weapons. The group was an ideal forum for exploring my sense of their threat to the human mind even without their use: generating a vast societal numbing, creating doubts about our remaining part of the great chain of being, and seducing all too many to succumb to the dangerous spiritual affliction of *nuclearism*. By *nuclearism* I meant an exaggerated dependency on the weapons to keep the peace or even keep the world going, to the point of near worship of their godlike world-destroying power. I invited others to the meetings who had made notable contributions to nuclear consciousness.

Richard Falk, a close friend, brought a knowledgeable critique of the political and legal attitudes surrounding the weapons, and also a stellar tennis game (his accurate topspin forehand was too much for me, except in high altitudes as in Mexico and Arizona, where the outcome was mysteriously reversed). Later we would collaborate on the editing of two *Crimes of War* volumes, and also on an original book we called *Indefensible Weapons*, with the subtitle "The Political and Psychological Case Against Nuclearism." Over the years Richard and I would occasionally disagree on important issues: he initially saw Ayatollah Khomeini as primarily a third-world revolutionary, while I viewed him as a dangerous religious and political fundamentalist; and more recently he has encouraged conspiracy theories involving American collusion in 9/11 attacks, theories that in my view interfere with a more accurate exposure of the Bush administration's combination of belligerence and ineptitude. My hope is that, just as Richard was quick to change his mind about Khomeini, he will do the same about conspiracy theories, although I agree with Richard that we could learn much from further investigation of 9/11. And in another area of disagreement, that concerning problems of large-scale American interventions in the world, I have changed my mind in the direction of his sustained skepticism.

Others who came to Wellfleet taught me much about the extent to which nuclear weapons have created a "national security state." Richard Barnet, who had been a young advisor in the Kennedy administration and cofounded the important Institute for Policy Studies in Washington, D.C., was eloquent on this and related subjects, as was the writer Jonathan Schell. I've known Jonathan since his remarkable reporting on the Vietnam War and he brought to Wellfleet his developing mastery of all aspects of the nuclear weapons issue. His *The Fate of the Earth* was surely the most influential, and perhaps the best book on the subject yet written. I confess a tinge of envy, along with an element of regret that nothing I have written on the subject has had that kind of impact—all the more so since Jonathan has acknowledged some influence from my book *The Broken Connection* in his writing of *The Fate of the Earth*. His presentations at Wellfleet have been moving in their combination of scholarship and passionate advocacy of nuclear abolition. Dan Ellsberg also became a regular participant, and the group's only example of an activist who had been willing to risk a long jail sentence, notably in making public the top-secret Pentagon Papers. Dan has brought chilling accounts of nuclear danger made all the more plausible by his own prior history as a Pentagon planner. Though he tends to focus on worst-case scenarios, his presence at Wellfleet has kept us grounded in some of the terrible realities in the interactions of world-destroying weapons with human beings who are either catastrophically wrongheaded or generally unable to hold back the technology entrusted to them.

A high point in our nuclear deliberations was the presentation by Philip Morrison, the American physicist who had played a prominent role at Los Alamos in creating the weapon and then become a leading voice in warning America and the world about its danger. I'd always been fascinated by the psychology of the scientists who made those first weapons, and Morrison succeeded in bringing Los Alamos into my Wellfleet study. Phil conveyed in the most immediate way the atmosphere of good feeling that prevailed among the scientists, their shared dedication to beating the Nazis to a weapon that could determine the outcome of the war, and the beneficent leadership of the widely admired Robert Oppenheimer, the director of the project. But Phil was uncharacteristically vague about why he and other scientists continued their work, without even raising questions, when it became known that the Germans had failed in their efforts to produce the weapon. He spoke of the general sense of keeping to the task with the war not yet won, and of trust in the continuing guidance of Oppenheimer. (There was one scientist who did leave the project then, the Polish Jewish physicist Joseph Rotblat, who had been assigned to it from England, but there was little general awareness of a moral issue.) Phil went on to describe his physical connection with the weapon: riding in the jeep together with the plutonium core at the Alamogordo test, and three weeks later holding the components of the Nagasaki bomb in his hand on the island of Tinian, from which it was launched. He had no hesitation in carrying out these tasks.

Everything changed for him when he went to Hiroshima soon after the end of the war to help assess the effects of the bomb. At Wellfleet and then during an interview I had with him for a later book, *Hiroshima in America*, he stressed how distant people who made decisions could be from the deaths and suffering they caused—but "when you go there, you saw what it was like." Soon after that 1979 Wellfleet meeting, Phil's wife, Phyllis, always his close personal and scientific companion, sent a thank-you note to BJ and me in which she wrote: "Phil has now read *Death in Life* and come to understand how and why he put it aside with a cursory glance. Survivor guilt works two ways."

Much later (in 2003, two years before he died) Phil told more of his life story to a group I then convened in Cambridge, describing with sad irony his trajectory from a young pacifist to a scientist participating in creating the atomic bomb, and attributing that sequence to the way in which all of our behavior and worldviews can be profoundly shaped and reshaped by the power of prevailing historical circumstances.

I was especially affected by what Morrison said, as I had known him and admired his early and sustained antinuclear work, his extraordinary articulateness both in private conversation and in hosting science programs on public television, and his capacity to overcome permanent bodily impairment from childhood poliomyelitis. And I identified with Phil concerning our shared experience of the transformative power of Hiroshima. We had both started out with peace-minded idealism and then been socialized to a sense of the bomb's necessity before committing ourselves to antinuclear work. To be sure, I had no involvement in making the bomb, but had I been a physicist at that time I might well have shared that with Phil as well. What he conveyed to us was the collective momentum—technological, bureaucratic, and psychological—that contributed to what became for physicists and others an atrocity-producing situation. The historical circumstances Phil spoke of could bring almost anyone to participate in the creation and use of the weaponry—unless, of course, the full truth of its destructiveness is made part of those "circumstances."

The Holocaust at Wellfleet

The first to bring the Holocaust to Wellfleet was neither an American nor a Jew but an anti-Nazi German. Alexander Mitscherlich came in the early seventies, with America in the throes of Vietnam agonies, to talk about the impact of the Nazi era on Germans. We had an evening session called "Vietnam and Nuremberg" (the title Telford Taylor had given to a new book) in which we probed the relevance of Nuremberg judgments for post-Vietnam America. I had no idea that this would be a prelude to my later work with Nazi doctors, and also to important friendships with Germans. I was stirred by Alexander's continuing intellectual and ethical courage in confronting head-on what so many of his countrymen could not touch.

The most powerful Holocaust presentation came from my friend Raul Hilberg in the mid-eighties. He told of his family's escape from Vienna and of his later experience as an American soldier given access to Hitler's library in the Munich chancellery. He described in his resonant baritone the vicious anti-Semitic epithets he uncovered—Jews were treacherous and murderous, fiendish in their lasting influence, dangerous to Germany and the world—and then asked us rhetorically "Were these quotations from Hitler or Goebbels?" and answered: "No, they were from Martin Luther." I had known something about Luther's anti-Semitism but had never heard it juxtaposed in this way with Nazi imagery. I found myself wondering about the relatively benign rendering of the great Reformation theologian by Erikson (who could by then no longer come to Wellfleet) in focusing mainly on Luther's spiritual and psychological breakthroughs (Erich Fromm came closer to what we were hearing in emphasizing Luther's later vicious authoritarianism, but it was the Erikson study as a whole that had so influenced my life). When listening to Raul in Wellfleet I joined him in Hitler's library and observed that moment of truth when this passionate young Viennese Jewish American soldier triumphantly commandeered the Führer's reading material and broadcast it to the world.

Raul recounted how, when pursuing his American education as a Holocaust scholar, his thesis advisors told him that it would be "academic suicide" to focus on the generally rejected view of a detached Nazi bureaucracy providing the key mechanism for the systematic killing. That brought into play his dogged persistence in uncovering evidence for his view, and what he wrote and described to us seemed to me to confirm what I learned about the medical bureaucracy, whether in Auschwitz or Berlin. He also told of his still more controversial position in accusing Jewish ghetto leaders of collusion with the Nazis in arranging deportations for killing. He was undoubtedly right in demonstrating how Nazi manipulation of those leaders contributed to the efficiency of the project, but here I thought it important to engage him in dialogue about the psychology of coerced collaboration, and the resulting situations in which there were no good choices. I could in fact point out parallel situations faced by Polish and Jewish inmate doctors in Auschwitz when pressed by Nazi doctors to help select a certain number of those on their medical blocks for the gas chambers, all of which Raul took in and appreciated but without, I suspect, much changing his views. Fervent and irascible, Raul had the demeanor of an atheist rabbinical prophet with something underneath I would only call sweetness. I learned much from him both about how the Holocaust worked and how a determined and probing scholar spent a lifetime re-creating that dreadful narrative.

Recent Decades

As Wellfleet approached and entered the twenty-first century, Chuck Strozier took an increasing part in all phases of the meetings. I'd met Chuck during the seventies when he was a young historian and editor of a small journal, *Psychohistory Review*. Over the years he has done exceptional work in a number of directions, including a book on Lincoln, a biography of Heinz Kohut, and interview studies of American fundamentalists and of survivors of 9/11. He became interested in my work in general, including my interview method, my ideas about nuclear weapons beginning with Hiroshima, and my explorations of proteanism and fundamentalism. I was able to help in arrangements for his appointment to John Jay College at City University, where he essentially ran our Center on Violence and Human Survival as codirector. A man of unusual intellectual range, Chuck also has a special capacity for friendship. Over the years we have become increasingly close as he brought admirable grace to his transition from following and extending my work to finding his own clear voice. Chuck began to come to Wellfleet in the late seventies and made a number of presentations, but two especially riveting ones on his 9/11 work and on the Bush "war on terror." He has also done much to help me put together recent Wellfleet meetings, always with appreciation of their special ambiance.

From the time of the September 11, 2001, Al Qaeda attacks, we brought considerable focus to the Middle East and explored Islamist violence and American totalism under George W. Bush. As always, my preference for the group was for hands-on experience, and we were able to invite such thoughtful journalists as Lawrence Wright, who had close and extensive knowledge of Al Qaeda, and Mark Danner, who as a war correspondent had done much work on the American use of torture. I was personally a bit saddened at reaching a stage where I no longer went out into the field to ask my own questions (my study of Aum Shinrikyo in the late nineties has been my last effort of that kind). But in listening to men like Wright and Danner, I could almost feel myself still out there talking to important actors in those conflicts. And with our group I was helping to provide an environment in which we could probe some of the meanings of the accounts others brought to us.

Israeli-Palestinian struggles had a long presence at our meetings. Over the years a number of Israeli friends came to Wellfleet, notably the sociologist Eugene Wiener, mostly people who love their country but in various ways contested its policies. In the early 2000s, a particularly compelling presentation was made by Guy Grossman, a young leader in an

Israeli group of army reservists called "Courage to Refuse." He told how soldiers like himself, when serving in such Palestinian areas as the West Bank and East Jerusalem, became confused and brutalized occupiers who found themselves humiliating, wounding, and killing Palestinian civilians. He told of his deep concern not only for abused Palestinians but for the souls of his own countrymen. Hence the stand his group took in which its members, while willing to fight to defend Israel, refused to serve in the occupied territories. It was he who told me that his group had been affected by the American experience in Vietnam, and by the work of the war's critics. The Wellfleet meetings could serve as a forum for writers and activists in expressing that sensibility.

We have also continued to explore more general war-peace issues— it would seem that America has had too many of these lately. One presenter was Rolf Ekeus, the knowledgeable Swedish diplomat who had participated in many international antinuclear undertakings and had then served as the first U.N. chief weapons inspector in Iraq following the Persian Gulf War. Rolf and his wife, Kim, who was originally a diplomat as well but subsequently a Jungian analyst, became our good friends and introduced us to U.N. secretary general Kofi Annan and his wife, Nane, with whom BJ and I could also enjoy an affectionate friendship.*

I was to be deeply disappointed, though, by Rolf's surprising public support for the Iraq War, undoubtedly influenced by his direct observation and personal experience of the crude and murderous beligerence of the Saddam Hussein regime. But Rolf and Kim remain our close friends.

In our war-peace sequence, Chris Hedges brought to the group his troubling observations on the emotional attractions of combat, which he noted in fellow journalists and in himself. Jim Carroll spoke movingly about his agonizing conflicts, on becoming an anti–Vietnam War activist, with his Air Force general father, whom he nonetheless loved (described in his powerful book *American Requim*). I later learned that Jim had been part of our first Redress act of civil disobedience in 1972,

---

*On one occasion our center sponsored a talk by Kofi at the City University, and it was quite remarkable to observe so high an international official fielding questions so knowledgeably and informally; another time, he and Nane came to our Central Park West apartment for dinner, preceded by security agents who staked out the area, and again Kofi was direct and compelling in his discussions with everybody present on his policies as secretary general.

after which his father refused to speak with him, though the two men eventually reconciled.

It was Howard Zinn who conveyed to us most indelibly the evil of war itself. I think of him at Wellfleet, talking to us in quiet tones about his experience as a bombardier in World War II. During the last days of the war his unit was ordered to carry out a bombing raid on the small city of Royan in western France. He noticed that they were given new incendiary material, and later learned that this was the first use of napalm. Howard later became skeptical of the purposes of the mission, and arranged to spend time in Royan to study all available documents, French and American, concerning that series of bombings. He discovered that they had killed about four hundred people, the great majority of them Frenchmen, and that the raids had no genuine military justification but resulted from the ambition of a few American officers. Howard's personal witness, gentle and angry, was for me an unforgettable moment of survivor wisdom. I could never again be insensitive to the effects of aerial bombing on human beings, or to the involvement during war of good people in that deadly enterprise. It was particularly powerful to experience such witness from the most compelling activist, the most dedicated advocate of peace and justice, of our generation. I had many lunches with Howard that were full of jokes and banter and baseball talk, but at bottom was his message of the evil that emanates from any war.

One of the most remarkable of all Wellfleet moments had to do with Norman Mailer's presentation of his last novel, *The Castle in the Forest*, in 2007. Norman had been a regular participant in the group since the early nineties. He had surprised many, who anticipated a rambunctious celebrity, a perhaps less than sober character, and encountered instead a very thoughtful and friendly intellectual who took ideas seriously and listened to other people. Norman became so enthusiastic about the group that he began to ask me months in advance what theme I had in mind that year, often providing bold (if unfeasible) suggestions of his own.

But he did put forth a few unusual ideas. The novel was based on a cosmology in which God existed but was limited in his influence and made many mistakes (and was hence nicknamed Dumkopf), always struggling with his more savvy adversary, the Devil (accordingly nicknamed Maestro). *The Castle in the Forest* was ostensibly a novelistic re-creation of Hitler's origins and childhood, in accordance with that cosmology. Indeed, Hitler's extraordinary evil was attributed to the intervention of the Devil, through one of his agents, from the time of conception. At the meeting Norman was to read passages from the novel but was by then in physical decline, and because both his voice and eyes had become weak, asked Mike Lennon, his dedicated Boswell and knowledgeable assistant, to read them instead. Indeed, given Norman's physical state, the novel was a heroic undertaking; he immersed himself in German culture and the Nazi era (including, he told me, rereading much of *The Nazi Doctors*) and made a trip to Bayruth to listen to the entire Wagner Ring cycle.

As Mike spoke the words of the Devil's agent and narrator—on how "devils live in both the lie and the truth, side by side, and both can exist with equal force," much like the demonstration by physicists that "light is both a particle and a wave"—I don't think that any others in the group, committed as they were to secular reason, took any of the philosophical argument (or for that matter the whole cosmology) very seriously. But they were engaged by what they understood to be a work of the imagination, asked Norman provocative questions about his characters, especially the diabolic ones, and generally got into the spirit of the session's playful intellectual ambiance. Norman responded with riffs on such matters as the nature of God and the poignancy of his struggles, the cunning of the forces of evil, and the richness of such a cosmology for a writer's imaginings. The result was one of the most animated and bizarre sessions ever held at Wellfleet. Its joyous mood extended into the champagne-lubricated farewell lunch that always follows our Sunday morning session along with my traditional virtue-mocking and sixties-reminiscent toast: "Up with us and down with the motherfuckers!" I could hardly allow myself any thought that this would be Norman's last Wellfleet meeting.

Mailer My Doppelgänger?

My bringing Norman into the Wellfleet group was a way of continuing and expanding our decades of conversation. He and I were what could be called unalike doppelgängers, and that had much to do with our friendship. We were Jewish boys (he three years older) from lower-middle-class families in the Crown Heights section of Brooklyn (I was horrified to learn later that Norman was actually born in New Jersey). When Norman introduced me to his mother at the National Book Award ceremony in 1969, as also from Brooklyn (and she responded by saying, "That's nice that you both won it"), mother and son were implying that he and I were similar offshoots of adjacent vines. More than that, Norman and I resembled each other in our preoccupation with extremities of human behavior and our opposition to any form of political oppression. We've also been Jews who, while identifying with our heritage, have resisted, in our embrace of the universal, being defined by an all-encompassing Jewishness (by the perennial question, "Is it good for the Jews?"). Otherwise the contrasts between us could hardly be greater. Norman prided himself on being a "psychic outlaw" while I remained a relatively well-behaved rebel. And there was the small matter of Norman's literary imagination, which the likes of me could only appreciate. Being with Norman, in fact, always reminded me of my literary limitations, though in a way that inspired me to take chances and be better.

I met Norman in Provincetown during the summer of 1965, when BJ and I were renting a house on the bay not far from his and were introduced by a mutual friend. He was a kind of king of Provincetown, having spent time there regularly since the 1940's, his presence reverberating at all levels of that former fishing village. Provincetown is at the geographical edge of the North American continent and the unconventional edge of American society in its hospitality to gays and general cultural openness.

Early in our friendship I witnessed one of Norman's uglier public transgressions. He (some time in 1968) invited a number of friends to his Brooklyn apartment for an Old Left/New Left exchange involving his daughter and her Columbia University SDS friends, which he effectively sabotaged with a drunken rant in his phony Texas accent. I was as offended as everyone else and doubtful about the possibility of a friendship with such a man. Still, BJ and I enjoyed the pseudo-wild parties he and his then wife Beverly Bentley gave in Provincetown in the seventies, during which he might play the part of a boxing dude (often present was a real boxing champion, José Torres, who was much more mild-mannered). Norman drank a lot but was still eloquent (though you had to catch him between his fifth and fifteenth drink, because before that he was edgy and after that a little incoherent). He was experimenting with himself as always, sometimes with his own and others' humiliation, and would be at his desk the next morning producing with his pencil those brilliantly convoluted sentences. I think I too was experimenting, in my case with the fantasy of becoming my doppelgänger, the psychic outlaw.

We became closer in approaching old age, which in his case meant a significant mellowing. Indeed Norman surprised and moved me with his capacity for affectionate friendship. He characteristically expressed his feelings with gentle teasing. Once, toward the end of a Wellfleet meeting, he said to me: "You are doubly heroic. You've struggled through two levels of trauma, the events themselves and the bad writing about them you have been obliged to read." But he also expressed himself in his actions. I have an image of his sensitive participation in about 1990 at a fund-raiser at our New York apartment for our Center on Violence and Human Survival (at a time when our financial survival was in doubt). His remarks were characteristically self-referential but in a way that could not have been more compelling: he asked himself why he had never really taken on the nuclear weapons issue, said he realized that it was because the subject had become so abstract and meaningless, and pointed to my Hiroshima work and the activities of the center as rendering the issue more real and connecting it with human beings. I don't know which pleased me more—the money we raised that evening to help keep the center going, or Norman's act of friendship.

Another evening that BJ and I spent with Norman, this one on the Cape the same year, taught me something about the connection between the ascetic and the orgiastic. Norman, BJ, and I arranged to go out to dinner at one of the Cape's few genuinely gourmet restaurants, and he insisted upon holding to the plan despite the fact that he was in the middle of one of his periodic bodily purifications in which he could imbibe only water and juices. He in fact ate nothing but instead experienced his dinner by advising us on each course and imagining in succulent detail the taste of each dish, exploring its harmony or disharmony with other dishes, and his reasons for choosing or rejecting it. BJ and I got into the spirit of things by saying more than we knew about gourmet nuances and expressing the anticipated experience of our own taste buds. As we devoured each course, Norman asked us about its specific attributes and the degree of success of the chef in its preparation. We praised Norman's epicurean sensibility and he responded by declaring that it had been the most delicious meal he'd ever eaten. I believed him. He had managed to create something close to an altered state of consciousness for all three of us by means of his rigorous replacement of physical culinary pleasure with a completely imagined version of it.

"All Memoirs Are Lies"

During the last few years of our conversations, we inevitably talked about memoirs. Norman said that none he had read ever seemed true, leading him to the conclusion that "all memoirs are lies." But then he contradicted himself by expressing pride in his accurate rendering of details in *The Armies of the Night*, his account of his experience in an antiwar march on the Pentagon, right down to the precise words of conversations with Robert Lowell and Dwight Macdonald (as confirmed later by each of them). But something else he told me was just as interesting, namely that he could not get going on the book until he realized he could make himself into a novelistic character, "Mailer," about whom he could write in the third person. The message I was getting from him was that there was indeed such a thing as historical accuracy but that characters in a memoir were not just "there" but had to be re-created, which was a manifestation of the all-pervasive symbolizing process. That did not mean I had to follow his lead, make myself into a third-person character ("Lifton" or "Robert" or "Bob"), but rather that any representation of myself, whether from memory or my library papers, would inevitably be newly imagined.

When I mentioned my sense of being responsible to the history I had been part of as recorded in my library papers, Norman made the suggestion that I inform the reader at every point whether I am making use of those papers or writing from memory. I thought the suggestion cumbersome and overly schematic, but it did alert me to the difference between immediate observation and the fallibility and imaginative openings of memory.

In terms of a writer's responsibility in such matters, Norman used the interesting word *scrupulousness*. What he meant by it was bringing to bear on his subject his most disciplined and painstaking effort, so that the word became a writer's manifesto of truth-telling. I've thought a lot since then about my own efforts at "scrupulousness" in probing individual and collective truths that can be uncomfortable for many (such as "survivor guilt" or what I call "death guilt"). There was a shared principle here for psychological researcher and writer of fiction, a relation between conscience and words offered.

One soft Provincetown summer evening, looking out at the bay at high tide from the lounge of the Red Inn, we talked of the pleasures of old age. Upon hearing that I'd recently celebrated my eightieth birthday, Norman offered a small but appreciated compliment, calling me "a young eighty" (he was an older codger by three years). What Norman valued about old age was the sense that "I finally know who I am." He said that he had been protected by his "guardian angel" from wrong turnings that undermined his essence as a writer ("I wanted to be a great lover and I was rejected by a woman. I wanted to be a filmmaker and made a couple of films that nobody thought much of"). He could also surrender unrealizable ambitions, the existence of one of which I found a bit frightening. He said, "I no longer expect to be president," explaining that he had anticipated being elected mayor of New York (for which he unsuccessfully ran in 1969) and then becoming a national figure who would win the presidency. That degree of grandiosity seemed to be on the edge of madness, but it occurred to me that it was necessary to his more grounded but still outlandish talent. Norman could give up that scenario because he felt realized in his writing, because, as he put it, "I know I've done it!" That guardian angel seemed also to provide him with new self-knowledge. Once in discussing his long-standing conflicts with feminists, he smiled at me and said quietly, "That was one I lost," perhaps at least partially recognizing that his public behavior toward women had been boorish.

It occurred to me that my own "guardian angel" had protected me against such missteps as pursuing a doctorate in Japanese studies or responding to exploratory offers to become chairman of the Department of Psychiatry at Yale or elsewhere, president of Physicians for Social Responsibility, or even a university president. And I too had surrendered an illusory ambition, that of bringing about a transformation of psychological thought. Like Norman I might have required such an illusion to achieve whatever I had in the way of original ideas. I couldn't quite declare, "I know I've done it!" but I have been aware of a quiet building of interest in my work from various sources, including a considerable number of documentary filmmakers approaching me in recent years concerning the four research studies described in this memoir. The guardian angel of all this is what we used to call one's inner voice, in my case never entirely without static or contradiction, but somehow moving toward clarity.

Evil and Good

Norman was much concerned about the issue of evil, and considered me a good conversational partner on it because of the extent to which I had been exposed to it in my work, most specifically with Nazi doctors. He had contempt for "liberals" because he thought they denied evil, and he made a point of calling himself a radical conservative. We had a disagreement about Hannah Arendt's concept of the "banality of evil," which Norman hated because it seemed to bypass the truly draconian nature of evil and "made everything easy" by seeing evil as readily expressed by anyone. But he was open to my insistence that the behavior of Nazi doctors and some American soldiers in Vietnam confirmed Arendt's thesis that ordinary people under certain circumstances could be capable of radical evil. We discussed how the banality applied to the people involved and not to the evil itself. He was interested in my description of Albert Speer's willed refusal to take in clear evidence of evil. These conversations helped me to formulate my own views on evil.

Norman and I were on the same side of an interesting question about evil that arose at the Wellfleet meetings. A young scholar named David Frankfurter made a presentation based on a new book he had written urging that we cease using the word *evil* altogether because it absolutizes everything and can lead to violent behavior in the claim to counter it (as in George W. Bush's depicting American enemies as an "axis of evil" and mounting a "war on terror" as a means of "eliminating evil"). Norman responded with his facetious humor: "If we're going to get rid of the word *evil*, then we should get rid of the word *good* as well." I felt that work with Nazi doctors in particular confirmed my view of the necessity for a word whose reverberations could suggest the degree of cruel and destructive behavior human beings were capable of, and that the idea of eliminating the word reflected a misguided view of what we require of language.

Norman did not want evil shortchanged, so to speak, as it was so central to his cosmology. I often talked with him about that cosmology, and BJ got into the spirit of things by asking Norman about God and the dinosaurs: why had God wasted so much time on them before eliminating them as a species? To which Norman replied, with a straight face but a certain impish delight: "Maybe God changed his mind, so that at first he "thought that dinosaurs would be great," and as he evolved "realized that they would not be and made his way to humans." As I listened to him I asked myself, "Does he really *believe* this stuff?" I sensed that Norman was spinning out a novelist's yarn, one that had to be playful and amusing and include characters that were vivid and memorable. I had no such defining spiritual narrative in my own life, and in fact resisted the idea, preferring to keep my ethical struggles secular with all the resulting questions and ambiguities.

But I too had to address spiritual needs, and Norman was fascinated by my account of how some Hiroshima survivors told of suffering more from the emperor's surrender speech than from the atomic bomb itself. He seized upon my term *spiritual annihilation* and proposed a related concept of more gradual and subtle *spiritual erosion* brought about by such influences as unmanageable technology, deadening modern architecture, and ubiquitous plastic. While I wouldn't have chosen those examples, I thought he had a point. For here he was confirming my emphasis on collective internalization of behavior, including psychic numbing and the experience of loss, all of which he could fit into his spiritualized cosmology.

I read *The Castle in the Forest* just before its publication and we talked about it at a Thanksgiving dinner at the Mailers' in Provincetown in 2006. To be sure, there were witty and even charming passages in the voice of the Devil's agent who could, at times, sound much like Norman. For me the problem was not the cosmology so much as the structure and the prose, which were erratic and uneven. I didn't say that, but he probably suspected that I was less than enthusiastic. He made the point that ordinary psychological explanations—parental and sibling relationships or early trauma—were insufficient to explain evil of Hitler's magnitude.

I didn't disagree with that but suggested the enormous power of ideology to contribute to evil, and the sense of virtue it provided those engaged in large-scale killing. Grim as the subject was, Norman and I could engage in a little friendly banter, in which I told him he was divesting people of responsibility for their bad behavior by laying it all on the Devil; and he countered by claiming his perspective was egalitarian because the Devil could inhabit anyone, so that each of us can feel that "there but for the grace of God go I."

I discovered only later that *The Castle in the Forest* contained another bit of Maileresque teasing at least partly directed at me. In an epilogue not included in the galleys I had read, he tells of a fictional American Jewish psychiatrist, "a pacifist by temperament," who interviews a former Nazi intelligence officer and then kills him. Norman was imagining the vengeful rage he thought I should have experienced, the "killer" who resides "in the depths of the average pacifist." Of course he understood that I could restrain my feelings because of my sense of carrying out an important professional project. But he also knew of my strong aversion to violence (though I am not a pacifist), which was part of what he was mocking. Still, in terms of my underlying emotions, he may have been on to something.

Norman also told me that, whatever one thinks of his ideas, the novel is at least "a little different," unlike those of other writers who "mainly tell us what we know." It was certainly that, and when I later wondered about modern novels that might have influenced him I thought of Thomas Mann's *Doctor Faustus*, which drew upon the Faust legend of voluntarily surrendering one's soul to the Devil as a way of helping us grasp the Nazi effort to conquer time and death ("Dar[ing] to be barbaric, twice barbaric indeed"). I found Mann more convincing than Mailer. But I am certain that not even Mann could have brought the Devil and his associates to my study in a way that Mailer did in rendering our Wellfleet dialogue a transcendent moment.

Norman died a little more than a year after that Wellfleet meeting. BJ and I drove with our friends Larry Shainberg and Vivian Bower in the funeral cortege as it circled through and around Provincetown on the way to the grave. The night before, Norman's body had been displayed in an open casket. The embalming made him look ridiculously clean and pure, even beatific. Several people dismissed what they saw as having nothing to do with the actual person. But I felt it to be Norman nonetheless. This was what Norman would have looked like had he been a saint, Norman as a parody of sainthood, Norman still playing games. I was not ready to lose him. I looked at him and said—silently and impatiently—"Norman, get up and talk to me!"

20

_____

Full Circle

THROUGHOUT THE WELLFLEET meetings, and over the decades, the four studies described in this book have continued to reverberate within me. Insights from them have moved beyond Hong Kong and China, Hiroshima, the Vietnam War, and the Nazi movement. I have found them all too relevant for the unfolding history of the late twentieth and early twenty-first centuries, for interactions between individual psychology and larger history, and for our understanding of the far reaches of the human psyche.

I sought to make those larger connections in two theoretical books, *The Broken Connection* and *The Protean Self*. I began work on the issues they explore as early as the mid-sixties, though I did not publish them until years later. The two books became a bridge between my research and the world beyond.

The Broken Connection

The Broken Connection emerged initially from my efforts to make conceptual sense of what I had encountered in Hiroshima. But it grew to be something much more ambitious, close to a psychohistorical interpretation of our era. The title referred to ways in which rhythms between life and death had been severed by technological killing and by the confusions of historical change (what I called "psychohistorical dislocation"). Its subtitle, "On Death and the Continuity of Life," referred to the model or paradigm I suggested for psychological work—the organizing principle, the lens or prism, for behavior in general. That was a shift from the traditional psychoanalytic model of instinctual drives and psychological defenses against those drives. The subtitle also suggested the book's impossible reach, the application of my model to all levels of experience. I tried to show how death-and-life continuity, or related imagery, entered into basic emotions over the course of the life cycle, all of the major psychiatric syndromes, and the collective behavior of groups and nations.

I was saying that our struggle with the knowledge of death, and our need for connection and continuity in the face of that knowledge, provided the psychological motor for ordinary life, psychological disturbance, and the larger flow of history. At whatever level, we struggle with death or symbolic endings, and seek new beginnings that sustain individual and shared vitality. At the historical level I was concerned with lapses into totalism, victimization, and violence, as opposed to more open structures affirming life continuity. I also took my first systematic plunge into nuclear psychology: into ways in which the weapons affected individual psychology and threatened our sense of continuous human life (or symbolic immortality); and into motivations for using the weapons in Hiroshima and Nagasaki, including vignettes of such major actors as Robert Oppenheimer, Harry Truman, and Henry Stimson and their specific vulnerabilities to the psychological disorder I called *nuclearism*. My own inner doubts about my capacity to do all this were reflected in the epigraph I chose from Theodore Roethke: "Last night I dreamt of a jauntier principle of order; / Today I eat my usual diet of shadows."

I received help from a surprising direction. Freud made a prominent reappearance in my work with his pithy observations about death and its relation to cultural forces, even if I always had to translate from his instinctual language (the "death instinct" or "death drive") to one of symbolization, which is a language of creation and re-creation of images, ideas, forms, and feelings. Paradoxically, the master came most alive for me after I had left the Boston Psychoanalytic Institute, where he had been so slavishly adhered to. Now I no longer concerned myself with agreeing or disagreeing with his concepts and could instead engage him freely in terms of the relevance of his ideas to my own work. No wonder that my friend Cathy Caruth, a close student of psychoanalysis and its relation to trauma, could speak of *The Broken Connection* as "a post-Hiroshima dialogue with Freud." It was also an exploration of my general intellectual relationship to psychoanalysis and psychiatry.

Another figure who made a prominent appearance was Otto Rank. One of the few in the early Freudian circle concerned about death-related issues, Rank was later to write about "irrational immortality systems" and of man's need, in the face of death, "to maintain his spiritual self." While I disagreed with Rank about the "irrationality" of our need for a sense of immortality, his discussions of death and immortality were invaluable to me in developing ideas in an area of thought that has been strikingly neglected by psychological theorists.*

In learning more about Otto Rank I began to picture him with Beate (or "Tola," as her friends called her) as central figures in that odd assemblage of analysts surrounding Freud during the early decades of the twentieth century. No one was closer to Freud than Otto, while Beate, whom I had only known in her sixties, was also much admired by Freud as a knowledgeable, lively, and beautiful young woman whom he sometimes called upon to serve as his hostess. That image gave me a sense that my analyst had been, so to speak, present at the creation, which in turn meant that I had a certain relationship to those psychoanalytic origins. My sense of pride was mixed with a feeling of being ancient (Do I really go back that far into prehistory?).

The cosmic reach of *The Broken Connection* led to another standing joke between BJ and myself. She and I could be discussing a psychological or historical issue, whether separation anxiety in children or collective social confusions, and I would mention what I wrote about it in that book. Soon, in response to just about any question that arose, large or small, one

---

*Of course I wondered how much my interest in Rank had been influenced by my having been analyzed by his former wife and the mother of his daughter. The matter was a bit more complicated as they had divorced and gone their separate ways psychoanalytically: she had remained a classical Freudian while he had rebelled from Freud's nurturing control in a way painful to both men and had gone on to create an important body of original work. Given the paucity of psychoanalytic concepts having to do with death-and-life continuity, I might well have come to Rank in any case, but having shared my intimate thoughts over a couple of years with a woman who bore his name had to enter into the equation.

of us would grandly declare: "Just look it up in *The Broken Connection*!" The little joke, at least from my side, represented a mixture of pride (in having at least attempted the cosmic undertaking) and self-mockery (in realizing the absurdity of the attempt).

The Broken Connection was in some ways a more professional book than my others, and was reviewed mostly by psychiatrists, psychoanalysts, and social theorists. Though it was well received and has never gone out of print, I've had the sense that it's been more respected than read. I have thought of trying to publish a somewhat reduced version, though I have also wondered whether that wouldn't be a cowardly retreat from the very boldness of the book's projection. I know of course that these are little more than the ruminations of a would-be innovator who wants his work to be more influential than it has been.

Throughout *The Broken Connection* I was trying to apply what Ernst Cassirer called the "new dimension of reality," that of the symbolizing principle, of inwardly re-creating all we perceive, to the ultimate psychological and historical arena of life and death. That is what I told Jacques Lacan when the eccentric French psychoanalyst made a visit to Yale in the seventies, during which his hosts found themselves divided as to whether he was a genius or a madman. At a small dinner seminar, midst a bilingual babble of tongues, Lacan consistently stressed the centrality of symbolization. I suggested that the logic of his emphasis should lead him away from the Freudian paradigm of instinct and defense as an organizing principle for human behavior, and toward the more encompassing model of symbolization of life and death.

Lacan turned to the attractive young woman who served as translator and helper, asked who I was, and when told my name declared histrionically, "Je suis Liftonian!" He explained that he completely agreed with me about symbolization and the life-death dimension but that his "intellectual formation" still held him to Freud's model. Lacan was of course a considerable performer and there was playfulness, mockery, and self-mockery in his declaration—but also, I thought, an element of enthusiasm about what I had said.*

---

*There was a sequel to the conversation. Since Lacan had achieved high guru status in Paris and elsewhere, all such exchanges were duly recorded more or less verbatim in a widely circulated newsletter, and that resulted in periodic visits from Lacanians who

The "new dimension of reality" I tried to express in *The Broken Connection*, then, had to do with both the symbolizing process and the centrality of death imagery in the way we live our lives. Although I explored patterns of totalism, violence, and nuclearism, the book was not without hope. I wrote also of the formidable human struggle for a sense of human continuity, our efforts at life-symbolizing behavior that involved connection, movement and change, and integration. And at the book's completion I spoke of our ever-present potential as human beings for awareness, which at its most profound means "the ability to anticipate and realize danger on the one hand and the capacity for knowledge and transcendent feeling on the other." When I added that "our increasing capacity for awareness gives direction to our life-symbolizing process," and that "we live on images and the images shift," I was initiating the argument of *The Protean Self.*

The Protean Self

I first used the word *protean* to describe the self-fluctuations of Japanese university students I interviewed in the early sixties, with reference to Proteus, that notoriously shape-shifting Greek sea god. But as far back as the mid-fifties I had noted impressive combinations of dislocation and resilience in Chinese whom I interviewed in Hong Kong after their fleeing the Mainland. I thought it striking that such fluidity could occur in people from East Asian cultures, which we tend to think of as highly traditional and unyielding in their institutions and symbol systems. I had a lot to learn about the vulnerability of every kind of culture to the psychological as well as physical assaults of the twentieth and twenty-first centuries—but also about sources of resilience.

I came to understand three dimensions of proteanism: the self's capacity to change and transform itself; its potential for "odd combinations" of seemingly unlikely or even antithetical elements; and its overall varia-

---

assumed that he and I had more in common than we actually did—that if Lacan were a "Liftonian," then Lifton must be a Lacanian.

tions, so that particular cultures, subcultures, or groups can be made up of very different kinds of people. None of that now seems remarkable, but these tendencies have been far from prominent in much of human experience. I came to understand proteanism as itself historically created, a product in our time of the dislocations of change, the mass media and information revolutions, and our reaction to imagery of extinction. In that sense I came to see proteanism as a modus vivendi for the historical and psychological flux of our era.

But as proteanism came to inhabit my work, I was constantly learning more about its nuances and how it functioned. For instance, I returned regularly from Yale to Cambridge, Massachusetts, to discuss proteanism in sessions of David Riesman's course on American society. At the end of one such session, while sitting and talking in Dave's office, he surprised me by saying: "Bob, I've been thinking about what you say about prote-anism, and find it an interesting concept. But looking at you personally, I wonder. You're a dedicated scholar, consistent in your work habits and in your development of ideas, you have a long marriage and a regular fam-ily life—so where's the proteanism?" I had to smile, and then answered, "It's in my imagination, Dave." (I could have mentioned my unorthodox research studies and idiosyncratic career, but I didn't.) It was serious ban-ter, and I realized that Dave was on to something important, having to do with seeming contradictions as well as limits in connection with pro-teanism. Not long after that I had another encounter that raised similar questions for me. At a large reception during a conference, a graduate student I didn't know confronted me in a New York/sixties manner so brash as to be almost charming: "Hey, Lifton, I tried to be a protean man, and it doesn't work." Again I smiled, this time perhaps with a little more uneasiness. I told him that proteanism was not an absolute—one didn't have to be changing or reconfiguring one's psyche every day—but rather a *tendency* of the self. That was true enough, but I knew it to be only the beginning of an answer.

I thought of an essay I had read some time before by Lewis Mumford, the American critic and humanist, on the subject of Freud and Jung. He told how each man in lonely isolation (Freud late at night in his study, Jung in his mystical tower) spun out the wildly imaginative ideas that were to have so profound an impact on the twentieth century. Yet each of them, Mumford emphasized, met with his patients the next day. Mumford was saying what had come out in my conversations with Dave and the graduate student. To innovate and carry through one's proteanism, to maintain a grounded imagination, one requires a certain core of stability within the self. Considering Freud in particular, it would be hard to find a greater creature of habit, whether in his Victorian family life, his systematic work with patients, his compulsive letter writing during brief breaks in his schedule, his late-night literary efforts, and even in his August walking and working vacations. Rather than conflict with his more fluid imagination, that orderliness and conventionality helped make it possible.

As for me, my plunges into unusual studies have required a more orderly component for reimagining my material through many redraftings for each of my books, and an otherwise anchored life. Conflicts in going about that tandem have never disappeared, but over time have mattered less.

There is another relevant essay, this one by the art historian John Berger, who spoke of "the moment of cubism" to describe the remarkable dialogue that took place from 1907 through 1914 between Pablo Picasso and Georges Braque and gave rise to that movement. That dialogue was also, at least for painting, a "moment of proteanism." I experienced two such historical moments of proteanism characterized by broad social and political experimentation and change: that of the sixties and seventies as mentioned earlier; and that of the "Velvet Revolution" in 1989–91 in Czechoslovakia, a term often used to include related uprisings in Eastern Europe and the Soviet Union.

BJ and I were able to make trips to Czechoslovakia in 1990 and 1991 to talk to people about their experience in the nonviolent transformations that had occurred in their country, and I included a brief segment titled "Proteus in Prague" in my book on the protean self. Those I interviewed told of expanding as individuals, of engaging in activities they had never imagined themselves able to perform, in mounting a collective rebellion while innovating every step of the way. A young journalist, and sometime musician, previously footloose and undependable, gained great general respect by steadily and courageously editing and publishing a leading underground journal. A writer was left without a livelihood when her magazine was shut down by the regime; she found a job in a mental hospital, where the uninhibited expression of patients inspired her to write more freely and reenergize her commitment to the opposition; she eventually became an advisor to Václav Havel, the leader of the opposition movement and eventual president. Of course, the Velvet Revolution required a man like Havel, who combined many-sided literary gifts with great personal courage and endured four years of imprisonment. But many in Prague, like him (as I wrote at the time), "could realize aspects of the self that had before only been potential and, in the process, carve out new combinations of content and capacity."

I've always been drawn to twentieth-century novels, and that sensibility is surely bound up with my interest in proteanism. The novels themselves have taught me much more about the phenomenon. In *The Protean Self* I quote widely from James Joyce (who began his breakthrough novel *Ulysses* in 1914, chronicled in it a single day in 1904, and included a specific "Proteus episode") as having set a protean tone for twentieth-century literature. I referred also to subsequent American writers including Saul Bellow and Don DeLillo, and Indian-born novelists working in the West such as Bharati Mukherjee and Salman Rushdie. Bellow (in *Herzog* and other books) provided hilariously melancholy depictions of mid-twentieth-century protean (and antiprotean) Jewish seekers; DeLillo (in *White Noise* and *Mao II*) told of shifting realities and what he called "ambiguities, contradictions, whispers, hints" of existence; and Mukherjee (in *Jasmine*) wrote of how coming to America took her "out of God's sight" to a place where "we could say or be anything we wanted." The powerful proteanism of Rushdie's *Satanic Verses* has been almost overlooked in the ugly drama of the death threats it evoked, but the book, in Rushdie's own words, "celebrates hybridity, impurity, intermingling, the transformation that comes of new and unexpected combinations of human beings, cultures, ideas, politics, movies, songs." Indeed it was his spoof on religious fundamentalism that was responsible for those death threats.

My daughter Natasha (no mean novel devourer herself) couldn't help teasing me a bit about working on *The Protean Self*. Then in her early twenties, she said: "Dad, I think I understand why you are enjoying writing this book so much. It's mainly because you *really* like reading novels."

After all it was she who, some years earlier, had said to me (referring to the four studies featured in this volume): "Dad, have you ever considered taking up more cheerful subjects?" Well, now I finally had; proteanism was not always joyous, but a big improvement in that direction, notably in its stress on resilience and potential change. To be sure, I did draw upon interviews that Eric Olson and I had done in another context with people we called "innovative professionals," but now much of my research data could come from the kind of novels I was especially fond of. And the general focus of my book was that of life-enhancing imagination.

Still, not everyone was thrilled by the concept of the protean self, especially if my views on it were applied sympathetically to the rebellious young. As early as 1970, Dan Bell wrote to me that he had "come to a very opposite conclusion about youth," and preferred to view them through a "pathographic trajectory," one that interprets their behavior as psychologically abnormal and that he misleadingly attributed to Erik Erikson. And I can remember, when presenting the concept of proteanism at Suffolk University in England at about that time, a senior faculty person rising from the audience in anger and declaring that people with ideas like mine were responsible for the decline of Western civilization.

Erikson and Proteanism

Erik's responses were both more nuanced and more personal. His identity theory was meant to allow for considerable nonpathological search, but some of what I described as protean struggles could be viewed as troubled confusions surrounding identity that needed to be rectified. He undoubtedly perceived in my ideas on proteanism a critique, however respectful, of his more structured identity requirement. This bothered him more than my post-Hiroshima need to look elsewhere for concepts about death and death symbolism.

Characteristically, Erik spoke only indirectly. For instance, at the Wellfleet meetings he would often say something on the order of "You know, some time we must reexamine Bob's ideas"—which I and others understood to mean, recast them to become Eriksonian. And when I sent him, probably in the mid-seventies, a manuscript copy of an early paper on "protean man" (so titled prior to the days of gender sensitivity), I was told that he crossed out "man" and wrote "boy," to suggest that what I was describing applied only to adolescent psychological experiment.

But we remained friends, and Erik came to Wellfleet every year. A breakthrough in our relationship occurred when I articulated more carefully the connection of my work on proteanism to Erikson's identity theory in a little book I published in 1976, *The Life of the Self.* I described a shift in paradigm from Freud's theme of instinct and defense, to Erikson's focus on identity and the life cycle, to my own (and a few others') emphasis on death and the continuity of life. For me proteanism, with its continuous reconfiguring of life-death images, was part of that paradigm. I said, "While the enterprise requires that I emphasize points of departure from Erikson, his extensive influence on my work will be strongly evident," and also that I offered the volume "in a nonpolemical spirit of inquiry and acknowledgement, and in the belief that fidelity to one's mentors lies in the receptive confrontation and imaginative re-creation of their legacy."

Erik responded to the galleys I sent him with a long, thoughtful letter in which he praised the book, clarified some of his own views, and pointed to the few places where he thought I had misinterpreted his work. I was moved by the letter because I could perceive him to be transcending his own hurt and writing not only as a friend but as a generous colleague. A couple of years later, when I was visiting him at his California home in Tiburon (in Marin County, outside San Francisco), he stunned me by saying: "You know, Bob, I've been assigning your work on protean man to my students. I think it's one of the best things you've done." I felt like embracing him on the spot, but instead simply muttered something about being pleased that he felt that way and being aware that the work followed upon his own.

Indeed, I had always believed that identity theory was necessary to my concept of proteanism, even if the concept questioned some of that theory. Similarly, Erikson's work on identity required the existence of the very Freudian theory that he himself questioned. Freud's own early intellectual proteanism had given way, among many of his followers, to static antiprotean dogma. That sequence is always possible, and there were glimmers of it in connection with identity theory. And yes, even ideas about proteanism could become antiprotean in spirit if rendered a dogma (which is partly what that graduate student was trying to tell me). Here

I think of the words of the jazz clarinetist, saxophonist, and composer Sidney Bechet: "You know, there is this mood about the music, a kind of need to be moving. You just can't set it down and hold it. . . . You just can't keep the music unless you move with it."

"Moments of proteanism" always emerge from the circumstances of history (there were such moments earlier in the West in the Weimar era, the Enlightenment, and the Renaissance, and in East Asia in the Meiji Restoration and precommunist China). But I was also to discover that psychological *theory* about the self has had, and is still having, its historical moment: a movement away from traditional notions of fixity and stability toward an emphasis on multiplicity, psychic action, and change. When I first began writing about the protean self in the sixties, the concepts seemed to many a very radical psychological idea. But by the time I came around to publishing my book in 1993, American thinkers were in the midst of debates on modern and postmodern thought, and some were advocating that we jettison the concept of self altogether. So I was pleased when the cultural anthropologist Richard Shweder, in a *New York Times* review, characterized *The Protean Self* as a "responsible" version of postmodernism (a movement to which he was committed) in its focus on many-sidedness and even fragmentation while finding a way to retain a useful concept of self.

The psychologist Howard Gardner, reviewing the book elsewhere, did not agree, calling it bold and imaginative but unconvincing in its view of the self. Ten years later, however, Gardner made a point of telling me that he had changed his mind and had come to believe that the protean phenomenon very much existed. Putting aside modern and postmodern categories, I have long viewed proteanism as a kind of rescue operation for the self: a way of adapting to and sustaining imaginative thought amid the chaos of historical change and avoiding the attractions of fundamentalism. That view has been affirmed by the happy discovery that Internet theorists are invoking the protean concept to describe both the individual behavior of Web users and the kinds of communities they form. One pointed to my statement "Not just individual emotions but communities may well be free-floating, removed geographically and embraced temporarily and selectively, with no promise of permanence," and then added: "This is precisely the appeal of online social networking." Proteanism hardly resolves the great psychological dilemmas that surround online networking, but it does have something to say about our participation in it.

The Stuff of Dreams

Protean theory inevitably extended to dreams. Shifts and odd combinations of the self are bound to be reflected in that important realm. Some of my own dreams that I have mentioned have been protean in moving in a number of different directions while revealing what I think of as "the state of the mind" and its varied inclinations. In that sense Freud was only partially right in emphasizing hidden impulses and unacceptable desires, leaving out the prospective or forward-looking dimension of dreams. Free as they are from conscious requirements of logic, narrative, or "reality," their uninhibited symbolizing can take us to places where the waking mind is not ready to go. (Hence the tendency in many premodern cultures to associate dreams with shamanistic magic in foretelling the future.)

It is no surprise that I would view dreams in a multilevel fashion. One's dreams tend to confirm one's psychological worldview, so Freudians have Freudian dreams, Jungians Jungian dreams, and protean theorists protean dreams. But what may be surprising is the tendency of a protean theorist like myself to emphasize as well the primordial, physiological aspect of dreams. Neuroscientists have observed the REM (rapid eye movement) states associated with dreams in newborn infants and prehuman animals. Dreams are bound up with rudimentary physiology and represent the most primitive kind of mental function as well as the most advanced. That suggests to me an inherent biological basis for dreaming and for the open-ended symbolization that takes place in dreams.

That biological basis certainly exists for symbolization in general; with the development of the forebrain, human beings have no choice but to symbolize. As Langer and Cassirer have shown, we take nothing, so to speak, nakedly, from the environment but recast all that we perceive in endless psychic action. And contemporary neuroscientists have made similar points in discussing the phenomenon of "representation," of changing images created by the human forebrain and other brain areas.

I came to see the self as "an engine of symbolization as it continuously receives, recreates, and extends all that it encounters." That symbolizing engine can give rise to proteanism, to the construction and reconstruction of images in the service of multiplicity and change. The overall process takes place within a cultural matrix, but here as elsewhere biology and culture are so inseparable as to raise questions about two distinct categories. Given its link with both forebrain function and cultural shifts, proteanism is an ever-present potential in human behavior.

Proteanism includes a quest for moments of transcendence, so it was appropriate for me to complete my manuscript of the book during a half-year sabbatical in Hawaii in 1991–92. There I could experience something close to a continuous high state that included: my view of the Pacific from my study in our apartment near Diamond Head on Oahu, daily swims in a warm ocean, and ever available tennis matches on excellent public courts. BJ and I had long enjoyed a special relation to Hawaii, beginning with stops there during trips to Asia during the pre-jet era of the fifties and extending to intermittent talks at the university from the early seventies (including an intersession lectureship in 1971–72 on my work with antiwar veterans). We made trips to the various islands and experienced the whole area as a zone of pleasure.

Now that pleasure included outdoor dinners by the water with friends we made there: Reuel Denney (Dave Riesman's coauthor of *The Lonely Crowd*) and his wife, Ruth; Leon Edel (the Henry James biographer and student of life narratives) and his wife, Marjorie; and most especially John Holt, a part-Hawaiian writer deeply committed to preserving the culture and mythology of the islands, in which he still imaginatively dwelled, a man BJ and I had grown to love. John regaled us with stories of Polynesian gods and the exploits of the great king Kamehameha, while also asking us to share the sufferings of Queen Liliuokalani when she and her people were victimized by American imperialism and economic exploitation. But John could also combine his commitment to Hawaiian culture with an awareness of its contemporary proteanism, its blending of those origins with every imaginable expression of Polynesian, Asian, and Western influence, as immediately evident on the streets of Honolulu.

The Broken Connection, The Protean Self, and *The Life of the Self,* concerned as they are mainly with theory, have been more or less eclipsed by my more dramatic books on the destructive events described in this volume. All too understandably, I've been seen as a person who simply deals with such extremity and much less one with a love of ideas. In actuality I have been a psychological witness with a strong aspiration toward creating an interpretive narrative—a set of ideas—for that witness. Perhaps I fall among that fairly large contingent of people who would like the world to view them differently from the way it has: the journalist who wants to be a novelist, the classical actor with a longing to do farce—in my case, the recorder of disaster bent on creating a new psychological and historical perspective on the world. The larger truth, I believe, is that witness requires theory, but such theory must take shape from direct experience.

Reverberations from my four studies have never ceased. Unsurprisingly, most of those reverberations have been far from pleasant, but insights from the studies themselves have mattered. Consider first a few events, mostly in my own country, relevant to thought reform.

The Scourge of Totalism—American Thought Reform

There is an ugly coda to my thought reform work, and it has to do with an American embrace of what we are supposed to be against. Much has been written about this but I'll mention only situations in which I personally encountered American hunger for its own mind control.

In late 1962, soon after returning from Hiroshima and moving into our house in Woodbridge, Connecticut, I received a strange telephone call. The caller identified himself as a member of a "government agency" speaking from Fort Detrick, Maryland. He said that hc had read and admired my book *Thought Reform and the Psychology of Totalism* (which had been published the previous year) and thought it would be useful if I would consult with his agency about my work because "we often take prisoners ourselves." He was making it quite clear that what was wanted from me was instruction on how to apply thought reform to people taken into American custody.

I knew that American military and intelligence groups could be drawn to my work for that purpose but found it upsetting to receive an abrupt request to participate in Americanized thought reform. I had no hesitation about declining the caller's offer to consult with his agency (which I assumed to be the CIA) but was less certain about the words and tone with which to do that. So I behaved like an irritated academic, which in a sense I was. I chastised the caller for not having read my book carefully, telling him that if he had done so he would be aware of my opposition to thought reform–like practices on the part of anyone. I probably should have said more about ethical questions related to mind manipulation, but it was not the kind of phone call that encouraged reflective conversation. Indeed, once I made it clear that I would reject his invitation, we had little to say to one another and the phone call quickly ended. I was left with an unpleasant image of Americans seizing upon my work to make the cruelties I exposed in others their own.

I had a much more painful encounter with CIA mind manipulation through a person whose family had suffered grievously from it. Eric Olson, a psychologist and a man of great intellectual gifts, was my assistant in the early seventies, became a close colleague and friend, and collaborated with me on three books. He also did original work on a collage method of psychological evaluation and therapy, and a collage theory of the mind. Eric's father, Frank Olson, had worked in the bacteriological warfare program at Fort Detrick and had died suddenly and mysteriously in 1953. One day in 1975 Eric telephoned me in an agitated state with the news that the Rockefeller Commission investigating the CIA's domestic activities had revealed that his father had been made an unwitting subject of an LSD experiment by the CIA and had soon afterward jumped to his death from a New York City hotel room.

Eric has since spent decades pursuing information about what was actually done to his father, and has found convincing evidence that he did not jump but was pushed to his death by a CIA operative. In any event, the CIA was surely responsible for the death of Frank Olson and made use of a crude experiment that was part of its quest for methods of mind control. Much has subsequently been documented about this CIA project called "Operation Artichoke" and then "MKULTRA," whose activities represented what has been called "the search for the Manchurian Candidate," for all-powerful "brainwashing" techniques. Eric's findings also suggested that his father had a CIA connection but had become disillusioned with American behavior and wanted to leave government work, creating fears in the agency that he would reveal damning information. The Ford administration, through an act of Congress, made a monetary settlement with the Olson family along with a public apology (arranged by Donald Rumsfeld and Dick Cheney, then running the White House) for having subjected Olson to the LSD experiment, all of which served to cover up the details of CIA behavior and its connection to Frank Olson. Eric's pain brought me much closer to the grotesque extremes of the CIA infatuation with mind control.

In 1988 I was able to reconnect with the issue as it arose in my own profession by testifying against the CIA in a case involving its support of the "brainwashing experiments" of the psychiatrist D. Ewen Cameron in Canada in the 1950s and '60s. I had been in touch with Harvey Weinstein, a young Canadian psychiatrist who had taken up the issue because his father, while ostensibly being treated for a mild depression, had been victimized by these experiments and had his life virtually destroyed. I would later write an introduction for the American edition of Weinstein's book *Psychiatry and the CIA: Victims of Mind Control.*

The case in which I participated, mounted by the civil rights lawyer Joseph Rauh and his associate James Turner, involved nine Canadian plaintiffs, and there was more than enough documentation of their experience for me to find parallels between Cameron's experiments and thought reform. Cameron's work, encouraged and financially backed by the CIA, featured four components: "depatterning" by means of frequent severe electroshocks; "psychic driving" in the form of exposure to relentless repetition (sixteen hours a day for six to seven days) of portions of tapes containing painful experiences revealed by the patient and interpretations by psychiatrists; varying degrees of sensory deprivation; and the use of heavy narcotics to induce continuous sleep over seven to ten days in order to bring about repression of the overall process. I could refer not only to my work on thought reform but to that on Nazi doctors as well, pointing to the aura of legitimacy physicians could create while participating in highly destructive behavior.

The CIA lawyer took my deposition in my Wellfleet study and did not contest anything I said, as the agency sought to end its bad press on the issue by making a financial settlement. The atmosphere was sufficiently friendly for the CIA lawyer to ask my advice on a local seafood restaurant, but when he returned the next morning to complete the deposition he looked as though he himself had just been through Cameron's brainwashing experiments—pale, sluggish, and suffering from indigestion. I felt badly because I had recommended the restaurant (a good one that had never before made anyone I knew sick), but a side of me took a certain pleasure in this small embodiment of a CIA collapse. The settlement of $750,000 was made with the former patients later that year.

Details about Cameron himself suggested the corruptibility of psychiatric colleagues in the highest places when it came to the lure of thought reform. Cameron, who was born in Scotland but worked mostly in the United States and Canada, was at one time or another president of the American Psychiatric Association, the Canadian Psychiatric Association, and the World Psychiatric Association. He also had been part of the Nuremberg medical tribunal that examined the crimes of Nazi doctors, and one wonders whether he justified some such methods for himself if applied against a totalitarian system such as Soviet communism. Cameron was just one of a cadre of CIA-connected psychiatrists enlisted for Cold War–related mind control projects. I found it particularly satisfying to make use of my own work on thought reform to confront the abuses of those who sought their own version of the procedure.

Finally, there was a "smoking gun" brought to my attention in 2008 by journalists, a document revealing the direct use of Chinese "brainwashing" techniques by American interrogators at the Guantanamo Bay prison in Cuba. The briefing paper for the interrogators contained a completely unaltered list of Chinese communist methods as described in 1956 by an American social scientist, Alfred D. Biderman. To be sure, there had been earlier evidence of that policy reported in a series of *New Yorker* articles by Jane Mayer, who told how an American military program called SERE (Survival, Evasion, Resistance, Escape), initially used in preparing American soldiers for what they would encounter if captured, was turned on its head in teaching these techniques to American interrogators to break down "terrorist" prisoners.

Psychologists belonging to or consulting with the military were key designers of the turnabout. What was new was the verbatim copy of the Biderman summary of brainwashing techniques, which he characterized as torture, now meant specifically for American use. And what brought the matter especially close to home was my having been part of the symposium (the proceedings of which were published in the *Bulletin of the New York Academy of Medicine* in 1957) in which Biderman's original paper as well as one of my own were presented. The whole sequence was a melancholy confirmation of the interpretive point I expressed in my 1961 book to the effect that totalism and thought reform methods could be anyone's temptation. But I would still insist on the urgency of making use of our democratic right to expose such tendencies in our midst.

Religious Cults and the Eight Deadly Sins

My work on totalism could pop up in surprising places. In the late sixties and early seventies, about ten years after its publication, I began to hear that chapter 22 of my book on thought reform was emerging as an underground document for young people making their way out of American religious cults. They found the eight deadly sins discussed in that chapter to apply to the cultic environments. All of those themes—*milieu control, mystical manipulation, the demand for purity, the cult of confession, the sacred science, loading the language, doctrine over person,* and the *dispensing of existence*—could be present with suffocating intensity. I was told that the chapter was also used by "deprogrammers" hired by their parents to help the younger people extricate themselves mentally from these cults, partly by convincing them that they had been subjected to mind control rather than true Christianity. While I considered these themes to be fundamental, I had given little thought to where they might land.

In fact, those themes became an important part of an "anticult movement." I had considerable sympathy for the movement but could observe it to have excesses of its own. These included the promiscuous use of the label "cult" for idiosyncratic religious and secular groups, and the use of force by some deprogrammers to remove an unwilling person from a cultic group. That of course raised questions of civil liberties of young adults, and of the cultic groups themselves. I felt myself under a certain amount of pressure from both sides: from former cult members and their parents and the anticult movement in general to denounce the "brain-washing" that occurred in cults; and from members of cultic groups and civil libertarians to denounce the misuse of my work by those depro-grammers who violated the rights of young people. I had my own inner conflicts. My allergy to totalism had not diminished, and I was aware of the danger of cultic coercion and violence. I also detested the thought reform–like measures in cults that produced robotlike behavior in many members. But the issue of civil liberties always loomed large with me in a personal way, having taken activist public stands on behalf of small and vulnerable antiwar and antinuclear movements.

My struggles with the problem were reflected by strong friendships on each side of the divide. Margaret Thaler Singer became what could be called the dean of the anticult psychologists, generous and nurturing in her work with people who had been damaged by cultic involvements. I had known Margaret since the late fifties as not only an authority on thought reform or "brainwashing" (she and I testified together at the Patricia Hearst trial) but also a leading researcher in the use of psycho-logical tests to detect schizophrenia. Margaret went a bit further than I did in some of her anticult advocacies—perhaps understandably, as she and her husband had to take elaborate security measures for their home in the face of threats of violence from members of fanatical cults—but I admired her work, trusted her, and wrote an introduction to her impor-tant book on the subject, *Cults in Our Midst*.

At the same time I have been equally friendly with the theologian Har-vey Cox, who has been a leading figure among supporters of "new reli-gions," insisting on full freedom of spiritual practice, all the more so when eccentric or unpopular. In our continuous dialogue, we have not so much disagreed as had different emphases: mine on the dangers of totalism, his on the dangers of suppressing religious experience by labeling it as cultic. But we have been supporters of each other's work, and Harvey has been a periodic participant at the Wellfleet meetings. In 2007 he and I gave a course at Harvard Divinity School on the subject of evil (my contribution of course having much to do with my work on Nazi doctors) in which we could explore together nuances as well as extremes in ethical violations.

Cultic behavior during the 1970s touched off waves of social hysteria, containing as it did primal struggles between parents and their children, and fanaticism that could lead to fatal violence in the name of absolute virtue. Whatever my concerns about totalism, I did not want to be consumed by that hysteria to a degree that would interfere with my work on Vietnam, nuclear weapons, and later Nazi doctors. So I avoided formal connection with either anticult groups or new-religion advocates. But it was important for me to spell out my position, which I was able to do in an article I wrote in the late seventies for a Berkeley conference on "The Law and the New Religious Movements." On the much disputed question of terminology, I argued that groups should be called *cults* when they met three specific criteria: the increasing transfer of worship from original spiritual principles to the person of an omnipotent guru; the extensive use of thought reform–like methods; and a tendency toward idealism from below and extreme exploitation, mostly economic and sexual, from above. I applied my eight totalistic principles but urged that both psychiatrists and theologians "avoid playing God" in imposing simple solutions to what was a large social issue. I stressed that civil liberties were "as necessary for people who do nasty things as for those who do nice things"—as long as those nasty things did not involve lawbreaking in the form of fraud, violence, or bringing about physical or psychological harm. Concerning the spread of cultic behavior in America and elsewhere, I suggested as causes the broad "psychohistorical dislocation" accompanying the breakdown of many cultural forms as well as widespread imagery of extinction associated with nuclear weapons.

Over time, thoughtful people in both camps came to common ground, recognizing that idiosyncratic expressions of religious worship had to be protected but that intervention was necessary when cultic groups harmed their members or engaged in violence. Of course confusions remained, as did various forms of excess, but the whole issue was cruelly clarified in November 1978 when a charismatic, sometimes mad guru of an American cult called People's Temple orchestrated the suicide and murder (more the latter, as it turned out) of more than nine hundred members in a jungle clearing in the South American state of Guyana to which the group had fled from California. The poison, a mixture of cyanide and Kool-Aid, was prepared by the group's physician, evoking images of both

Auschwitz and counterculture extremity. After that it was hard to ignore my and others' emphasis on the potentially lethal expressions of the totalism of such cultic groups.

But there could be nuances, as in the case of a poignant young man I'll call George who had spent about a year in a cultic group on the West Coast. His parents had played an important part in his leaving the group, and all three had been influenced by my chapter 22. I talked to George separately and made it clear that I would focus on his needs and struggles. He plunged quickly into a detailed description of the appealing life he led in the cult—close communal existence in the form of eating and praying together, participating with the group in various kinds of religious study and practice as well as physical work, and the presence of an omniscient guru who cared for everyone and answered all questions. He said he had left mainly because of his parents' persuasion, but that did not mean he was without his own doubts. He seemed to want to suppress those doubts but at the same time was eager to explore with me his overall experience with the group.

Toward the end of our talk he asked me, quite simply, what I thought about all he had told me. Now I experienced a certain conflict of my own. I abhorred the cultic components he described, but I could perceive his deep satisfaction in an environment he mostly portrayed as idyllic. So I told him that I could understand the attraction of the strong communal support he received there, but that I was wary of any group or guru that exerted such control over individual minds. We had a brief additional discussion about the nature of totalism and the possibilities for more open environments. And he responded enthusiastically to my suggestion that we have a few more sessions together during which we could explore these matters more fully.

But that was never to happen. I learned from his parents that they had taken him, more or less against his wishes, to an intense debriefing meeting of former cult members, where he felt confused, agitated, and resentful. He then fled back to his cult, and I was told further that, when boarding his bus, he was observed by a friend to be carrying my thought reform book in his hand. That made the narrative sound almost too melodramatic, but I was learning that movements of young people in and out of cults were full of just that kind of melodrama.

George's in-between state resembled that of the French physician who, in his confused transition between a Chinese Communist prison and the noncommunist world outside, asked me whether I was "standing on the people's side or the imperialists' side." Deprived of the space he required to inwardly absorb the transition, George took the direction he associated with safety. But that did not mean that the doubts that had been previously intensified by chapter 22 would not surface again in his mind, or that the cult would be his last stop. I did hear from many others over the years that the chapter had opened their eyes to what they had been put through, helped them leave a particular cult, changed their lives. It was gratifying to discover that a chapter in my book on Chinese thought reform could serve as a lifeline for people making their way out of a very different but nonetheless totalistic environment.

Living the Apocalyptic—and Destroying the World

My forays into the psychology of extremity came to include Aum Shinrikyo, the Japanese religious cult, which was not the most murderous group I have encountered in my work (though it did kill people) but surely the weirdest. I began to hear a lot about Aum when I was in Japan in the fall of 1995 (for the purpose of giving workshops to Japanese psychological professionals on helping victims of the Kobe earthquake). I found the media to be obsessed with the shock this small group had caused the entire Japanese nation with its outbreak of terror and violence, including the release of deadly sarin gas on five Tokyo subway trains earlier that year. How could I not be fascinated by a group that managed to incorporate strong elements of all four of the earlier studies discussed in this memoir? Aum was not only totalistic in the extreme but its members lived in an apocalyptic realm in which Armageddon was more real than anything in the present; they were obsessed with nuclear and other ultimate weapons, not just as they existed in the world but as potential possessions of their own, and a contingent of young scientists among them succeeded in producing crude versions of chemical and biological weapons; their approach to the world at large echoed the notorious statement by an American soldier in Vietnam after the burning down of a Vietnamese village, "We had to destroy it in order to save it"; and they had parallels to the Nazis (whom the guru openly admired), including the enlisting of physicians and other professionals to apply their skills to killing.

The sarin release killed just thirteen people, but had the Aum scientists produced a more purified form of the deadly gas, casualties could have been in the hundreds of thousands. While the sarin attack was a reaction to police closing in on the violent cult, it was also part of Aum's larger apocalyptic scenario: producing a great catastrophe in Tokyo, which would involve Japanese and then American military forces and initiate World War III; which would in turn bring about a postnuclear biblical Armageddon, with the world and its inhabitants entirely destroyed except for an Aum remnant; which would give rise to a new and spiritually puri-fied humanity. Aum's guru, Shōkō Asahara, and his disciples were suf-ficiently bound to this mad apocalyptic logic for them to plunge into a mini-version of world destruction.

In my work on Aum I learned that the ancient rabbis encountered such apocalyptic activism on the part of groups who wished to hasten the com-ing of the messiah by contributing to the violence that would precede his appearance. This behavior was called "forcing the end" and the rabbis had the good sense to reject it with the argument that only God could set the messiah's timetable. But Asahara and Aum showed no such restraint. Their behavior suggested to me a new temptation, created by the very existence of nuclear weapons, for megalomaniac gurus or politicians to "force the end."

Interviews with ten former Aum members gave me a direct sense of the bizarreness of the "mystical experiences" that they underwent while in an altered state of consciousness, induced by the guru either through the deoxygenation of heavy breathing exercises or by drugs such as LSD. A soft-spoken young man I called "the gentle Armageddonist" described to me in detail how he found himself "actually going through reincarna-tion," experiencing "what is called nothingness," merging with the guru to the extent that he could no longer tell who was asking and who was answering questions, and witnessing Armageddon itself with "great fires" and "parts of the earth sinking into the ocean" while he and a few Aum comrades calmly performed their religious practices. A young woman told me how her merger with the guru was brought about by using a headset that gave her access to his brain waves, and how her mystical experiences convinced her of the Aum principle of *Poa*, in which the killing of a person of low spiritual attainment by one who is spiritually evolved was justified because it rid the world of the "bad karma" of the person killed, who would in any case benefit by receiving a more favorable rebirth. Neither of these young people could be called mentally ill. They both functioned quite efficiently in living out the moral insanity of the guru-centered Aum vision, including involvement not just in religious practices but also in varied commercial enterprises of the cult. Asahara too was quite functional during most of Aum's existence, displaying in fact considerable talent in his teaching of early Buddhism and yoga and in organizing and manipulating followers during most of Aum's ten years of existence. Like other extremist gurus, he was vulnerable to paranoid psychotic breakdown, which could be precipitated by his rejection by former followers. From the interviews I was struck by how extreme the imposed norms of a totalistic environment could become.

Throughout the work I benefited from and greatly enjoyed close collaboration with Manabu Watanabe, an eminent Japanese religious scholar who did everything from interpreting interviews to guiding me through the complexities of old and new Japanese religion. During one of the five trips I made to Japan to conduct the research, we even found time to take advantage of a meeting close to the world-renowned pottery center at Mashiko to indulge ourselves in a passion we shared for this remarkable Japanese artistic cum folkcraft tradition.

I found awakened in me a special form of energy I seemed to experience in connection with intense interview work. When I presented some of my findings at our City University center, Chuck Strozier commented that he had not seen me so galvanized by research since my work on Nazi doctors. Aum made me aware of the apocalypticism—the impulse toward world destruction in the service of renewal—that could lurk behind any totalistic movement. I also retain a sense of dark wonder at the far reaches of the human psyche.

Proteanism Versus Totalism

Aum's self-enclosed environment was the essence of totalism, or of its religious manifestation of fundamentalism. It was the very opposite of the fluidity, multiplicity, and changeability of proteanism. But I was interested to learn that, despite their totalism, Asahara and his disciples could themselves be innovative and many-sided, whether in their combining Hindu, Buddhist, and Christian doctrine, their use of imaginative business practices, or their ways of blending science and religion. That suggested to me—and there was much evidence elsewhere—that there could be back-and-forth tendencies of proteanism and fundamentalism, in groups and within the individual psyche. There is also much evidence that fundamentalist impulses are responses to protean experimentation: the term *fundamentalism* itself, which appeared early in the twentieth century in connection with American Protestantism, emerged from efforts of some church leaders to stem the tide of religious liberalism in order to retain what they considered the "fundamentals" of Christianity. Such fundamentalist impulses can readily give rise to an ideology of return to a utopian past in which no such threats to fundamentals existed, a past of perfect harmony that never was. That same response to protean experiment can include fear, a hunger for order, and violent anger at those who are seen as threats to or destroyers of "fundamentals."

The Hiroshima Imprint—and the World of Survivors

If my research on thought reform and totalism established my way of living and working, my Hiroshima study was the shock that permanently changed my way of relating to the world. Images from that city became the prism through which I viewed everything else—whether it was conflicts between nations and groups, political violence of any kind, and even psychological struggles of individual people. Hiroshima's imprint led me in two related directions. The first was that of envisioning and combating nuclear annihilation and joining others in efforts to do so. The other direction had to do with the psychology of survivors and the special knowledge they may have acquired. I did not mean knowledge to be applied to "survivalism," a movement advocating preparations to live through an anticipated nuclear holocaust. That movement seemed futile in the extreme and could itself become associated with apocalypticism and violence (as in the case of Aum Shinrikyo and various American survivalist groups). Rather, I became concerned with the effects upon people of experiencing destructive events and how their understanding of their ordeal might help us to avoid the recurrence of such events and contribute more generally to our knowledge of human behavior.

All this began with *hibakusha* and they became my template for survivor explorations. But for some time I had difficulty integrating the various aspects of their experience and generalizing from it. I can remember a key moment when things seemed to come together. I was at a midwestern airport back in 1966—probably O'Hare in Chicago but I'm not sure—making a connection to Detroit to speak at a Wayne State University symposium on "massive psychic trauma." The other participants had mostly worked with Jewish survivors of the Holocaust, and having read much of their work I was to compare the two experiences. I sat down in the airport waiting room and looked over my notes but found them lacking in the kind of unifying principles I was after. As I reimagined the experience of Hiroshima survivors and of inmates in Nazi death camps, five general themes came to mind—none of them starkly new but all contributing to a general structure or grid of survivor response. I quickly wrote them down on the back of an envelope and then transferred them to the notes for my talk. Those five themes, however quirkily arrived at, came to anchor my work on survivors: the comparison of the effects of the two holocausts I was to make at the end of *Death in Life*, as well as subsequent work I did with survivors of such varied events as the Vietnam War, the man-made flood at Buffalo Creek, West Virginia, in 1972, the leak of nuclear materials at Three Mile Island in Pennsylvania in 1979, and even the experience of individual people in the death of someone close to them.

The themes have always seemed quite obvious to me, and do not surprise those who have worked with survivors. But they may be unusual in that each includes residual pain as well as potentially useful experience. The first, the *death imprint*, is an indelible image that condenses the full horror of the disaster but can also be a source of energy in pursuing life-enhancing goals. The second theme, that of *death guilt*, has to do with self-blame or even self-condemnation for remaining alive or failing to do more to help others (however impossible that might have been), but can be transformed into a sense of responsibility or what I call animating guilt. The third, *psychic numbing*, is necessary for remaining physically and mentally alive, but can also lead to longer-term struggles with feeling and not feeling, sometimes associated with withdrawal or depression. It can also enable the survivor to be a student of his own disaster. The fourth, that of *suspicious vigilance* (I've sometimes called it *suspicion of counterfeit nurturance*), can significantly impair human relationships but can also clarify what is authentic and basic in one's own life. I have especially emphasized the fifth theme, *the quest for meaning*, the need for a significant narrative of one's experience. That quest can be impaired and leave one stuck in a permanent sense of victimization—but can also give rise to a commitment to bear witness and to other life-enhancing efforts. These can include a *survivor mission* of combating disease or destructiveness. I found the struggle for meaning to be the most encompassing theme in the survivor experience and to contain its potential wisdom. The bodily knowledge survivors acquire is inseparable from the meaning they give to their ordeal.

In connection with Hiroshima I myself started out as what I came to call a "historical survivor," one affected by large events from a distance. But taking in the suffering of *hibakusha* brought me closer to the actual experience. Only later did I come to realize how much the survivor ethos has continued to inhabit me. It has led me to join the survivor mission of *hibakusha*, former Auschwitz inmates, and Vietnam veterans in writing and agitating against nuclear weapons, genocide, and American warmaking. Erik Erikson once told me that I was "a Jew who has heard the Christian message." While he may have been ignoring a Jewish tradition of social justice, he was picking up on my participation in the kind of survivor mission often associated with Christian religious narratives having to do with passionate expression of individual conscience on behalf of universal goals.

I was also to discover that the survivor experience could be a source of proteanism. Vietnam veterans in particular, as they revealed in our rap groups, could emerge from grotesque death encounters to experiment boldly with their sense of self, with new beliefs and attitudes toward their country, and with their changing love relationships. Putting it simply, survivors undergo a breakdown of inner form and meaning and can respond by either opening out or closing down. Those Vietnam veterans who managed to open out were encouraged by the overall experimental atmosphere of the sixties and the seventies. I had to remind myself that two thousand years earlier, a warrior named Ulysses had done pretty much the same thing. No wonder that James Joyce chose that warrior as a model and namesake for his very protean protagonist; and that Primo Levi, whose nuanced writings as an Auschwitz survivor have meant a great deal to me, closely identified himself with Ulysses as a kind of alter ego or second self.

Prophetic Survivors

Survivors can also experience their death encounter as a source of artistic energy. In an essay I wrote in the late seventies called "Survivor as Creator," I gave the examples of Albert Camus (in the French Resistance), Kurt Vonnegut (witnessing the Allied bombings of Dresden), and Günter Grass (experiencing the Nazi era). That is what Heinrich Böll meant by his maxim (mentioned earlier) "The artist carries death within him like a good priest his breviary."

But I have had a special interest in a particular group of survivors, not usually considered such, the scientists and military men who experienced together the test explosion of the atomic bomb at Alamogordo, New Mexico, on July 16, 1945. Their reaction was essentially that of profound awe frequently expressed in religious terms: "the brightest light . . . anyone has ever seen"; "The sun can't hold a candle to it!"; and Robert Oppenheimer's associations to the Hindu epic the Bhagavad Gita in recalling "the radiance of a thousand suns" and the phrase "I am become death, the shatterer of worlds." There was awe even in the irreverent responses, "Now we are all sons of bitches!" and "What a *thing* we've made!"

Those earliest atomic witnesses experienced a form of conversion in the desert, which could take them either way. A few (notably Edward Teller) became acolytes of the weapon itself, embracing the "thing" as a deity and succumbing to ardent forms of nuclearism. But others (Leo Szilard, Philip Morrison, and George Kistiakowsky) were converted to a mission of heading off world destruction and sustaining human life, spurred by their own culpability in having produced the dreadful entity. Or they could picture a world-destroying explosion in their minds, as in the case of Eugene Rabinowitz, who later wrote: "In the summer of 1945, some of us walked through the streets of Chicago vividly imagining the sky suddenly lit up by a giant fireball, the steel skeletons of skyscrapers bending into grotesque shapes . . . until a great cloud of dust rose and settled onto the crumbling city." From such survivor-like experiences, these men created what became known as the "scientists' movement," which initiated antinuclear sentiment throughout the world and was the inspiration for the later doctors' movement. I came to see that the first atomic bomb test, in actuality and in prior imagination, led to the beginnings of survivor wisdom. I thought of that group as prophetic survivors of the weapon they themselves had created.

Vietnam and Knowledge of War

For me and for many Americans, Vietnam was a terrible example of a wrongheaded war that took our country to a realm of murderous atrocity. But over time it also became a more general model of war-making, especially American war-making. Howard Zinn had addressed us at Wellfleet in connection with opposition to the Vietnam War, but his message was that even World War II, a "good war" (opposing evil and ending in victory), produced atrocity. I heard the same message after giving a talk in New York in the seventies on Vietnam. A tall, middle-aged man whom I had never met but who somehow looked familiar came up to me and said: "Look, I was a Marine in the Pacific in the Second World War. There were lots of atrocities in that war, too—on both sides. We killed people we captured—they did, too—and there were many other terrible things that happened." He went on to say that those war experiences transformed his spiritual life and led him to become a clergyman. The man was Paul Moore, the Episcopal bishop who gained public prominence with his strong opposition to war and advocacy of social justice. (Years later he would become my friend, and I retain a powerful image of him in the pulpit of the Cathedral of St. John the Divine delivering a Christmas Eve sermon in which he declared, "America is the most dangerous country in the world!")

I came to think of World War II and Vietnam in this way. World War II veterans could feel: Our war was more filthy than people at home realized and we ourselves did ugly things. But it was a war we had to fight and win. Vietnam veterans, in contrast, were likely to feel: Ours was a grotesque war—everyone did ugly things. And it was all for nothing—a war that didn't have to be fought. These all-important differences in survivor meanings had to do with purpose and purposelessness, and they strongly affected the outlook of both groups of veterans. Looking closely at what war was like for Americans in Vietnam opened me to a more unsparing—and accurate—view of what has been called "America's last good war."

Of course Hiroshima became an important part of the equation. With Hiroshima the atrocity lay both in the dimensions and characteristics of the weapon and in its relation to the Allied policy of extensive victimization of civilians as part of "strategic bombing." I agreed that World War II had to be won. But I couldn't avoid the recognition that, in fighting the war those with the greater moral claim used a weapon so extreme that it threatens human civilization. I also realize that war, any war, creates a climate for genocide: World War II made possible the Nazi genocidal project just as World War I had facilitated the Turkish genocide of Armenians, and the Vietnam War had much to do with the Cambodian genocide.

Home from the War turned out to be my volume about not only Vietnam but also its larger significance for war and peace. For the 1985 edition I emphasized in a new introduction the healing power of the Vietnam Veterans Memorial in Washington, D.C., that four-hundred-foot-long, V-shaped wall of polished black granite sunk into the landscape next to the Lincoln Memorial and containing the names of some fifty-eight thousand Americans killed or missing in Vietnam. I found the Wall to be stark, heartbreaking, and completely appropriate—just the names, a place where veterans could go to quietly mourn.

By the time *Home from the War* was reissued in this century, I found myself applying its lessons to American war-making in the Persian Gulf. In my introduction to the 2005 edition I emphasized the enormous significance of survivor meanings that a country gives to any war, and the sustained conflict over such meanings that still existed for Vietnam. There was the broad understanding of it as strategically disastrous, morally wrong, and an argument for future military restraint—the meaning antiwar veterans were putting forward, and which I joined in disseminating. But an opposite meaning was provided by more belligerent historical survivors who viewed such military restraint as an expression of American weakness or what they called the "Vietnam syndrome." Hence, at the end of the Persian Gulf War in 1991, President George H. W. Bush's most ringing words had nothing to do with American virtue and glory but were "By God we've kicked the Vietnam syndrome once and for all." (Ironically, those of us who did psychological work with Vietnam veterans in the early seventies used a similar term, "post-Vietnam syndrome," to emphasize the pain and alienation that went with rejection of their war. But in contrast to Bush, we recognized the considerable wisdom in that "syndrome.") George W. Bush and his advisors were also intent on reversing American "Vietnam syndrome" and weakness when they initiated both a broad invasion of Afghanistan (instead of a limited action against Osama bin Laden), and the Iraq War itself. This focus on survivor meaning was a way of understanding the source of the truism that war begets war.

From the very beginning of the Iraq invasion of 2003, I thought of Vietnam. The key connection for me was that of the atrocity-producing situation. As different as the Iraq War was from that in Vietnam, there were striking parallels in the experience of American soldiers. Once the first round of military victories had occurred and the American occupation began, Iraq also became a counterinsurgency war in an alien, hostile environment where it was difficult to track down the enemy or to delineate combatants from civilians. As buddies were blown up by explosive devices and by the relatively new phenomenon of suicide bombers, soldier-survivors longed for a chance to get back at this hidden enemy, even to the extent of imagining his presence in almost any ordinary Iraqi civilian. I wrote about the part played by the atrocity-producing situation in American torture at Abu Ghraib prison and elsewhere, and in the overall experience of Americans in Iraq no less than it had in Vietnam.

I experienced a personal form of déjà vu in connection with Vietnam but it was a different historical moment and I was a different man. To be sure, there had been large protests in this country and throughout the world even prior to the 2003 invasion, but this was not the sixties or seventies when such protests could rend the whole society. That was partly because there was no military draft and the Iraq War was fought by volunteers, narrowing and limiting the group of immediate soldier-survivors, and partly because we were living less in an era of rebellion than one of historical backlash. Yet the emotions aroused in me felt eerily similar to those I had experienced in connection with Vietnam thirty-five years earlier.

Talking to Iraq veterans and to family members opposed to the war confirmed my sense of the relevance of the atrocity-producing situation, but also left me feeling a bit guilty. Something in me believed I should be again participating actively in rap groups and devoting my full energies to opposing the war. But by then I was in my late seventies, and while by no means standing quietly on the sidelines (I did write a few angry pieces), I was much less inclined to initiate such undertakings.

Yet I did engage in one project that was a direct sequel to the Vietnam days. In a conversation with Richard Falk, we decided that we would once again edit a volume on American crimes of war, this one to be called *Crimes of War: Iraq*. As our other collaborator we now called upon Irene Gendzier, a committed political scientist and authority on the Middle East. I had a melancholy feeling about confronting the same kind of criminal behavior on the part of my country in a new war thirty-five years later. Whether at age forty-five or close to eighty, I was still outraged by slaughter and impelled toward some kind of action against it. This new volume (in which I included several of my own essays) did not seem to have the impact of our earlier *Crimes of War*, but it may still be too early (in 2010) to make any such comparison. Who can say how much this Iraq volume will turn out to have had useful reverberations, how much it might have influenced attitudes toward the disastrous, and atrocity-producing, American war in Afghanistan?

The Vietnam War had its impact on my profession in a way that I was able to participate in. During the early eighties I was part of a small committee of psychiatrists mobilizing support for the concept of post-traumatic stress disorder (PTSD), to be included in the bible of the profession, the *Diagnostic and Statistical Manual of Mental Disorders III*. That effort succeeded, largely through the efforts of Chaim Shatan, who had also been a key person in the rap groups. I managed to have inserted some of the language I used, such as the concept of psychic numbing. Whatever the confusions that came to surround the concept of PTSD, it did at least provide a diagnostic category that honored the suffering of people involved in war or experiencing other forms of significant trauma. I wish I had been able to include the concept of an atrocity-producing situation, but that does not qualify as a psychiatric disorder. Rather, such a situation reflects war-related moral disorder that can affect a small or large group, even a society.

I'm hardly alone in my generation when I say that Vietnam continues to inhabit me. That presence is mostly painful, but at the same time I have found it to be a valuable source of cautionary knowledge in every situation having to do with war and peace. For me its lessons have been embodied and best articulated by antiwar veterans. I recall a small meeting with a few of them in 1973 just after the cease-fire. They told me how that ending confirmed their sense of the war's pointlessness. But in discussing their future one of them said, "I'm going to be a Vietnam veteran against the war for the rest of my life." My parallel sentiment is that, for the rest of my own life, I'm going to be a critical student of what happened to Americans in the Vietnam War and of what that experience tells us about the dreadful overall phenomenon we call war.

Nazi Doctors and Return Visits

The sense of coming full circle has taken shape for me more in connection with my work on Nazi doctors than with any other project. Return visits I've made to Germany have been important to me in affirming my continuing connection with people I care about and with events in that country. The connection becomes all the more meaningful in the face of the ambivalence I originally brought to the entire German enterprise—as a Jew, and as an advocate of victims and survivors.

Nazi doctors revisited me in connection with the Iraq War and the revelations that American doctors and psychologists were participating in torture. It was bad enough to discover that America embraced Chinese Communist methods of interrogation and thought reform in our treatment of prisoners. It was worse to find parallels with Nazi doctors—not equivalents but troubling enough reminders—in the behavior of American medical and psychological professionals. That behavior included failing to report wounds that could only have been caused by torture, delaying and falsifying death certificates, and colluding with interrogators—indeed, doing much to create the procedures that spilled over from coercive interrogation to systematic torture. And as I complete this manuscript (in 2010), documented evidence has just appeared to the effect that these same American professionals participated in the second great area of Nazi transgression, that of coercive experimentation (or "research") on those same Iraqi prisoners in relation to the torture to which they were being subjected. Yet perhaps I should not have been surprised at this development. After all, my work on Nazi doctors emphasized their socialization to atrocity. As I wrote in my article "Doctors and Torture," which I published in the *New England Journal of Medicine* in 2004, Nazi doctors were mostly "ordinary people who had killed no one before joining murderous Nazi institutions." Like them, American doctors' later collusion in torture resulted from their having been subjected to a version of an atrocity-producing situation. They adapted to their role in torture because torture had become a prevailing American policy in Iraq and elsewhere. Their transgressions in no way approached those of Nazi doctors but what they did was nonetheless shocking, as they too were professionals committed to healing.

At the end of my article I urged that these American doctors and psychologists speak out on what they had experienced and done, as a way of providing insight about what went wrong and at the same time "reclaiming their role as healers." I was in effect urging that we assert our democratic distinction from Nazi behavior precisely in such a candid self-examination. That may have been a bit overidealistic on my part (though here too the returns are far from in), but I was asking that we extend the same democratic prerogative expressed by American and international human rights organizations (most notably the Physicians for Human Rights) in their detailed investigations of the scandal. Still, we have to pause, as citizens of the nation that did most to bring Nazi doctors to judgment in Nuremberg, at the significance of our own ostensible healers joining the ranks of torturers.

I keep thinking of the words of an Israeli dentist and long-term Auschwitz prisoner whom I interviewed in his comfortable sitting room overlooking the beautiful Haifa harbor. As we were completing our demanding discussion of medical misbehavior in that camp, he sighed deeply and exclaimed: "This world is not this world!" Whatever our apparent comfort, he was saying, underneath can lie the hidden menace of corrupted healers.

There are other professionals involved with torture in ways that even more closely resemble Nazi counterparts. I have in mind Bush administration lawyers who prepared the notorious "torture memos" that blithely argued that systematic application of extreme pain and deprivation, contrary to all previous understanding, was not a form of torture because it did not damage major bodily systems. Their behavior suggested an American version of what the Nazis called *Gleichschaltung*, or "coordination" or "regearing" of professionals to subsume their standards to the prevailing Nazi line, whether legalizing killing or torture.

This perspective was so prevalent during the George W. Bush administration that Chuck Strozier proposed to me that we create an annual "Nazi Doctor Award" for the American professional, whether psychologist or physician or lawyer, whose behavior has most resembled that of Nazi counterparts. I saw what he was getting at, and there is something to be said for injecting gallows humor into the issue. But I resisted the idea because I felt uneasy about the public "joke," and responsible to more sober assessments and comparisons. I was undoubtedly being a bit of a stuffed shirt, but I believe that humor about evil requires precision and a modicum of awe. Having said that, I am aware that the Nazi doctors who remain in my head evoke feelings less of awe than morally derailed ordinariness.

Armenian Echoes

Reverberations from *The Nazi Doctors* could come from people concerned with other genocides. My exploration of a more general psychology of genocide, toward the end of the book, led to an odd series of events involving Armenians and Turks and a lasting American friendship. In that exploration I referred a few times to the Turkish genocide of Armenians in 1915–17 as having certain parallels with Nazi genocide, including active involvement of doctors. I knew about the extensive Turkish efforts to deny their genocide, but I was still shocked to receive a letter in October 1990 from the Turkish ambassador to the United States, Nuzhet Kandemir, doing just that. He chastised me for "references in your work . . . to the so-called 'Armenian genocide,' allegedly perpetrated by the Ottoman Turks during the First World War." He called the event a "tragic civil war . . . initiated by Armenian nationalists" and urged me to make the appropriate changes in future editions of my book. There was another surprise: the enclosure, apparently inadvertently, of two in-house documents, both written by Heath Lowry, an American Ph.D. who had spent most of his professional life in Turkey and was now director of the Institute of Turkish Studies in Washington, D.C., mainly funded by the Turkish government. One was a draft of Kandemir's letter to me, identical to the version I received. The second document was a memo in which Lowry listed the exact references I made in my book to the Turkish genocide, and said that the real problem lay in the Turkish failure to respond more promptly and aggressively to countering the works of other scholars on the Armenian genocide, and that I was "simply the end of a chain." It seemed clear that Lowry was advising the Turkish government on how to be more effective in their denial of the genocide.

My first reaction was simple anger, and I composed in my mind the nasty reply I would send to Kandemir, questioning an ambassador's use of his position to attack reputable scholarship and falsify history. But then I had a better idea, that of making the whole sequence public in a thoughtful statement about genocide and Turkish denial. So I collaborated with my close friend Eric Markusen, long involved in genocide studies, and Roger W. Smith, a scholarly authority on the Armenian genocide and its denial, in an article published in 1995 in *Holocaust and Genocide Studies*, the journal of the United States Holocaust Memorial Museum in Washington, D.C. To head off legal or other difficulty from Turkey, we backed up our assertions of Turkish denial with a carefully referenced summary of the history of the actual genocide. We also brought out the wider academic scandal of Lowry's involvement in an institute promoting Turkish denial, and his having been appointed to an Atatürk Chair of Ottoman and Modern Turkish Studies at Princeton, which was financed by the

Turkish government as part of a plan to set up similar chairs at major American universities. We included facsimiles of the two Lowry memos and considered some of the motivations of American scholars in their participation in such historical distortions. Roger, a soft-spoken man with a great capacity for outrage, drafted most of the article. I wrote a concluding discussion in which I asserted that when scholars deny genocide in the face of decisive evidence they contribute to a false historical consciousness, send a message that "murderers did not really murder . . . that victims were not really killed," and thereby support "a deadly psychohistorical dynamic in which unopposed genocide begets new genocide."

The impact of the paper astonished us. It was widely reported on in a way that few articles in serious journals are, especially by publications concerned with issues involving academia. The *Chronicle of Higher Education*, for instance, ran a detailed account of our article and the issues raised, and there were shorter pieces in major newspapers such as *The New York Times* and *Washington Post*. The article had an electrifying effect on the Armenian community in America, which had felt itself beleaguered by bullying Turkish falsifications that were more or less encouraged by U.S. State Department policy (to avoid alienating a NATO ally). We heard that the community ordered more than a thousand reprints, and before long an exuberant Peter Balakian appeared at my CUNY office.

Poet, memoirist, professor of literature and genocide studies, indefatigable activist on Armenian issues, Peter seems to be everywhere doing everything, his high energy matched only by his personal warmth. It did not take long for us to become close friends who shared many ethical and political concerns, along with a passion for sports. We could joke about similarities between Armenians and Jews, their world-weary perseverance and their gallows humor. And I found it natural to join with Peter in his sustained efforts to combat Turkish denial and infiltration of American universities, including a particularly influential international petition he spawned, signed by major writers, scholars, and Nobel laureates.

Over time, I came to moderate, always with Peter's prodding help, a number of seminars and workshops among Turkish, Armenian, and Armenian-American scholars and activists, sometimes including Holocaust scholars, dealing with the genocide and with Turkish-Armenian reconciliation based on recognition of historical truth. I also wrote an introduction to a new edition of one of the classic volumes on the Armenian genocide, *Ambassador Morgenthau's Story*, the remarkable firsthand account by Henry Morgenthau, American ambassador to Constantinople from 1913 to 1916.

Looking back on these efforts, Peter is convinced that the article Roger, Eric, and I wrote was a turning point for the Armenian-American community in confronting Turkish denial and influencing American consciousness. He may be exaggerating, but I did welcome this added impact of my work on Nazi doctors and the important personal friendship to which it led.

Time's Arrow

There was another rewarding reverberation of *The Nazi Doctors*, also having to do with a friendship, this one with Martin Amis, the British novelist. Having married into a Cape Cod family notable for its beautiful daughters, Martin sought me out in Wellfleet because of our common interest in nuclear weapons. But the weapons were almost forgotten as we quickly discovered that we were both tennis zealots, and within days we were on the court together. At forty, Martin was twenty years younger than I and by far the stronger player. But in a series of fiercely competitive (ridiculously so, as I look back on it) matches, I could—through steadiness, guile, and an aggressive net game—play beyond my means, while with Martin the opposite was true. His erratic play and self-lacerating temper (what he called his "bad character") undermined his skills. So over the course of that first summer I managed to win a slight majority of matches. And when he learned my age, Martin's displeasure at this outcome turned to horror. Back in London he worked hard on his game, including added lessons, and the following summer in Wellfleet he so dominated our play that I was fortunate to win any matches at all.

But in our tennis encounters there was a nice sequence from our brutal contest on the court to our gentle conversation immediately after each match. We talked about our work, our sense of what was going on in the world, and what each of us was reading and thinking. I felt that I made contact with a tenderness in Martin, underneath his bad-boy bravado, along with a lively and discerning intellect. During one of those post-tennis conversations, Martin asked me about my study of Nazi doctors, and at the next dinner BJ and I had with him and his wife, Antonia Phillips, I presented him with a copy of the book. He quickly became obsessed with the volume, immersed in it to the exclusion of everything else, and questioned me persistently about Auschwitz doctors: what an actual day was like for them, how they felt about friends, wives, and lovers. Taking shape in Martin's mind was a novel, not just about a Nazi doctor but about the life of one lived backward, from death to birth. While I was pleased that my book could connect so intensely with his novelistic imagination, I was more than a bit worried about the kind of product that would result from this odd approach.

He wrote the novel quickly—we first talked about it during the late eighties and in early 1991 I was sent proofs of *Time's Arrow*. Soon after that a BBC television crew appeared at my Wellfleet study to record my views on the book, as Martin had clearly acknowledged its inspiration from *The Nazi Doctors*. Much to my relief, I liked the book a great deal and was moved by Martin's way of evoking Auschwitz. In fact I felt a little possessive about *Time's Arrow*, troubled when some reviewers found its structure heavy going, pleased when more of them praised Martin's dedication and skill, and delighted when it was short-listed for the important Booker Prize.

After a few summers Martin and Antonia separated and divorced, and he abruptly ceased coming to the Cape. I've seen him only occasionally in recent years, and my impression is that our sensibilities are less congruent than they used to be. When I ask myself whether it is the heroic tennis contests or the thoughtful dialogue I miss, my answer is neither alone but the unique constellation of them both, the seamless flow from tennis to talk, resulting finally in the literary bonding involving *The Nazi Doctors* and *Time's Arrow*.

Back to Germany

I returned to Germany in 1989 when I gave the Alexander Mitscherlich Memorial Lecture at the Sigmund-Freud-Institut in Munich on my work with Nazi doctors, and also received an honorary degree from the University of Munich (undoubtedly promoted by Fritz Friedmann and his colleagues at the Amerika-Institut there). It happened to be the time of the dismantling of the Berlin Wall, which I could observe together with friends on Munich television, so that a joyous event in their recent history could become a doubly exciting German moment for me.

In 2007 I was back in Germany to give the keynote speech at a conference held in Nuremberg celebrating the sixtieth anniversary of the medical trials in that city. By then Nuremberg had been long restored to its striking medieval appearance, and the conference took place in its opulent opera house, now part of a large state theater complex. That felt a little strange, but it did provide an opportunity for leaders and institutions in Nuremberg to confront and renounce its particularly fervent Nazi past. There was also an antinuclear cast to the conference, sponsored as it was by the German chapter of the International Physicians for the Prevention of Nuclear War, and I especially admired this juxtaposing of anti-Nazi and antinuclear sentiments. The speeches (by civic leaders and educators) and performances (by talented musicians) went on a bit long, but the audience fought off its fatigue sufficiently to hear me out, and I felt happy to be in that opera house with them.

Talking Head

BJ and I returned to Germany in November 2009 for previews in Frankfurt and Berlin of a film about me and my work on Nazi doctors. It was a documentary that two German filmmakers—Wolfgang Richter and Hannes Karnick—had been making and not making for almost a decade, and one that I thought would never find completion. They had spent ten days with me in Wellfleet in 2001, interviewing me in meticulous informal detail on how I went about the work, what I observed and what I felt, and about my developing understanding of how Nazi doctors could do what they did. It was my most extensive rendering of my personal and professional experience in the research. After intermittent e-mail correspondence about possible additional visual material—footage of Nazi doctors or Jewish victims, of killing centers or death camps—Wolfgang informed me that he had made the radical decision to use none of these by-now-conventional materials. In mid-2009 he wrote to say that they had completed the film and received enthusiastic responses from showings to fellow filmmakers, medical school audiences, and representatives of the Sigmund-Freud-Institut in Frankfurt. With the help of government funds, the institute agreed to cosponsor the trip BJ and I made to help launch the film, with its first preview arranged to coincide with a national psychoanalytic conference in Frankfurt.

Filmmakers are rightly warned to avoid relying on talking heads. Yet this ninety-minute film relies almost entirely on just one talking head, me. It did have an additional element that Wolfgang and Hannes had the wisdom to feature, staggeringly beautiful shots of the Atlantic Ocean, which provided relief from my words and conveyed a greater cosmic truth. In discussions I had with audiences in Frankfurt and Berlin, I was repeatedly asked how it felt as a Jewish psychiatrist to be working with German filmmakers on the criminal behavior of Nazi doctors. I found myself saying that it did not seem so remarkable to me because from the beginning of the study in the late seventies I had been working closely with concerned Germans who did a great deal to make the whole enterprise possible. But as I think about it now, there was something different this time. In the past I had been doing the interrogating—of the doctors themselves of course, as well as survivors and knowledgeable scholars and writers. In the film I myself was being interrogated, skillfully and sympathetically, to evoke a conversational tone in which viewers are not talked down to but invited to join me on a rather strange journey. Viewers in art theaters in various parts of Germany—and then in the United States as well—did seem to become engaged, and reviewers have noted that the absence of the usual Holocaust images contributed to the film's starkness and clarity. The result is what one friend called a "meditation" on my overall experience of studying Nazi doctors.

Superpower Syndrome

The extremities of the George W. Bush administration could be particularly inspiring to a scholar-activist, especially one whose head was filled with reverberations of work on totalism, nuclearism, atrocity-producing war-making, and on professionals lending their skills to killing. I called the book I wrote *Superpower Syndrome* and when I sent an advance copy to my friend Takeo Doi in Tokyo, he wrote back saying that it seemed especially appropriate for me to complete my career by applying my work to my own country. I had of course confronted American culpability in earlier studies on Hiroshima and Vietnam. But now I was doing something different: taking a psychohistorical look at the United States as an aberrant force that endangered everyone. My subtitle was "America's Apocalyptic Confrontation with the World," and I argued that the American vision of remaking the world in our own image was bound up with apocalyptic impulses of our own, by no means the same as those of Islamist extremists but more or less in tandem with them. By making use of the medical metaphor "superpower syndrome," I meant to suggest behavior that was not just random but part of a larger ideological constellation, a collective claim to omnipotence and to the ownership of history in which inner doubt could be masked by military belligerence. But I also argued that the omnipotence and the historical "ownership" were illusory, that the syndrome was a treadmill we would do best to step off as soon as possible. And even in those dark days, I was hopeful that we could and would.

It was a radical argument. A couple of media interviewers were shocked by my finding any parallel between our behavior and that of Bin Laden and Al Qaeda. While many Americans had soured on the Bush administration, it was quite another thing to attribute to our country a consistent pattern of violent extremism carried out in the name of a democratic mission, of a "war on terror." But I wished to hold nothing back, all the more so since I believed that *Superpower Syndrome* would be my last book, having not yet begun this memoir.

With all of the American angst during the first year or so of the Obama administration, one may readily forget the power of the historical moment of his election in 2008. BJ and I had a few friends in to watch the returns on the sleek television set in our living room, which we had purchased four years earlier for a similar gathering that had resulted in a roomful of despair and suspicion of fraud in relation to the Bush victory. But this time, in 2008, the television set did not betray us, and my reaction of not just joy but ecstasy, including tears, was hardly mine alone. What was special to me, though, was the quick realization that the outcome meant an end to the country's superpower syndrome. But was that the case? Only partly, it turns out. Certainly Obama and his administration have renounced the principle of American omnipotence in favor of more modest claims about our capacities and influence in the world. Apocalypticism and totalistic behavior have given way to something closer to Camus's "philosophy of limits," with an acceptance of ambiguity, nuance, and complexity. And most important, there has been a specific rejection of nuclearism and a call for abolition of the weapons.

Yet despite all that, the syndrome lingers in crucial areas that specifically connect with my work. Concerning nuclear abolition, Obama has not followed through with clear American policies, despite an impressive convocation of world leaders on the subject of nuclear danger. On revelations of torture, and more recently of illegitimate medical experiments in relation to torture, Obama has mostly tried to sidestep the issue and avoid legal culpability of those involved. Finally, his decision to send added troops to Afghanistan seems to me to be the stuff of war-making, and atrocity-producing, blunder. In all three cases there is a certain clinging to the very American omnipotence being renounced. I have found myself torn between joining a considerable segment of the left in a condemnation of shortcomings that perpetuate elements of the superpower syndrome, and an alternative inclination to defend Obama as an incremental reformer who needs more time.

I took the latter position in a series of discussions with Howard Zinn, who denounced Obama as "a Chicago politician" and a hypocrite. I still don't agree with that judgment but I am also willing to take a public stand of strong opposition to Obama policies on Afghanistan and on American torture and recently revealed experimentation. Yet I remain sensitive as well to the importance of supporting the Obama administration in the face of new waves of right-wing American totalism and potential violence in the backlash over the election of our first African-American president.

I have the feeling that if one lives long enough one can be witness to just about every variation of American domestic and foreign policy, good and bad. What I can best do, I believe, is to sustain a critique of residual features of the superpower syndrome, always connected with work I have done in areas that have contributed to that syndrome.

I think often of that lonely walk I took in the Kowloon section of Hong Kong in 1953, with which I began this memoir. Now, in 2010, it does not seem all that long ago. But I also think of another, much more recent walk, on the beach in Wellfleet with my daughter, Natasha, my son, Ken, and two of our grandchildren, Jessica and Kimberly. Kimberly, then eleven years old, asked questions about the beach and the dunes, and I could tell her that they had not changed much since BJ and I walked the same beach for the first time just four years after that Hong Kong stroll. I would like to believe that what I've done in the world all those years in between might somehow contribute to the lives of Kimberly and Jessica and those of our other grandchildren, Lila and Dmitri. There can be no certainty about such things, but for BJ and me the effort, at every step, continues to matter.

EPILOGUE

I T IS NO SECRET to the reader that BJ has been with me as a vital presence throughout the events described in this book. But as I completed
the volume and sent it to the copyeditor, she was suddenly stricken with a
virulent form of pneumonia that did not respond to antibiotics. She died
a few days later, on November 19, 2010, in Massachusetts General Hospital with Natasha, Ken, and myself at her side. While she had experienced
various medical problems before that, including a serious immune system
condition, she had been completely active until a week before her death.
She was counseling adoptees and speaking at meetings, having exuberant
talks with friends, and taking afternoon walks with me along the beach
in Wellfleet or to the Longfellow House in Cambridge. She had been an
elegant host at the Wellfleet Meetings in late October.

As I write this six weeks after she died, I am far from recovered from
the most painful experience I have ever known. BJ and I spent nearly six
decades together as intimate partners. Her support and belief in me made
all of my work possible, made possible the life I lived. When we had conflict, its resolution led to greater closeness. We were a couple, as people
have told me, that was greater than the sum of its parts.

The first reader of this memoir told me that it is, in its way, a love
poem to BJ. I was pleased to agree. She had written a similar love poem
to me, thirty-five years earlier, contained in her memoir of her search for
and reunion with her birth mother. She told of feeling, when deciding to
marry me, "Go with him. Make new dreams." We made them.

BJ also carved out a life of remarkable individual accomplishment.
Tributes to her have come from all over the world, from adoptees, birth

mothers, and adoptive parents in response to her books, speeches, interviews, and counseling; and from people in the adoption triad whom she had never met but who had exchanged e-mails and phone calls with her about dilemmas in their lives. The recurrent theme of these tributes: "She changed my life!" Indeed BJ did much to change national consciousness about adoption, to identify the "ghosts" she spoke of as haunting everyone in the triad and showing the way to exorcising them.

Wellfleetians write of her as the soul of the meetings, and have planted trees in Wellfleet and Provincetown in her honor. Readers of her many children's books have told of the lasting impact of her highly imaginative stories. And her biography of Janusz Korczak, while an important part of Holocaust literature, transcends that literature in its portrait of an extraordinary man. Beyond all that, BJ fiercely loved her children and grandchildren. And she had a remarkable talent for friendship, bringing to it endless loyalty and generosity.

As for me, I've learned what it costs when a long and profound human tie is severed. Having studied grief and loss for many decades, only now have I come close to a full realization of what those costs really are. When BJ died the hardest rooms for me to enter were her studies in Cambridge and Wellfleet, because the objects left in each of them—books, files, manuscripts, pictures, puppets, statues, dog dish, cat tree, reptilian stuffed animals—displayed her essence, her completely idiosyncratic combination of involvements in the world, which made the rooms her special universe. I think constantly of our little rituals and shared humor, the scrambled eggs I made every Sunday morning from the time our kids were small, the irreverent notes we left one another on the second-floor landing about the state of the cosmos in which she addressed me with a drawing of a bird and I her with my version of a dolphin.

I have of course become a survivor, and my work on that subject offers me some help after all. I have in mind my emphasis on survivors' need for meaning in connection with the death they have experienced. I cannot deny that the strongest meaning for me so far of BJ's death has been the shock and pain of loss. But as the days pass, I find myself gradually beginning to understand that the death itself is a part of the glorious life we shared—an end of that life but a part of it nonetheless. No wonder that a wise friend could speak of my participation in the family ritual of burial as a completion of my love for her. And so it was for our children, Ken and Natasha, and for our grandchildren as well.

I think of the first time I saw BJ, across the room in a nondescript Upper West Side apartment, in 1951, and could simply not take my eyes off this beautiful and charismatic young woman; and then of posing for a portrait with her after the Wellfleet meeting in October 2010, resulting in a photograph that made us look (as BJ and I later agreed) "like Grant Wood figures but with smiles." In between has been the witnessing referred to in the title of this book, witnessing always together.

ACKNOWLEDGMENTS

I T IS HARDLY possible to list all who have contributed in various ways to a volume that spans a lifetime. I refer to many such people in the book itself. Here I'll only mention those who did most to help me bring this specific book into being.

Melanie Yolles, Manager, Archives and Manuscripts, of the New York Public Library, skillfully and devotedly ordered my papers in a way that made the whole project possible. My agent Richard Morris of Janklow & Nesbit has been a supporter, facilitator, and friend throughout. Jane Isay provided key early guidance about the book's structure and principles of selectivity.

Emily Loose at Free Press has been what an author most needs, an editor as demanding as she was empathic and dedicated. She was ably assisted by Alexandra Pisano and (as copyeditor) Tom Pitoniak.

Chuck Strozier engaged in a beginning dialogue with me that helped release the book from its mental fetters. He and Peter Balakian read the manuscript and responded in ways that affirmed my efforts and greatly improved the volume. Mary Kolodny, my assistant, did further research and editing and coordinated everything in her painstaking preparation of the manuscript.

My dedication suggests the overriding importance to the work of my children, Ken and Natasha, and grandchildren, Kimberly, Jessica, Lila, and Dmitri. My wife BJ was my loving partner and muse throughout the writing and living of this book.

ABOUT THE AUTHOR

———

Robert Jay Lifton is a psychiatrist, author, and activist who has long been concerned with the interaction of psychology and history. He has written widely on such subjects as Nazi doctors (their killing in the name of healing) and genocide; nuclear weapons and their impact on our sense of life and death; the survivors of Hiroshima and the general psychology of survivors; the Vietnam War and its veterans who turned against it; Chinese "thought reform" and the Chinese Cultural Revolution; the nature of apocalyptic violence; and the psychology and potential of the contemporary self. Confronting some of the most destructive events of our era, he has also explored our more resilient and hopeful capacities for responding to immediate and more distant threats.

He has received numerous honorary degrees and professional and literary awards.

Among his books are *The Nazi Doctors: Medical Killing and the Psychology of Genocide*, winner of the Los Angeles Times Book Prize and the National Jewish Book Award; *Death in Life: Survivors of Hiroshima*, recipient of the National Book Award and the Van Wyck Brooks Award; *Home from the War: Vietnam Veterans—Neither Victims Nor Executioners*, nominated for the National Book Award; *Thought Reform and the Psychology of Totalism: A Study of "Brainwashing" in China*; *The Protean Self: Human Resilience in an Age of Fragmentation*; and *Superpower Syndrome: America's Apocalyptic Confrontation with the World*.

Lifton has also been a leading figure in the physicians' antinuclear movement and has taken strong public stands, including that of civil disobedience, in opposing American participation in wars in Vietnam, Iraq, and Afghanistan. He is a cartoonist by avocation and stresses the overriding necessity of humor in our lives, often gallows humor.

He is presently Lecturer in Psychiatry at Harvard Medical School and the Cambridge Health Alliance. He is Distinguished Professor Emeritus in Psychiatry and Psychology at the City University of New York, where he was also director of the Center on Violence and Human Survival. Prior to that he held the Foundations Fund research professorship in psychiatry at Yale Medical School.

He was born in New York City in 1926, attended Cornell University, and received his medical degree from New York Medical College. He divides his time between Cambridge and Wellfleet, Massachusetts.